Global and Domestic Public Health and Neuroepidemiology

Editor

DAVID S. YOUNGER

NEUROLOGIC CLINICS

www.neurologic.theclinics.com

Consulting Editor
RANDOLPH W. EVANS

November 2016 • Volume 34 • Number 4

ELSEVIER

1600 John F. Kennedy Boulevard • Suite 1800 • Philadelphia, Pennsylvania, 19103-2899

http://www.theclinics.com

NEUROLOGIC CLINICS Volume 34, Number 4
November 2016 ISSN 0733-8619, ISBN-13: 978-0-323-47690-4

Editor: Lauren Boyle
Developmental editor: Donald Mumford

Neurologic Clinics (ISSN 0733-8619) is published quarterly by Elsevier Inc., 360 Park Avenue South, New York, NY 10010–1710. Months of issue are February, May, August, and November. Periodicals postage paid at New York, NY, and additional mailing offices. Subscription prices are $300.00 per year for US individuals, $578.00 per year for US institutions, $100.00 per year for US students, $375.00 per year for Canadian individuals, $701.00 per year for Canadian institutions, $415.00 per year for international individuals, $701.00 per year for international institutions, and $210.00 for Canadian and foreign students/residents. To receive student/resident rate, orders must be accompanied by name of affiliated institution, date of term, and the *signature* of program/residency coordinator on institution letterhead. Orders will be billed at individual rate until proof of status is received. Foreign air speed delivery is included in all *Clinics* subscription prices. All prices are subject to change without notice. **POSTMASTER:** Send address changes to *Neurologic Clinics*, Elsevier Health Sciences Division, Subscription Customer Service, 3251 Riverport Lane, Maryland Heights, MO 63043. **Customer Service: Telephone: 1-800-654-2452 (U.S. and Canada); 314-447-8871 (outside U.S. and Canada). Fax: 314-447-8029. E-mail: journalscustomerservice-usa@elsevier.com (for print support); journalsonlinesupport-usa@elsevier.com (for online support).**

Reprints. For copies of 100 or more of articles in this publication, please contact the Commercial Reprints Department, Elsevier Inc., 360 Park Avenue South, New York, New York, 10010-1710; Tel.: +1-212-633-3874; Fax: +1-212-633-3820, and E-mail: reprints@elsevier.com.

Neurologic Clinics is also published in Spanish by Nueva Editorial Interamericana S.A., Mexico City, Mexico.

Neurologic Clinics is covered in *Current Contents/Clinical Medicine, MEDLINE/PubMed (Index Medicus), EMBASE/Excerpta Medica, and PsycINFO, and ISI/BIOMED.*

Contributors

CONSULTING EDITOR

RANDOLPH W. EVANS, MD
Clinical Professor, Department of Neurology, Baylor College of Medicine, Houston, Texas

EDITOR

DAVID S. YOUNGER, MD, MPH, MS
Division of Neuroepidemiology, Department of Neurology, New York University School of Medicine; College of Global Public Health, New York University, New York, New York

AUTHORS

JAYDEEP M. BHATT, MD
Clinical Associate Professor, Department of Neurology; Director, Division of Global Health, New York University School of Medicine, New York, New York

XIAOLING CHEN, MPH
Division of Neuroepidemiology, Department of Neurology, New York University School of Medicine, New York, New York

ARLINE FAUSTIN, MD
Departments of Pathology and Neurology, The Center for Cognitive Neurology, New York University School of Medicine, New York, New York

ALBERT S. FAVATE, MD
Division of Neuroepidemiology, Department of Neurology, New York University School of Medicine, New York, New York

REBECCA M. GILBERT, MD, PhD
Department of Neurology, New York University School of Medicine; Marlene and Paolo Fresco Institute for Parkinson's and Movement Disorders, New York University Langone Medical Center, New York, New York

DAVID R. GOLDMANN, MD
Perelman School of Medicine, University of Pennsylvania, Philadelphia, Pennsylvania

SALLY GUTTMACHER, PhD
College of Global Public Health, New York University, New York, New York

RICHARD A. HICKMAN, BMedSc (Hons), MBChB (Hons), MRCSEd
Department of Pathology, New York University School of Medicine, New York, New York

JONATHAN HOWARD, MD
Division of Neuroepidemiology, Department of Neurology, Comprehensive Care Center, New York University, New York, New York

ANDREA LEE, MD
Department of Neurology, New York University School of Medicine, New York, New York

KATHARINE A. McNEILL, MD
Division of Neuroepidemiology, Department of Neurology, Laura and Isaac Perlmutter Cancer Center, New York University School of Medicine, New York, New York

MIA T. MINEN, MD, MPH
Division of Neuroepidemiology, Department of Neurology, New York University School of Medicine, New York, New York

JOYCE MOON-HOWARD, DrPH
College of Global Public Health, New York University, New York, New York

TATYANA A. SHAMLIYAN, MD, MS
Elsevier Clinical Solutions, Evidence-Based Medicine Center, Philadelphia, Pennsylvania

ANURADHA SINGH, MD
Clinical Associate Professor; Chief, Department of Neurology, Director, Bellevue Epilepsy Center, Bellevue Hospital Center, New York, New York

STEPHEN TREVICK, MD
Senior Resident, Departments of Neurology and Psychiatry, New York University Langone Medical Center, New York University School of Medicine, New York, New York

THOMAS WISNIEWSKI, MD
Lulu P. and David J. Levidow Professor of Neurology; Professor, Departments of Pathology, Neurology, and Psychiatry; Director, The Center for Cognitive Neurology, New York University School of Medicine, New York, New York

ADAM P.J. YOUNGER, MPH
Public and Nonprofit Management and Policy, The Wagner Graduate School of Public Service, New York University, New York, New York

DAVID S. YOUNGER, MD, MPH, MS
Division of Neuroepidemiology, Department of Neurology, New York University School of Medicine; College of Global Public Health, New York University, New York, New York

Contents

Section I - Epidemiology

David S. Younger and Xiaoling Chen

> Epidemiology is the study of the distribution and determinants of health-related states and in specified populations and the application to control health problems. Classified as either descriptive or analytical, a variety of epidemiologic approaches can be used to allow assessment of hypothesized risk factor exposure with disease outcomes. This article reviews salient aspects of epidemiologic research methods that are used repeatedly in articles in this volume on public health, neuroepidemiology, and health systems.

Anuradha Singh and Stephen Trevick

> The International League Against Epilepsy defines epilepsy as at least 2 unprovoked seizures more than 24 hours apart. It is a wide-reaching and complex illness affecting more than 70 million people worldwide and can take on a variety of forms, patterns, and severities. Geographic differences in the illness are often related to its etiology. A host of endemic illnesses and parasitic infections can lead to epilepsy syndromes. Management varies by region due to the availability of diagnostic modalities and medications. Treatment gaps in epilepsy care often are related to social and cultural factors that must also be understood.

Mia T. Minen and David S. Younger

> Headache disorders cause significant disability. The public and most health professionals tend to perceive migraine as a minor or trivial complaint. In the past decade, important epidemiologic studies enjoining extensive surveys, pathophysiologic and genetic insights, and revised headache classification paradigms have produced clear evidence of the public health importance of headache disorders. The Global Campaign to reduce the burden of headache worldwide known as "Lifting the Burden" was launched in 2004 by the World Health Organization, the International Headache Society, the World Headache Alliance, and the European Headache Federation. This paper reviews salient progress in the neuroepidemiology of migraine headaches.

Alzheimer disease (AD) represents one of the greatest medical challenges of this century; the condition is becoming increasingly prevalent worldwide and no effective treatments have been developed for this terminal disease. Because the disease manifests at a late stage after a long period of clinically silent neurodegeneration, knowledge of the modifiable risk factors and the implementation of biomarkers is crucial in the primary prevention of the disease and presymptomatic detection of AD, respectively. This article discusses the growing epidemic of AD and antecedent risk factors in the disease process. Disease biomarkers are discussed, and the implications that this may have for the treatment of this currently incurable disease.

Parkinson disease (PD) is a common progressive neurodegenerative condition, causing both motor and non motor symptoms. Motor symptoms include stiffness, slowness, rest tremor and poor postural reflexes, whereas nonmotor symptoms include abnormalities of mood, cognition, sleep and autonomic function. Affected patients show cell loss in the substantia nigra pars compacta, and accumulation of aggregated alpha-synuclein into intracellular structures called Lewy bodies, within specific brain regions. The main known non modifiable risk factor is age. The neuroepidemiology of PD is complex with susceptibility genes and a number of modifiable risk factors that can increase and others that can mitigate risk and outcome.

Ischemic stroke is a heterogeneous multifactorial disorder recognized by the sudden onset of neurologic signs related directly to the sites of injury in the brain where the morbid process occurs. The evaluation of complex neurologic disorders, such as stroke, in which multiple genetic and epigenetic factors interact with environmental risk factors to increase the risk has been revolutionized by the genome-wide association studies (GWAS) approach. This article reviews salient aspects of ischemic stroke emphasizing the impact of neuroepidemiology and GWAS.

Brain tumors are the commonest solid tumor in children, leading to significant cancer-related mortality. Several hereditary syndromes associated with brain tumors are nonfamilial. Ionizing radiation is a well-recognized risk factor for brain tumors. Several industrial exposures have been evaluated for a causal association with brain tumor formation but the results are inconclusive. A casual association between the common mutagens of tobacco, alcohol, or dietary factors has not yet been established. There is no clear evidence that the incidence of brain tumors has changed over time. This article presents the descriptive epidemiology of the commonest brain tumors of children and adults.

 Video content accompanies this article at http://www.neurologic. theclinics.com.

Neuromuscular disorders as a group are linked by anatomy with significant differences in pathogenetic mechanisms, clinical expression, and time course of disease. Each neuromuscular disease is relatively uncommon, yet causes a significant burden of disease socioeconomically. Epidemiologic studies in different global regions have demonstrated certain neuromuscular diseases have increased incidence and prevalence rates over time. Understanding differences in global epidemiologic trends will aid clinical research and policies focused on prevention of disease. There is a critical need to understand the global impact of neuromuscular diseases using metrics currently established for communicable and noncommunicable diseases.

The global burden of adult neuropsychiatric illness and childhood mental disorders is enormous, accounting for a significant burden of disability in adults and a major factor of overall health that continues throughout the lifespan of children and into adulthood.

The role of vaccination in the control and prevention of endemic and emerging diseases cannot be overemphasized. Induction of host protective immunity may be the most powerful tool and effective strategy in preventing the spread of potentially fatal disease and emerging illnesses, in particular in susceptible immunologically naive hosts. The strategy for vaccination programs is engrained in population studies recognizing benefit for the health and economic welfare of at-risk indigenous populations. Worldwide collaboration is a necessary aspect of vaccine-preventable diseases recognizing that even a small number of wild-type cases of an eradicated disease in one region presents opportunities for re-emergence of the disease in geographically remote areas.

Zika virus is an arbovirus belonging to the *Flaviviridae* family known to cause mild clinical symptoms similar to those of dengue and chikungunya. Zika is transmitted by different species of *Aedes* mosquitoes. Nonhuman primates and possibly rodents play a role as reservoirs. Direct interhuman transmission has also been reported. Human cases have been reported in Africa and Asia, Easter Island, the insular Pacific region, and Brazil. Its clinical profile is that of a dengue-like febrile illness, but recently associated Guillain-Barre syndrome and microcephaly have appeared. There is neither a vaccine nor prophylactic medications available to prevent Zika virus infection.

Section II - Health Systems

minority of the available subsidies, whereas the richest obtain more than a third, fostering a divide in health care infrastructure across the rich and poor in urban and rural settings. This paradigm has implications for domestic Indian public health and global public health.

China has recently emerged as an important global partner. However, like other developing nations, China has experienced dramatic demographic and epidemiologic changes in the past few decades. Population discontent with the health care system has led to major reforms. China's distinctive health care system, including its unique history, vast infrastructure, the speed of health reform, and economic capacity to make important advances in health care, nonetheless, has incomplete insurance coverage for urban and rural dwellers, uneven access, mixed quality of health care, increasing costs, and risk of catastrophic health expenditures.

The South African health care system is embedded in a background of racial subordination and sexual violence against girls and women and of hierarchical male authority from youth to adulthood. Low wages, unemployment, urban overcrowding, inadequate sanitation, malnutrition, crime, and violence have contributed to economic and health inequality. With more health-insured whites than blacks and the proportion of gross national product spent on health care slowly increasing, two-thirds of health expenditures have been consumed by the private sector at a time when the cost of health insurance has risen to more than 3 times the rate of the consumer price index.

Special Article

NEUROLOGIC CLINICS

Preface

Public Health, Neuroepidemiology, and Health Systems

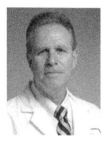

David S. Younger, MD, MPH, MS
Editor

I was trained to critically analyze human disease; however, it was not until I embarked upon formal training in public health and epidemiology that I appreciated the importance of a rigorous approach to understanding and addressing domestic and global health issues. In this *Neurologic Clinics* issue entitled, *Global and Domestic Public Health and Neuroepidemiology*, I have translated my professional medical experience in the academic and private practice sectors to the most pressing public health issues facing practicing neurologists and trainees in the United States and abroad. The faculty joining me, all experts in their respective fields, have been drawn from NYU Department of Neurology, Division of Neuroepidemiology, and the College of Global Public Health, to carefully frame their articles to make them relevant to researchers, clinicians, students, allied health providers, and policymakers.

I wish to express my appreciation to Ken Langone, Chair of the Board of Trustees of NYU Langone Medical Center, and the leadership of the Department of Neurology, expressly to Steve L. Galetta, MD and Laura J. Balcer, MD, MSCE, for supporting my work in this field. I am also grateful to epidemiology colleagues at Columbia University Mailman School of Public Health, notably Judith Jacobson, MBA, MPH, DrPH, who encouraged me to think critically as a student and to apply rigor to epidemiologic analysis. I dedicate this issue to my family, who inspired me to find the higher meaning of this project and for whom I try to be a role model. Randolph W. Evans, MD, *Neurologic*

Clinics Consulting Editor, encouraged me to pursue this volume, and Donald Mumford, Senior Developmental Editor for Elsevier, provided support throughout its preparation. I would like to express my thanks to Ms. Jessica Chen, NYU Clinical Research Coordinator, for her assistance and support in the handling of manuscripts and deliverance of proofs.

David S. Younger, MD, MPH, MS
Division of Neuroepidemiology
Department of Neurology
New York University School of Medicine
College of Global Public Health
New York University
333 East 34th Street, 1J
New York, NY 10016, USA

E-mail address:
david.younger@nyumc.org

Erratum

Benjamin Greenberg has been removed as an author of "Neurotherapeutic Strategies for Multiple Sclerosis", an article in the August issue of *Neurologic Clinics*.

Neurol Clin 34 (2016) xv
http://dx.doi.org/10.1016/j.ncl.2016.08.001
0733-8619/16/© 2016 Elsevier Inc. All rights reserved.

neurologic.theclinics.com

Section I - Epidemiology

Research Methods in Epidemiology

David S. Younger, MD, MPH, MS[a,b,*], Xiaoling Chen, MPH[a]

KEYWORDS

• Research • Epidemiology • Statistics

KEY POINTS

- Measures of disease frequency include incidence, prevalence, odds and mortality rates.
- Summary measures of disease and disability have relevance to global health and have been used successfully by the Global Burden of Disease Study.
- Measures of effect and association include risk difference, risk ratio, relative excess, null state and counterfactual, and prevalence ratios.
- Epidemiologic estimation examines validity and error through estimation of P values, hypothesis testing, confidence intervals, and confidence limits.
- The major types of epidemiology study designs are randomized controlled trials, and nonexperimental study types including cohort, case control, cross-sectional and ecological study types.

INTRODUCTION

Neuroepidemiology is a branch of epidemiology involving the study of neurologic disease distribution and determinants of frequency in human populations. It includes the science of epidemiologic measures, estimation, hypothesis testing, and design of experimental and nonexperimental studies. This article reviews basic aspects of epidemiology that will be useful for articles relating to the neuroepidemiology of diverse neurologic disorders. Those interested in reading more deeply into the area of research methods of epidemiology are directed to general texts and monographs on the subject.[1–8]

MEASURES OF DISEASE FREQUENCY

Greenland and Rothman[9] review measures of occurrence elaborated further below.

The authors have nothing to disclose.
[a] Division of Neuroepidemiology, Department of Neurology, New York University School of Medicine, New York, NY, USA; [b] College of Global Public Health, New York University, New York, NY, USA
* Corresponding author. 333 East 34th Street, 1J, New York, NY 10016.
E-mail address: David.younger@nyumc.org

Neurol Clin 34 (2016) 815–835
http://dx.doi.org/10.1016/j.ncl.2016.05.003   neurologic.theclinics.com
0733-8619/16/$ – see front matter © 2016 Elsevier Inc. All rights reserved.

Incidence

Incidence is defined as the occurrence of new cases of disease that develop in a candidate population over a specified time period. Cumulative incidence is the proportion of candidate population that becomes diseased over a specific time period mathematically expressed as follows:

$$\text{Incidence (I)} = \frac{\text{number of new cases of a disease}}{\text{number of candidate population}} \text{ over a specified time period.}$$

Note that the numerator is a subset of the denominator and thus the possible value of cumulative incidence ranges from 0 to 1, or if expressed as a percentage, from 0% to 100%. Time is not an integral part of this proportion, but rather is expressed by the words that accompany the numbers. Thought of as an average risk of getting a disease over a certain period of time, cumulative incidence is a commonly cited measure such as the "lifetime risk" currently estimated at 1 in 8, among United States men for the occurrence of stroke. Cumulative incidence is mainly used in fixed populations when there are no or only small losses to follow-up.

Epidemiologists have recognized that outcome events are not inevitable and may not occur during the period of observation; hence, the set of incidence times for a specific event in a population may not be precisely timed or observed. One way to deal with this complication has been to develop a measure to account for the length of time each individual contributes to the population at risk for the event during the period of time during which the event was a possibility and would have been counted in the population had it occurred. The sum of the person-times over all population members, termed the *total person-time at risk* or the *population-time at risk*, is the total of time during which disease onsets could occur in the population of interest. The incidence rate (IR), person-time rate, or incidence density of the population is defined as the number of new cases of disease (incident number) divided by the person-time over the period:

$$\text{Incidence rate (IR)} = \frac{\text{number of disease onsets}}{\sum_{\text{persons}} \text{time spent in population}}$$

When the risk period is of a fixed length equal to Δt, the proportion of the period that a person spends in the population at risk is their amount of person-time divided by Δt such that the average size of the population over the period of time is represented by:

$$\overline{N} = \sum_{\text{persons}} \frac{\text{time spent in population}}{\Delta t}$$

The total person-time at risk over the period is equal to the product of the average size of the population over the period $\overline{N}$, and the fixed length of the risk period Δt. If the incident number is denoted by A, it follows that the IR equals $A/(\overline{N} \times \Delta t)$. This formulation shows that the IR has units of inverse time that can be rewritten as $year^{-1}$, $month^{-1}$, or day^{-1}. The outcome events that can be counted in the numerator of an IR are those that occur to persons who are contributing to the denominator of the IR at the time that the disease onset occurs. Likewise, only time contributed by persons eligible to be counted in the numerator if they suffer such an event should be included in the denominator. An alternative way of expressing a population IR is as a time-weighted average of individual rates. An individual rate is either 0/(time spent in population) = 0 if the individual does not experience the event, or 1/(time spent in population) if the individual does experience the event. One then has the number of disease onsets A shown as follows:

$$A = \sum_{\text{persons}} (\text{time spent in population}) \, (\text{individual rate})$$

and so

$$IR = \frac{\sum_{\text{persons}} (\text{time spent in population}) \, (\text{individual rate})}{\sum_{\text{persons}} (\text{time spent in population})}$$

Although a central one in epidemiology, the IR has certain limitations. First, it does not capture all aspects of disease occurrence as illustrated by the analogy of noting that a rate of 1 case/(100 years) = 0.01 year^{-1} could be obtained by following 100 people for an average of 1 year and observing 1 case, but could also be obtained by following 2 people for 50 years and observing 1 case. To distinguish these situations, more detailed measures are needed, such as incidence time. Second, the numeric value lacks interpretability because the IR ultimately depends on the selection of time in which it is presented to give it significance. This is illustrated by the fact that an IR of 100 cases per 1 person-year might be expressed as: $100\dfrac{\text{cases}}{\text{person} - \text{year}}$, $8.33\dfrac{\text{cases}}{\text{person} - \text{month}}$, $1.92\dfrac{\text{cases}}{\text{person} - \text{week}}$, or $0.27\dfrac{\text{cases}}{\text{person} - \text{day}}$. Likewise, the IRs of 0.15, 0.04, and 0.009 cases per person-year could be multiplied by 1000 to be displayed as 150, 40, and 9 cases per 1000 person-years, regardless of whether the observations are made over 1 year of time, 1 week of time, or over a decade, just as one could measure the speed of a car in miles per hour even regardless of whether it is measured for only a few seconds.

Although the IR often includes the first occurrence of disease onset as an eligible event for the numerator of the equation, in many diseases there may be repeated events particularly in neurologic disorders such as multiple sclerosis and chronic inflammatory demyelinating polyneuropathy, both of which are characterized by relapses and remissions in which there may even be a disease-free period between recurrences. When the events tallied in the numerator of an IR are the first occurrence of disease, then the time contributed by each person in whom the disease develops should terminate with the onset of disease, meaning that further information would be obtained from further observation. Thus, each person who experiences the outcome should contribute time to the denominator until the occurrence of the event, but not afterward. In studies of both first and subsequent occurrences of a disease in which it is not important to distinguish between the first and subsequent occurrences, then the time accumulated in the denominator of the rate would not cease with the occurrence of the outcome event. A useful approach is to define the "population at risk" differently for each occurrence of the event, such as studies of individuals restricted to the population of those who have survived the first event of a given disease such as chronic inflammatory demyelinating polyneuropathy. The distinguished populations may be closed or open, with the former adding no new members over time and lost only to attrition. The term *cohort* is sometimes used to describe a study population, although typically it is reserved for a narrower concept as that of a group of persons for whom the membership is defined by a single event. If the number of people entering a population is balanced by the number exiting, the population is said to be stationary or in a steady state. In a stationary population with no migration, the crude IR of an inevitable outcome such as death will equal the reciprocal of the average time spent in the population until the outcome occurs such that a death rate of 0.04 year^{-1} would translate into an average time from entry until death of 25 years.

Within a given time interval, the incident number of cases can also be expressed in relation to the size of the population at risk such that in the absence of immigration or emigration, such a rate becomes the proportion of people who become cases among those in the population at the start of the interval. The latter is defined as the proportion of a closed population at risk that becomes diseased within a given period of time. Thus, the number of disease onsets A is then the sum of the individual proportions:

$$A = \sum_{persons} \text{individual proportions}$$

And thus,

$$\text{Incidence proportion (IP)} = \frac{\sum_{persons} \text{individual proportions}}{\text{initial size of the population}} = A/N$$

So, defined as individual risks, this formulation illustrates that the IP is an average risk, ignoring the amount of person-time contributed by individuals but with a more intuitive interpretation than the IR. With a range from 0 to 1, it is dimensionless however an IP of disease of 3% means something very different when it refers to a 40-year period than a 40-day period.

With regard to their numerical value, a cumulative incidence and rate can only be compared if they are based on the same time unit, for example, cumulative incidence over a 1-year period and rate per person-year. Under this circumstance, the general rule is that in absolute value, the rate will always be larger than the cumulative incidence notably when x cases are lost to follow-up with or without censoring (C).

In the absence of censoring:

$$I = \frac{x}{N} \text{ and } IR = \frac{x}{N - \frac{1}{2}x}$$

While in the presence of censoring with I and IR can be, respectively, represented as:

$$\frac{x}{N - \frac{1}{2C}} \text{ and } \frac{x}{N - \frac{1}{2C} - \frac{1}{2x}}$$

As long as $x > 0$, the denominator of the rate will always be smaller than that of the cumulative incidence, explaining the greater absolute value of the rate. This occurs because the cumulative incidence is based on the number of individuals at risk at the beginning of the interval whereas the rate is based on person-time of observations over the follow-up period, subtracting person-time lost by cases.

The hazard rate (H) is an alternative definition for an instantaneous IR also called instantaneous conditional incidence. It is defined as each individual's instantaneous probability of the event at precisely time t or at a small interval $[t, t + \Delta t]$ given or conditioned on the fact that the individual was at risk at time t. Thus the hazard rate is defined for each particular point in time during the follow-up in mathematical terms for a small time interval, assuming Δt is close to zero as follows:

$$\frac{P \text{ (event in interval between } t \text{ and } [t + \Delta t] \mid \text{alive at } t)}{\Delta t}$$

The H is analogous to the conditional probability of an event that is calculated at each event time using the Kaplan-Meier approach however because its denominator is "time at risk," it is instead a rate measured in unit of time^{-1}. Moreover, in contrast with the Kaplan-Meier conditional probability, the H cannot be directly calculated as it is defined for an infinitely small time interval; however, the H function over time can be estimated using available parametric survival analysis techniques.

Prevalence

Unlike incidence measures, which focus on new events or changes, prevalence focuses on existing states. Although incidence measures the frequency with which new disease develops, prevalence measures the frequency of existing disease. It is simply defined as the proportion of the population with the disease. Point prevalence and period prevalence refer to 2 types of prevalence measures. The first refers to the proportion of the population that is diseased at a single point in time, thought of as a snapshot of the population, and the latter as the proportion of the population that is diseased during a specified duration of time. Mathematically, point prevalence and period prevalence are expressed respectively as follows:

$$\frac{\text{Number of existing cases of disease}}{\text{Number of total population}} \text{ At a point } or \text{ in a period of time.}$$

Prevalence depends on the rate at which new cases of disease develop and the duration (D) or length of time that individuals have the disease. The duration of disease starts at the time of diagnosis and ends when the person either is cured or dies. Mathematically, the relationship between prevalence and incidence is as follows:

$$P/(1 - P) = IR \times D$$

where P is prevalence (the proportion of the total population with the disease), 1-P is the proportion of the total population without the disease, IR is the incidence rate, and D is the average duration (or length of time) that an individual has the disease. This equation assumes that the population is in steady state of inflow equals outflow, and that the IR and duration do not change over time.

If the population at risk and the prevalence pool are stationary and everyone is either at risk or has the disease, then the number of people entering the prevalence pool in any time period will be balanced by the number exiting from it. Supposing there is no immigration into or emigration from the prevalence so that no one enters or leaves the pool except by disease onset, death, or recovery, the size of the population at risk will be the size of the population (N), minus the size of the prevalence pool (P); and during any time interval of length Δt, the number who enter the prevalence pool would be $IR (N - P) \Delta t$ and the outflow of the prevalence pool would be $IR'P \Delta t$ where IR' is the IR of exiting the prevalence pool. In the absence of migration, the reciprocal of IR' will equal the mean duration of the disease, $\overline{D}$; and so it follows that:

$$\text{Inflow} = IR (N - P) \Delta t = \text{outflow} = (1/\overline{D}) P\Delta t \text{ which yields } \frac{P}{N - P} = IR \times \overline{D} \text{ where } P/$$

($N - P$) is the ratio of diseased to nondiseased people in the population or equivalently the ratio of the prevalence proportion to the nondiseased proportion, or the prevalence odds. If the prevalence is small (<0.1), then P approximates $IR \times \overline{D}$.

Although incidence is most useful for evaluating the effectiveness of a program that seeks to prevent diseases from occurring in the first place, researchers who study the cause of disease and prefer to examine new cases (incidence) over existing ones (prevalence) because they are interested more in exposures that lead to developing the disease in question.[2] Prevalence obscures the relationship because it combines incidence and survival. On the other hand, prevalence is most useful for estimating the needs of medical facilities and allocating resources for treating individuals who already have a disease.

Odds

Odds are the ratio of the probability of an event of interest to that of the nonevent and can be defined both for incidence and for prevalence. When dealing with incidence probabilities, the odds are simply:

$$\frac{I}{1-I}$$

And while knowing the odds allow the calculation of probability:

$$\frac{odds}{1+odds}$$

The point prevalence odds are similarly expressed as:

$$\frac{Point\ prevalence}{1 - Point\ prevalence}$$

Both odds and proportions can be used to express the frequency of a disease and can approximate a proportion when the disease is very small (eg, <0.1). If the proportion of a disease is known in a population to be 0.20, the odds of the disease can be expressed as:

$$\frac{proportion\ of\ the\ population\ with\ disease}{1 - proportion\ of\ population\ with\ disease} = \frac{proportion\ of\ the\ population\ with\ disease}{proportion\ of\ the\ population\ without\ disease}$$

Although as an isolated measure epidemiologists rarely if ever use odds to express disease occurrence, the odds ratio (OR) is a useful measure of association because it estimates the relative risk (RR) in case-based studies.

Mortality Ratios

Other measures of risk are generally expressed using mortality ratios (MR) to estimate the frequency of this occurrence of death in a defined population over a specified interval, whether expressed as crude mortality for all causes in a population or a single cause. MRs can be studied in reference to infant and maternal deaths, or adjusted for sex, age, race, and ethnicity, or by particular conditions or the proportion thereof to provide insight into public health responses to the leading causes of mortality and health disparities. Crude mortality generally refers to the total number of deaths from all causes based on raw data per 100,000 population per year. Cause-specific mortality is the number of deaths from a specific cause per 100,000 population per year. Age-specific mortality or the death rate is the total number of deaths from all causes among individuals in a specific age category per 100,000 population per year in the age category. Often divided into neonatal deaths occurring during the first 27 days after birth and postneonatal deaths occurring from 28 days to 12 months, the infant mortality rate is the number of number of deaths of infants less than 1 year of age per 1000 live births per year. The morbidity rate represents the number of existing or new cases of a particular disease or condition per 100 population. The time period and the size of the population concerned may vary. The attack rate is the number of new cases of disease that develops usually during a defined and short time period, per the number in a healthy population at risk at the start of the period. This cumulative incidence measure is usually reserved for infectious outbreaks. The case fatality rate is the number of deaths per number of cases of disease. This is a type of cumulative incidence, so it is generally useful to specify the length of time to which it applies. Last, the survival rate is the number of living cases per number of cases of diseased. This rate is the complement of the case fatality rate, and is also a cumulative incidence measure.

Disability and Summary Measures

The term *premature mortality* was originally proposed to address the inadequacy of MR in measuring the burden of disease owing to tuberculosis and has since proved to be a particularly useful way to describe other diseases.[10] In choosing an arbitrary limit to life, the calculation of the difference between the age at death and an arbitrary designated limit measured in years of life lost (YLL) owing to premature mortality is a useful assessment of the impact of premature mortality in a given population. The YLL rate, which represents years of potential life lost per 1000 population below an arbitrary endpoint age such as 65 years, is more desirable in comparing premature mortality in different populations because the YLL does not take into account differences in population sizes.[11]

Another measure of the burden of disease in a population termed disability-adjusted life years captures in a single figure, health losses associated with mortality and different nonfatal outcomes of diseases and injuries.[12] Summary measures used by the Global Burden of Disease Studies[13,14] such as Healthy Adjusted Life Expectancy (HALE) are derived from YLLs and years lived with disability (YLDs) to compare assessments of broad epidemiologic patterns across countries and time, and to quantify the component of variation in epidemiology related to sociodemographic development. Calculated by adding YLLs and YLDs, disability-adjusted life years add disability to the measure of mortality, and based on the universal measure of time in life years, provides a common currency for health care resource allocation and the effectiveness of interventions assessed one relative to another across a wide range of health problems. YLDs, equal to the sum of prevalence multiplied by the general public's assessment of the severity of health loss, has been used as a primary metric to explore disease patterns over time, age, sex, and geography, and in recognizing that the aging of the world's population has led to substantial increases in the number of individuals with sequelae of diseases.[15] Because YLDs have been declining much more slowly than MRs, the nonfatal dimensions of disease require more and more attention from health care systems. Neurologic disorders accounted for 7.7% of all cause YLDs in 2013, a 5% increase in age-standardized YLDs from 1990 to 2013 (2.4%–7.9%) with the leading causes being Alzheimer disease, Parkinson disease, epilepsy, multiple sclerosis, migraine, tension and medication overuse headaches, and other neurologic disorders.[14]

MEASURES OF EFFECT AND ASSOCIATION

Measures of effect compare what would happen to 1 population under 2 possible but distinct life courses or conditions, of which at most only 1 can occur. In contrast, a measure of association compares what happens in 2 distinct populations, although the 2 distinct populations may correspond to one population in different time periods. Subject to physical and social limitations, one can observe both populations and so can directly observe an association. Greenland and colleagues[16] review measures of effect and measures of association further detailed below.

Risk Difference

Consider a cohort followed over a specific time or between a given age interval under 2 different conditions, some of whom who are exposed to a potentially harmful factor, and others who are not and one asks the question of the alternative potential outcomes in each of the 2 cohort groups. The IR of each potential outcome could be expressed as a difference in IR or *causal rate difference*, alternatively as a difference in incidence proportions to derive an absolute effect per se of a treatment intervention to derive an absolute effect on the incidence proportion. Supposing that we have a cohort of size N defined at the start of a fixed time interval and that anyone alive without the disease is at risk of the disease, everyone is exposed throughout the time interval leading to A_1 cases over a time T_1. A_0 cases will also occur over a total time risk noted as T_0. Thus the causal rate difference will be written as:

$$\frac{A_1}{T_1} - \frac{A_0}{T_0}$$

whereas the casual risk difference will be expressed as:

$$\frac{A_1}{N} - \frac{A_0}{N}$$

And the causal difference in average disease-free time would be noted as:

$$\frac{T_1}{N} - \frac{T_0}{N} = \frac{T_1 - T_0}{N}$$

When the outcome is death, the negative of the average time difference ($T_0/N - T1/N$) is often called the YLL.

Risk Ratio

Effect measures are most often calculated by taking ratios notably the rate and risk ratios terms RRs. The casual rate ratio can be expressed as:

$$\frac{\frac{A_1}{T_1}}{\frac{A_0}{T_0}} = \frac{I_1}{I_0}$$ where $I_1 = A_1/T_1$ is the IR|1 = exposed and 0 = unexposed, and the

caused risk ratio can be expressed as: $$\frac{\frac{A_1}{N}}{\frac{A_0}{N}} = \frac{A_1}{A_0} = \frac{R_1}{R_0}.$$

Relative Excess

A RR of greater than 1, reflecting an average effect that is causal, can be expressed as an excess RR. The excess casual rate ratio is written as:

$$IR - 1 = \frac{I_1}{I_0} - 1 = \frac{I_1 - I_0}{I_0}$$ where $IR = I_1/I_0$ is the causal rate ratio.

The excess causal risk ratio can be expressed as:

$$RR - 1 = \frac{R_1}{R_0} - 1 = \frac{R_1 - R_0}{R_0}$$ where $RR = R_1/R_0$ is the casual risk ratio.

The excess rate can be expressed relative to I_1 or R_1, respectively, as:

$$1 - \frac{1}{IR} \text{ or } 1 - \frac{1}{RR}$$

The measures that arise from interchanging I_1 with I_0 and R_1 with R_0 in attributable fractions, also termed *preventable fractions*, can be interpreted easily. The expression fraction of the risk under nonexposure that could be prevented by exposure can be written as:

$$(R_0 - R_1)/R_0 = 1 - R_1/R_0 = 1 - RR$$

In vaccine studies, this measure is also known as the *vaccine efficacy*.

Null State and Counterfactual in Relation to Effect Measurement

When the occurrence measures being compared do not vary with exposure, then the measures of effect will equal 0 if expressed as a difference, or 1 if expressed as a ratio. A null effect or null state does not depend on the way an occurrence measure is compared. Counterfactual refers, as its name implies, to the effect measure contrary to fact such that if a cohort is exposed or treated, then the untreated state will be the counterfactual. The important feature of counterfactually defined effect measures is that they involve 2 distinct conditions: an index status, which usually involves some exposure or treatment, and a reference condition, such as no treatment against which the exposure or treatment will be evaluated. Although unapproachable in practical terms, the counterfactual can be thought of as the outcome if the exposed or treated group had not been exposed.

Prevalence Ratios

It was shown previously that the crude prevalence odds (PO) equals the crude IR, I, multiplied by the average disease duration, $\overline{D}$ when both the population at risk and the prevalence pool are stationary and there is no migration in or out of the it. Restating this relation between a single population under exposure and another unexposed, or separate exposed and unexposed populations:

$$PO_1 = I_1\overline{D}_1 \text{ and } PO_0 = I_0\overline{D}_0,$$

where subscripts 1 and 0 refer to exposed and unexposed respectively.

If the average disease duration is the same regardless of exposure $(\overline{D}_1 = \overline{D}_0)$, the crude prevalence OR (POR), will equal the crude IR:

$$POR = \frac{PO_1}{PO_2} = \frac{I_1}{I_0} = IR$$

EPIDEMIOLOGY ESTIMATION

Rothman and colleagues[17,18] review validity, precision, and statistics in epidemiologic studies discussed further.

Validity and Error

The epidemiologic estimate is the end product of the study design, the conducted study, and the data analysis. The goal of an epidemiologic study is to obtain a valid and precise estimate of the frequency of a disease or of the effect of an exposure on the occurrence of a disease in the source population under investigation. This entails consideration of all the possible threats to internal and external validity. Taken to an extreme, however, epidemiologic studies designed to sample subjects from a target population of particular interest such that the study population is a probability sample from that population through oversampling subgroups in an effort to enhance *internal validity*, may fail to identify causal relationships, thereby limiting the external validity or generalizability of study. Most violations of internal validity can be classified into 3 general categories: confounding, selection bias, and information bias. Accuracy in estimation necessitates that statistical measures are estimated with little error, failures of which can be either random or systematic. Although random errors in the sampling and measurement of subjects can lead to systematic errors in the final estimates, important principles of study design emerge from separate considerations of sources of random and systematic errors. Random error or variation can detract from accuracy and has many components, but the major contributor is the process of selecting study subjects. Referred to as sampling error or variation, it factors more heavily in case control studies that involve a physical sampling process than it does in cohort studies. At least conceptually, the subjects in the study population selected to represent the population of broader interest may not satisfy the definition of a random sample for which strict statistical tools will be used to measure random variation. Other sources of random error include unexplained variation in occurrence measures such as observed IRs or prevalence proportions, mismeasurement of key study variables, and variance of the measurement or estimation process. Common approaches to reduce random error and to increase precision in epidemiologic estimation include increasing the study size, modification of the study design to increase precision, stratification of data to examine effects in subcategories, and significance and hypothesis testing using confidence intervals (CI) and interval estimation.

Systematic errors in epidemiologic estimation commonly referred to as *biases*, threaten the internal validity of a study. They are classified primarily into 3 general categories: confounding, selection bias, and information bias. Confounding occurs when the apparent effect of the exposure of interest is distorted because the effect of extraneous factors and is mistaken for, or mixed with, the actual exposure effect. The distortion introduced by a confounder may lead to overestimation or underestimation of an effect, toward or away from the null, depending on the direction of the association that the confounder has with exposure and outcome; or even change the apparent direction of an effect. By definition, confounders are extraneous risk factors for the outcome, associated with but not affected by the exposure or disease in the source population under study, and not an intermediate in the causal path between the exposure and outcome.

By contrast, selection biases are distortions resulting from procedures used to select subjects and from factors that influence study participation. The common element is that the relationship between exposure and outcome is different for those who participate, and all those who should be theoretically eligible for study, including those who do not participate. Bias in estimating an effect can be caused by measurement errors termed *information bias*, the direction and magnitude of which depends on whether the distribution of errors effect discrete variables with a countable number of possible values (misclassification errors), the values of 1 or more variables (nondifferential or differential misclassification), and its impact on binary variables. Misclassification can lead to alterations in the sensitivity or specificity of the measurement method. Although correctly classifying someone who is truly exposed as exposed, enhancing sensitivity, will be offset by falsely categorizing another unexposed and who is truly exposed; conversely, categorizing someone correctly as unexposed, strengthening specificity, will be lessened by misclassifying another as exposed.

Predictive probability positive is the probability that someone who is classified as exposed is truly exposed, whereas predictive probability negative is the probability that someone who is classified as unexposed is truly unexposed.

P Values

There are 2 types of P values: upper and lower, and accurate definitions of the associated statistics are often not considered rigorously in epidemiologic literature. An upper 1-tailed P value is the probability that a corresponding quantity computed from the data known as the test statistic, such as a t-test or χ^2 statistic, will be greater than or equal to its observed value, assuming that the test hypothesis is correct and there is no source of bias in the data collection or analysis. Similarly, a lower 1-tailed P value is the probability that the corresponding test statistic will be less than or equal to its observed value, again assuming that the test hypothesis is correct and that the underlying statistical model is correct. The 2-tailed P value, however, is usually regarded as twice the smaller of the upper and lower P values; however, being a probability, a 1-tailed P value must fall between 0 and 1, whereas the 2-tailed P value as defined, may exceed 1. Although equally regarded as a level of significance,[19] this term is usually avoided because it may be used in reference to alpha levels. In significance testing, small P values are supposed to indicate that at least 1 of the assumptions used to derive it is incorrect, but all too often, the statistical model is taken as a given so that a small P value is taken as indicating a low degree of compatibility between the test hypothesis and the observed data.

Hypothesis Testing

The use of P values and references to statistically significant findings highlights the dominant role that statistical hypothesis testing has occupied. Based on a value less than or greater than an arbitrary cutoff value, usually .05, called the *alpha* (α) level of the test, statistical significance testing of associations focuses on the null hypothesis, which is usually formulated as a hypothesis of no association between 2 variables from a population in which the observed study groups have been sampled in a random fashion. One may test for example the hypothesis that the risk difference in the population is 0 or the risk ratio is 1.0; alternatively, that the former is 0.1 and the latter equal to 2.0. The use of a fixed α cutoff is the hallmark of statistical hypothesis testing with both the alpha level and P value called the significance level of the test. This usage has led to misinterpretation of the P value as the alpha level of a statistical hypothesis test. A common misinterpretation of significance testing is to assert that there is no difference between 2 observed groups because the null test is not statistically significant and because the P value is greater than the cutoff for declaring statistical significance. Another misinterpretation of P values is that they represent probabilities of test hypotheses. A P value for a simple test hypothesis that exposure and disease are unassociated is not a probability of that hypothesis. The P value includes not only the probability of the observed data under the test hypothesis, but also the probabilities for all other possible data configurations. Although the P value is a continuous measure of the compatibility between a hypothesis and data, the alpha level is used to classify an observation as either significant, as when the $P \leq \alpha$, such that the test hypothesis is rejected, or not significant at the level α if $P > \alpha$, in which case the test hypothesis is accepted, or at least not rejected.

To avoid confusion, one should recall that the P value is a quantity computed from the data, whereas the alpha level is a fixed cutoff, usually 0.05, that can be specified without even seeing the data. Formal hypothesis testing avoids use of the P value in the formulation of hypothesis testing, instead defining the test based on whether the value of the test statistic falls into a rejection region for the test statistic. An incorrect rejection is called a type 1 error or alpha error. A hypothesis testing procedure is said to be valid if, whenever the test hypothesis is true, the probability of rejection ($P \leq \alpha$) does not exceed the alpha level, provided there is no bias and the statistical model is correct. Hence, a valid test with $\alpha = 0.01$ (a 1% alpha level) will lead to a type 1 error with no more than 1% probability, provided there is no bias or incorrect assumption. However, if the test hypothesis is false but is not rejected, the incorrect decision not to reject is called a type II or beta error. If the test hypothesis is false, so that rejection is the correct decision, the probability that the test hypothesis is rejected is called the *power* of the test. The probability of a type II error is related to the power (*Pr*) by the equation: *Pr* (type II error) = 1 - *Pr*. The trade-off between the probabilities of type I and II errors depends on the alpha level chosen in that reducing the type I error when the test hypothesis is true requires a smaller alpha level, because a smaller *P* value will be required to reject the test hypothesis. Unfortunately, a lower alpha level increases the probability of a type II error if the test hypothesis is false while, increasing the alpha level reduces the probability of type II error when the test hypothesis is false, thus increasing the probability of type I error if it is true.

Confidence Intervals and Limits

Estimation measurement may benefit from more detailed statistics performed on a continuous scale with a theoretically infinite number of possible values than the simple dichotomy produced by statistical hypothesis testing of a simple parameter such as a risk or rate ratio, IR or another epidemiologic measure. Although one way to account for random error in the estimation process is to compute *P* values for a broad range of possible parameters in addition to the null value, if the range is broad enough, it is possible to calculate a confidence interval (CI) for which the *P* value exceeds a specific alpha level typically 0.05 as an example of interval estimation. The endpoints of the CI are termed *confidence limits* and the width of the depends on both the amount of random variability inherent in the data collection process and an arbitrary selected alpha level that specifies the degree compatibility between the limits of the interval and the data wherein one minus the alpha level (0.95 if alpha is 0.05) is called the confidence level of the CI and expressed as a percentage. Considering the relation of the CI to significance and hypothesis testing, consider a test of the null hypothesis with an $\alpha = 0.10$ If the 90% CI does not include the null point, then the null hypothesis would be rejected for $\alpha = 0.10$. On the other hand, if included in a 95% CI, then the null hypothesis would not be rejected for $\alpha = 0.05$. Because the 95% CI incudes the null point and the 90% did not, it can be inferred that the 2-sided *P* value for the null hypothesis is greater than .05 but less than .10. Thus, although a 2-sided *P* value instead indicates only the degree of consistency between the data and a single hypothesis, confidence limits provide an idea of the direction and magnitude of the underlying association as well as the random variability of point estimation.[20]

Because a given CI is only one of an infinite number of ranges nested within one another, points nearer to the center of the ranges are more compatible with the data than points distant from the center; thus, to see the entire set of possible CI, one constructs a *P value function*, comprising all points for which the 2-sided *P* value exceeds the alpha level of the CI. It summarizes the 2 key components of the estimation process. The peak of the curve indicates the point estimate and the concentration of the curve around the point estimate indicates the precision of the estimate. A narrow *P* value function would result from a large study with high precision, whereas a broad function would result from a small study with low precision. A CI represents only 1 possible horizontal slide through the *P* value function. A *P* value function from which one can find confidence limits for a hypothetical study with a rate ratio estimate of 3.1, has a curve that reaches its peak corresponding to the point estimate for the rate ratio; while the 95% CI can be read directly from the graph as the function values where the right-hand ordinate is 0.95. The *P* value for any value of the parameter can be found from the left-hand ordinate corresponding to the height where the vertical line drawn at the hypothesized rate ratio that equals 1 intersects the *P* value function. Likelihood intervals, likelihood functions, and natural logarithms of the likelihood function or log-likelihood, which are beyond the scope of this article can be found in advanced epidemiology texts, have sought to replace CI.[21–23]

EPIDEMIOLOGIC STUDY DESIGN

Epidemiologic study designs comprise both experimental and nonexperimental types. The term *experimental* implies that the investigator manipulates the exposure assigned to participants in the study. In a randomized clinical trial (RCT), the gold standard for medical investigation, the investigator creates groups through random allocation of an exposure or treatment. However, when experiments are infeasible or unethical, epidemiologists design nonexperimental or observational studies that simulate what might have occurred had an experiment been conducted. In that regard, the researcher is an observer rather than an agent who assigned interventions. Rothman and colleagues[24–26] review the major types of epidemiologic studies further explained below.

There are 4 types of nonexperimental studies: cohort, case control, cross-sectional and ecological types. In cohort studies, the subjects of a source population are classified according to their exposure status and followed over time to ascertain disease incidence. In case control studies, cases arising from a source population and a sample of the source population are classified according to their exposure history. Cross-sectional studies include as subjects all persons in the population at the time of ascertainment or a representative sample, selected without regard to exposure or outcome status, usually to estimate prevalence. In ecological studies, the unit of observation is a group of people rather than an individual.

Cohort Studies

In principle, cohort studies can be used to estimate average risks, rates, and occurrence times, but to do so the entire cohort remains at risk and under observation for the entire follow-up period. Such measurements, however, are only feasible when there is little or no loss to follow-up. When losses and competing risks occur, IRs can be estimated directly, whereas the average risk and occurrence time can be estimated using basic survival analysis involving stratification on follow-up time using life-table analysis methods. The main guide to the classification of persons or person-time should be defined explicitly according to the study hypothesis and design to estimate appropriately the exposure effects and avoid implicit assumptions. Chronic exposures based on anticipated effects is more complicated than when exposure occurs only at a point in time, which can be conceptualized as a period during which the exposure accumulates to a sufficient extent to trigger a step in the causal process. The time at which an outcome event occurs can be a major determinant of the amount of person-time contributed by a subject to each exposure category. The method of calculation for cumulative incidence and IR in cohort studies is shown in the example below.

In a study, a researcher observed 2000 people in total with 1000 in each exposure status for 3 years to see whether they develop a disease. The result is shown in **Table 1**.

$$I = \frac{\text{number of new cases of a disease}}{\text{number of candidate population}}$$

$I_{exp} = 36/1000 = 0.036$, $I_{nonexp} = 10/1000 = 0.010$,
risk ratio = $I_{exp}/I_{nonexp} = 0.036/0.010 = 3.6$.

$$\text{Incidence rate} = \frac{\text{number of disease onsets}}{\sum_{persons}\text{time spent in population}}$$

$$IR_{exp} = \frac{\text{number of disease onsets}}{\sum_{persons}\text{time spent in population}}$$

$$= \frac{36}{0.5 \times 4 + 1 \times 5 + 1.5 \times 8 + 2 \times 6 + 2.5 \times 4 + 3 \times 973}$$

$$= \frac{36}{2960 \text{ person} - \text{year}}$$

$$IR_{nonexp} = \frac{\text{number of disease onsets}}{\sum_{persons}\text{time spent in population}}$$

$$= \frac{10}{0.5 \times 2 + 1 \times 1 + 1.5 \times 1 + 2 \times 3 + 2.5 \times 1 + 3 \times 992}$$

$$= \frac{10}{2988 \text{ person} - \text{year}}$$

Rate ratio = $IR_{exp}/IR_{nonexp} = 3.63$.

It is important to define and determine the time of the event in cohort studies as unambiguously and precisely as possible, incorporating the details of available data and the current state of knowledge about the study outcome. Cohort studies are expensive to conduct because stable estimates of incidence require a substantial number of cases of disease, and therefore person-time giving rise to the cases will be substantial. When studying a rare disease or one that has a long latency for development, especially when cost is a factor, a case control study design is preferable.

Table 1
Incidence and incidence rates

Years of Observation	No. of Cases in Exposed (1000)	No. of Cases in Nonexposed (1000)
0.5	4	2
1.0	5	1
1.5	8	1
2.0	6	3
2.5	4	1
3.0	9	2

Case Control Studies

The use and understanding of case control studies was an important methodologic advance in modern epidemiology as the field advanced from randomized to non-randomized cohort studies to case control studies. Although conventional wisdom holds that cohort studies are useful for evaluating the range of effects related to a single exposure, case control studies nested within a single population using several disease outcomes as the case series is possible with a case cohort study design. Recognizing that case control studies are most practical for rare diseases when expo-sure is rare, ordinary case control studies may likewise be inefficient unless selective recruitment of additional exposed subjects is performed. Ideally, a case control study should be conceptualized as a more efficient version of a corresponding cohort study. Rather than including all of the experiences of the source population that gave rise to cases, as would be the practice in a cohort study design, controls are selected from the source population. Therein lies the challenge of achieving random sampling of controls from the source population, and when it is not possible to identify explicitly the source population, and simple random sampling is not possible, secondary source populations become an option using neighborhood controls, random digit dialing, hospital- or clinic-based controls, and even friends with close attention to representa-tiveness, comparability of information accuracy, and the number of control groups needed.

Recognizing that the primary goal for control selection is that the exposure distribu-tion among controls is such that it is the same as in the source population of cases, OR calculations achieve this goal by using control cases in place of the denominator in measures of disease frequency to determine the ratio of the disease frequency in exposed relative to unexposed people. Using person-time to illustrate, the goal re-quires that exposed controls (B_1) has the same ratio to the amount of exposed person-time (T_1) as unexposed controls (B_0) have to the amount of unexposed person-time (T_0), apart from sampling error to compute control sampling rates:

$$\frac{B_1}{T_1} = \frac{B_0}{T_0}$$

If A_1 is the exposed cases and A_0 unexposed cases over a study period, the exposed and unexposed IR are computed as:

$$I_1 = \frac{A_1}{T_1} \text{ and } I_0 = \frac{A_0}{T_0}$$

Using the denominators of the frequencies of the exposed and unexposed controls as substitutes for the actual denominators of the rates to obtain exposure-specific case control rates or pseudo-rates, those rates can be rewritten as:

$$\text{Pseudo-rate}_1 = \frac{A_1}{B_1} \text{ and Pseudo-rate}_0 = \frac{A_0}{B_0}$$

By dividing the pseudorate for exposed by the pseudo-rate for unexposed, we obtain an estimate of the ratio of the IRs in the source population provided that the control sampling is independent of exposure.

The ratio of the 2 pseudo-rates in a case control study also known as the cross-product ratio or OR is written as:

$$OR = A_1 B_0 / A_0 B_1$$

It can be viewed as the ratio of cases to controls among the exposed subjects (A_1/B_1) divided by the ratio of cases to controls among the unexposed subjects (A_0/B_0) or as the odds of being exposed among cases (A_1/A_0) divided by the odds of being exposed among controls (B_1/B_0), in which case it is termed the *exposure OR*. Although either interpretation gives the same result, viewing this OR as the ratio of case control ratios shows more directly how the control group substitutes for the denominator information in a cohort study and how the ratio of pseudo-frequencies gives the same result as the ratio of IR, incidence proportion, or incidence odds in the source population, if sampling is independent of exposure. Further, it is not necessary to assume that the disease under study is rare.

Cross-Sectional Studies

Cross-sectional studies investigate the association between prevalence of diseases or mortality and prevalence of risk factors in a defined population at a certain time point. All the information is collected at the same time. Cross-sectional studies conducted to estimate prevalence are termed a *prevalence study*. Exposure is ascertained simultaneously with the disease and different exposure subpopulations may be compared with respect to their disease prevalence. Two potential limitations in cross-sectional studies are determining the time order of events and overrepresentation of cases with long duration and underrepresentation with short durations of illness, termed *length-biased sampling*. Because prevalence depends on incidence and duration, a high prevalence of disease or mortality may result from long duration of time despite a low incidence. Because cross-sectional studies investigate the status at one specific point in time, it may not be possible to determine whether the risk factors happened before disease. Cross-sectional studies may involve sampling subjects differentially with respect to disease status to increase the number of cases in the sample. Such studies termed *prevalent case control studies* are designed similar to incident case control studies except that the case series comprises prevalent rather than incident cases. Although significant associations may be found in a given cross-sectional study, it may not reflect the true causation.

Ecological Studies

Ecological studies focus on the association between the summary measure of disease or mortality and risk factors, and the unit of ecological studies is a group not an individual. The groups can be countries, states, regions, schools, or zip codes, among others. Ecological measures can be classified into aggregate, environmental, and global measures. *Aggregate measures* reflect characteristics of individuals within a group and *environmental measures* represent physical characteristics of the geographic location; *global measures* may be characteristics of the group or place without analogy to the individual. Such studies are able to examine a broad range of diseases and risk factors using demographic and consumption data, and are very useful in generating hypotheses on association in advance of epidemiologic studies on individual observations. In addition, ecological studies have other advantages, such as low cost and the convenience link of aggregate data, freedom from the measurement and design limitations of individual-level studies, and simplicity of analysis and presentation. For some risk factors, aggregate measurements may be more accurate than individual measurements. Data collection, disease definition, and treatment may vary across units, and this can introduce bias. A major limitation of ecological studies is bias, which can be interpreted as the failure of associations seen at one level of grouping to correspond with effect measures at the grouping level of interest. In other words, the association between risk factor and disease found on the group level may not hold true within individuals.

REGRESSION TECHNIQUES

Szklo and Nieto[6] review regression techniques.

Simple Linear Regression

The process of determining whether the relationship between the 2 variables is compatible with straight line begins with the visual inspection of a scatter plot followed by the calculation of the liner correlation coefficient, r. With a range of -1.0 to 1.0, inscribing perfectly straight lines of negative and positive 1.0 slopes, a value of 0 indicates instead no linear correlation. The correlation coefficient value contains no information about the strength of the association between the 2 variables that is represented by the slope of the theoretic line it inscribes that is further defined by 2 other parameters, β_0 and β_1, respectively, the y intercept when $x = 0$, and the regression coefficient as shown in the formula below:

$$y = \beta_0 + \beta_1 x$$

In linear regression, the method used to estimate the values of the regression coefficients is the least-squares method, which consists in finding the parameter values that minimize the sum of the squares of the vertical distance between each of the observed points and the line.[27,28] The notation traditionally used to represent the estimated linear regression line is as follows:

$$y = b_0 + b_1 x$$

The regression coefficient (b_1) estimates the average increase in the dependent variable per unit increase in the independent variable and like any other statistical estimate, it is subject to uncertainty and random error. Thus, it is important to estimate the standard error of the regression coefficient to evaluate its statistical significance and to calculate the confidence limits around its point estimate. The standard error estimate is provided readily by most statistical packages performing linear regression.

Multiple Linear Regression

Simple linear regression can be extended to multivariate regression using the same model adjusted when the outcome is a continuous variable as follows:

$$y = \beta_0 + \beta_1 x_1 + \beta_2 x_2 + \ldots + \beta_k x_k \text{ or } y = b_0 + b_1 X_1 + b_2 X_2 + \ldots + b_k X_k$$

The postulated risk factors (x or independent variables) can be continuous or categorical (dichotomous) with multiple levels that can be treated as ordinal or transformed in a set of binary variables. The estimated values of the regression coefficients are obtained by the least-squares method. An important assumption in the model is that there is no interaction between the variables in the model such that the change in y associated with a unit change in x for the entire range of x and vice versa. The regression coefficient (β_k) represents the average increase in outcome per unit increase in x_k, adjusted for all the other variables in the model. If interaction is present, stratified models can be used for each variable. Alternatively, interaction terms, known as *product terms*, can be used in the regression equation. The multivariate model enables one to study the effect of main exposure while adjusting confounders, mediators, and interaction at the same time. The traditional way, such as restriction or stratification, is limited if there are many confounders. The model can adjust both categorical and continuous variable as demonstrated in the study by Weinstein and colleagues[29] of the association between clinical stroke and subsequent cognitive function in initially nondemented individuals. Outcome can be expressed in natural log-transformed cognitive scores, as necessary, to reduce skewness. The primary independent variable was stroke status. The unadjusted model was expressed as: log-transformed cognitive scores $= b_0 + b_1 \times$ stroke. Model 1 was adjusted for age, sex, education level, cohort (original or offspring), and the Mini-Mental State Examination (MMSE) score. Model 2 was further adjusted for systolic blood pressure (SBP), diabetes, prevalent cardiovascular disease (CVD), prevalent atrial fibrillation and current smoking.

Model 1: log-transformed cognitive scores $= b_0 + b_1 \times$ stroke $+ b_2 \times$ age $+ b_3 \times$ sex $+ b_4 \times$ education $+ b_5 \times$ cohort $+ b_6 \times$ MMSE score; for model 2, add $b_7 \times$ SBP $+ b_8 \times$ diabetes $+ b_9 \times$ CVD $+ b_{10} \times$ atrial fibrillation $+ b_{11} \times$ smoke. There is a list of 1 domain of cognitive scores as an example in **Table 2**

Multiple Logistic Regression

For binary outcome variables, the logistic regression model offers a more robust alternative to binary multiple linear regression. The logistic regression model assumes that the relationship between a given value of a variable x and the probability of a binary outcome follows the logistic function:

$$P(y|x) = \frac{1}{1+e^{-(b_0+b_1 x)}}$$

where $P(y|x)$ denotes the probability (P) of the binary outcome (y) for a given value of x. The outcome of this equation, a probability, is constrained to values within the range of 0 to 1. By translating instead into OR estimation, the probability equation can be expressed in the equivalent equation:

$$\text{Log}\left(\frac{P}{1-P}\right) = \log(\text{odds}) = b_0 + b_1 x,$$ where P is the short notation for $P(y|x)$.

This expression is analogous to the simple linear regression function, except that the ordinate in now the logarithm of the odds or log odds, also known as *logit*, rather than the usual mean value of a continuous variable. Thus, if the relationship between exposure (x) and the occurrence of an outcome is assumed to fit the logistic regression model, that implies that the log odds of the outcome increases linearly with x. The multiple logistic regression model is shown as:

Table 2
Association of clinical stroke with cognitive performance

Outcome	Model 1		Model 2	
	$b_1 \pm$ SE	P Value	$b_1 \pm$ SE	P Value
LMi	-1.35 ± 0.52	.010	-1.27 ± 0.60	.035

Abbreviations: LMi, logical memory-immediate recall; SE, standard error.

$$\text{Log}\left(\frac{P}{1-P}\right) = \text{log(odds)} = b_0 + b_1 x_1 + b_2 x_2 + \ldots b_k x_k,$$ [where the regression coefficient (b_k) is the average increase in the log odds of the outcome per unit increase in x_k, adjusted for all other variables in the model].

The OR corresponding to a unit increase in the independent variable is the antilogarithm or exponential function of the regression coefficient b_1 as follows:

$$OR = e^{b_1}$$

Thus, the logistic regression model is a linear model in the log odds scale. What this means in practical terms is that, when a continuous variable is entered as such, the resulting coefficient and corresponding OR is assumed to represent the linear increase in log odds or the exponential increase in odds, per unit increase in the independent variable across the entire range of x values. Davydow and colleagues[30] studied whether depression, cognitive impairment without dementia (CIND), and/or dementia were each independently associated with risk of ischemic stroke. The outcome of interest was ischemic stroke. The primary independent variable was depression, CIND or dementia status at baseline defined categorically as no disorder, depression alone, CIND alone, dementia alone, cooccurring depression and CIND, or cooccurring depression and dementia. In unadjusted analysis, the model could be written as:

$$\text{Log}\left(\frac{P(\text{stroke})}{1-P(\text{stroke})}\right) = b_0 + b_1 \times \text{baseline status}.$$

Demographics, medical comorbidities, and health risk behaviors were treated as the possible characteristics to modify the association. In adjusted analysis the multiple logistic model is:

$$\text{Log}\left(\frac{P(\text{stroke})}{1-P(\text{stroke})}\right) = b_0 + b_1 \times \text{baseline status} + b_2 \times \text{demographics}$$
$$+ b_3 \times \text{comorbidities} + b_4 \times \text{health} - \text{risk behaviors}.$$

The OR are shown in **Table 3**.

The adjusted OR resulting from the exponentiation of the logistic regression coefficient obtained is often used as a surrogate of the RR or prevalence rate ratio, respectively. This interpretation is only justified for the analyses of rare outcomes, but when the frequency of the outcome of interest in high, the OR is a biased estimate of the RR

Table 3
Multiple logistic model

Baseline Status	Unadjusted OR (95% CI)	Adjusted OR (95% CI)
Depression alone	1.11 (0.88, 1.40)	1.09 (0.85, 1.38)
CIND alone	1.55 (1.27, 1.90)	1.37 (1.11, 1.69)
Dementia alone	1.36 (1.04, 1.77)	1.08 (0.81, 1.44)
Cooccurring depression and CIND	1.95 (1.48, 2.56)	1.65 (1.24, 2.18)
Cooccurring depression and dementia	1.51 (1.09, 2.10)	1.16 (0.82, 1.65)

Abbreviations: CI, confidence interval; CIND, cognitive impairment without dementia; OR, odds ratio.

or the prevalence rate ratio, because it tends to exaggerate the magnitude of the association. Thus, it is important to keep in mind the built-in bias associated with the OR as an estimate of the incidence or prevalence rate ratio when the outcome is common. An alternatives regression procedures to consider the log-binomial regression model, which results in direct estimates of the incidence or prevalence rate ratio.[31]

ACKNOWLEDGMENTS

The author (D.S. Younger) wishes to acknowledge the faculty of the Columbia University Mailman School of Public Health, New York, NY, who provided him the expertise in biostatistics and epidemiology to write this article and to provide it as a resource to neurology trainees and colleagues.

REFERENCES

1. Agresti A. An introduction to categorical data analysis. 2nd edition. Hoboken (NJ): John Wiley & Sons; 2007.
2. Aschergrau A, Seage GR III, editors. Essentials of epidemiology in public health. 2nd edition. Boston: Jones and Bartlett Publishers; 2008.
3. Hoffmann JP. Generalized linear models. An applied approach. New York: Pearson; 2004.
4. Hosmer DW Jr, Lemeshow S, Sturdivant RX. Applied logistic regression. 3rd edition. Hoboken (NJ): John Wiley & Sons; 2013.
5. Kleinbaum DG, Kupper LL, Nizam A, et al. Applied regression analysis and other multivariable methods. 4th edition. Belmont (CA): Thomson Brooks/Cole; 2008.
6. Szklo M, Nieto FJ. Epidemiology. Beyond the basics. 3rd edition. Burlington (MA): Jones & Bartlett Learning; 2014.
7. Rosner B. Fundamentals of biostatistics. 7th edition. Boston (MA): Brooks/Cole Cengage Learning; 2006.
8. Rothman KJ, Greenland S, Lash TL, editors. Modern epidemiology. 3rd edition. Philadelphia: Wolters Kluwer Health/Lippincott Williams & Wilkins; 2008.
9. Greenland S, Rothman KJ. Measures of occurrence. Chapter 3. In: Rothman KJ, Greenland S, Lash TL, editors. Modern epidemiology. 3rd edition. Philadelphia: Wolters Kluwer Health/Lippincott Williams & Wilkins; 2008. p. 32–50.
10. Dempsey M. Decline in tuberculosis. The death rate fails to tell the entire story. Am Rev Tuberc 1947;56:157–64.
11. National Center for Health Statistics. Health, United States, 2004. Hyattsville (MD): Department of Health and Human Services, National Center for Health Statistics; 2004. Available at: http://www.cdc.gov/nchs/hus.htm.
12. Murray CJ, Acharya AK. Understanding DALYs (disability-adjusted life years). J Health Econ 1997;16:703–30.
13. GBD 2013 DALYs and HALE Collaborators, Murray CJ, Barber RM, Foreman KJ, et al. Global, regional, and national disability-adjusted life years (DALYs) for 306 diseases and injuries and healthy life expectancy (HALE) for 188 countries, 1990-2013: quantifying the epidemiological transition. Lancet 2015;386:2145–91.
14. Global Burden of Disease Study 2013 Collaborators. Global, regional, and national incidence, prevalence, and years lived with disability for 301 acute and chronic diseases and injuries in 188 countries, 1990-2013: a systematic analysis for the Global Burden of Disease Study. Lancet 2013;2015(386):743–800.
15. Vos T, Flaxman AD, Naghavi M, et al. Years lived with disability (YLDs) for 1160 sequelae of 289 diseases and injuries 1990–2010: a systematic analysis for the Global Burden of Disease Study 2010. Lancet 2012;380:2163–96.

16. Greenland S, Rothman KJ, Lash TL. Measures of effect and measures of association. Chapter 4. In: Rothman KJ, Greenland S, Lash TL, editors. Modern epidemiology. 3rd edition. Philadelphia: Wolters Kluwer Health/Lippincott Williams & Wilkins; 2008. p. 51–70.

17. Rothman KJ, Greenland S, Lash TL. Validity in epidemiologic studies. In: Rothman KJ, Greenland S, Lash TL, editors. Modern epidemiology. 3rd edition. Philadelphia: Wolters Kluwer Health/Lippincott Williams & Wilkins; 2008. p. 128–47.

18. Rothman KJ, Greenland S, Lash TL. Precision and statistics in epidemiologic studies. In: Rothman KJ, Greenland S, Lash TL, editors. Modern epidemiology. 3rd edition. Philadelphia: Wolters Kluwer Health/Lippincott Williams & Wilkins; 2008. p. 148–67.

19. Cox DR, Hinkley DV. Theoretical statistics. New York: Chapman and Hall; 1974.

20. Bandt CL, Boen JR. A prevalent misconception about sample size, statistical significance, and clinical importance. J Periodontol 1972;43:181–3.

21. Goodman SN, Royall R. Evidence and scientific research. Am J Public Health 1988;78:1568–74.

22. Edwards AWF. Likelihood. 2nd edition. Baltimore (MD): Johns Hopkins University Press; 1992.

23. Royall R. Statistical inference: a likelihood paradigm. New York: Chapman and Hall; 1997.

24. Rothman KJ, Greenland S, Lash TL. Types of epidemiologic studies. In: Rothman KJ, Greenland S, Lash TL, editors. Modern epidemiology. 3rd edition. Philadelphia: Wolters Kluwer Health/Lippincott Williams & Wilkins; 2008. p. 87–99.

25. Rothman KJ, Greenland S. Cohort studies. In: Rothman KJ, Greenland S, Lash TL, editors. Modern epidemiology. 3rd edition. Philadelphia: Wolters Kluwer Health/Lippincott Williams & Wilkins; 2008. p. 100–10.

26. Rothman KJ, Greenland S, Lash TL. Case-control studies. In: Rothman KJ, Greenland S, Lash TL, editors. Modern epidemiology. 3rd edition. Philadelphia: Wolters Kluwer Health/Lippincott Williams & Wilkins; 2008. p. 111–27.

27. Armitage P, Berry G, Matthews JNS. Statistical methods in medical research. 4th edition. Oxford (United Kingdom): Blackwell Publishing; 2002.

28. Draper N, Smith H. Applied regression analysis. 3rd edition. New York: John Wiley & Sons; 1998.

29. Weinstein G, Preis SR, Beiser AS, et al. Cognitive performance after stroke-The Framingham Heart Study. Int J Stroke 2014;9:48–54.

30. Davydow DS, Levine DA, Zivin K, et al. The association of depression, cognitive impairment without dementia and dementia with risk of ischemic stroke: a cohort study. Psychosom Med 2015;77:200–8.

31. Spiegelman D, Hertzmark E. Easy SAS calculations for risk or prevalence ratios and differences. Am J Epidemiol 2005;162:199–200.

The Epidemiology of Global Epilepsy

Anuradha Singh, MD[a],*, Stephen Trevick, MD[b,c]

KEYWORDS

- Epilepsy • Seizures • Treatment gap • Taboos • Epidemiology • CNS infections

KEY POINTS

- Epilepsy, defined as a syndrome of at least 2 unprovoked seizures, affects more than 70 million people worldwide. Approximately 90% of those suffering from epilepsy are in developing regions.
- Causes of epilepsy include brain injury, genetic syndromes, brain masses, and a variety of central nervous system (CNS) infections.
- Approximately 75% of people with epilepsy in developing regions do not receive appropriate treatment.
- Complex financial factors limit treatment, along with a variety of cultural beliefs and taboos.
- Understanding of the variation in cultural understandings of epilepsy can help providers provide effective treatment.

INTRODUCTION

Epilepsy is a neurologic condition that affects people of all ages and has no geographic, social, or racial boundaries.[1] Descriptions of epileptic seizures and epilepsy date back to antiquity and were described in Mesopotamian writings[2] and Indian Vedas[3]; they are among the world's oldest recognized conditions, with written records dating back to 4000 BC. The word, *epilepsy*, comes from a Greek word that means to be taken, seized, or attacked. A seizure can have motor, sensory, psychic, or autonomic manifestations or a combination of these. A seizure is defined as a transient change in the clinical state of the patient due to excessive neuronal firing or depolarization. Seizures can be provoked or unprovoked. The

Disclosure Statement: The authors have nothing to disclose.
[a] Department of Neurology, Bellevue Epilepsy Center, Bellevue Hospital Center, NBV 7W11, New York, NY 10016, USA; [b] Department of Neurology, NYU School of Medicine, New York, NY, USA; [c] Department of Psychiatry, NYU School of Medicine, New York, NY, USA
* Corresponding author.
E-mail address: anuradha.singh@nyumc.org

Neurol Clin 34 (2016) 837–847
http://dx.doi.org/10.1016/j.ncl.2016.06.015
0733-8619/16/$ – see front matter © 2016 Elsevier Inc. All rights reserved.

neurologic.theclinics.com

operational revised 2014 definition of epilepsy by the International League Against Epilepsy is

1. At least 2 unprovoked (or reflex) seizures occurring greater than 24 hours apart.
2. One unprovoked (or reflex) seizure and a probability of further seizures similar to the general recurrence risk (at least 60%) after 2 unprovoked seizures, occurring over the next 10 years.
3. Diagnosis of an epilepsy syndrome
   a. Epilepsy is considered to be resolved for individuals who had an age-dependent epilepsy syndrome but are now past the applicable age or those who have remained seizure-free for the last 10 years, with no seizure medicines for the last 5 years.

EPIDEMIOLOGY

According to a recent study, 70 million people have epilepsy worldwide and nearly 90% of them are found in developing regions.[4] The study also estimated a median prevalence of 1.54% (0.48%–4.96%) for rural and 1.03% (0.28%–3.8%) for urban studies in developing countries.[4] Globally, an estimated 2.4 million people are diagnosed with epilepsy each year. In high-income countries, annual new cases are between 30 and 50 per 100,000 people in the general population. In low-income and middle-income countries, this figure can be up to 2 times higher. This is likely due to the increased risk of endemic conditions, such as malaria or neurocysticercosis (NCC); the higher incidence of road traffic injuries and birth-related injuries; variations in medical infrastructure; and availability of preventative health programs and accessible care. Approximately 90% live in resource-limited settings, which belong to low-income and middle-income countries, according to the World Bank income classification.[5] The prevalence of epilepsy in developed countries ranges from 4 to 10 cases per 1000.[6] Studies in the developing and tropical countries have reported higher prevalence rates of epilepsy, ranging from 14 to 57 cases per 1000 persons.[7,8] Higher prevalence rates of epilepsy in the developing countries is probably related to the methodological aspects of those studies, although in some regions in the world, specific infectious diseases, such as NCC, are frequent causes of epilepsy.[9] In developed countries, the incidence of epilepsy exhibits a U-shaped curve, with highest rates in the children and the elderly. In comparison, the incidence of epilepsy seems to peak in early adulthood in developing countries.

RISK FACTORS

There are many known risk factors for epilepsy, which range from head injuries at birth to those at any age, to chromosomal/genetic syndromes and various inborn errors of metabolism, CNS tumors or infections and so forth. The risk factors for epilepsy are listed in **Table 1**. The relative risk of developing epilepsy with different conditions in different populations is not known.

Epilepsy resulting from infection is a major cause of morbidity and mortality in low-income countries and the most preventable cause of epilepsy worldwide. Herpes simplex virus is the most common and most severe viral encephalitis in immunocompetent subjects (**Fig. 1**). Encephalitides due to arboviruses, Coxsackie virus, measles, rubella, Japanese encephalitis, chikungunya, and dengue fever are endemic in different parts of the world (**Table 2**). Patients may present with seizures during the acute encephalitic process but more often develop neurologic disability, including epilepsy, as a long-term complication. NCC is common in vast areas of South America, West Africa, and Asia. NCC is probably the most preventable form of epilepsy worldwide (**Fig. 2**). Approximately one-third of people with epilepsy living in regions

Table 1
Risk factors for epilepsy

Risk Factors	Comments
Febrile seizures	—
Family history of seizures	—
Congenital/developmental	Inborn errors of metabolism, Angelman syndrome, Prader-Willi syndrome, Rett syndrome
Neurophakomatoses	Tuberous sclerosis, Sturge-Weber syndrome
CNS infections	Meningitis; encephalitis; parasitic infections, such as NCC and *Plasmodium falciparum* in endemic areas, *Toxocara canis*, and *Onchocerca volvulus*
Head trauma	Subdural/epidural/intraparenchymal hemorrhage, dural penetrating injuries, skull fracture(s)
Neurodegenerative	Various dementias, Rett syndrome, progressive myoclonic epilepsies, neuronal ceroid lipofusinosis
Strokes	Congenital or acquired
Vascular malformations	Cavernomas, arteriovenous malformations
CNS tumors	Gangliogliomas, ganglioneurocytomas, DNETs, meningiomas, benign and malignant grades of tumors
Neuronal migrational disorders	Focal cortical dysplasia, lissencephaly, hemimegalencephaly, schizencephaly, periventricular nodular heterotopia, subcortical heterotopia
Other neurologic conditions associated with epilepsy	Autism, learning disabilities, migraine, depression, cerebral palsy

Abbreviation: DNET, dysembryoplastic neuroepithelial tumor.

endemic for *Taenia solium* were associated with NCC.[9] A large cohort of mesial temporal lobe epilepsy–hippocampal sclerosis patients were studied from a region in which it is endemic, and all patients were extensively evaluated by a team specialized in the treatment of NCC or epilepsy.[10] Cerebral malaria is a severe neurologic presentation of acute falciparum malaria, which can present as encephalopathy, seizures, or even status epilepticus. The neurologic sequelae may include residual epilepsy, hemiplegia, speech problems, cortical blindness, or cognitive deficits.

HIV infections may be complicated by a subacute cortical and subcortical encephalopathy and partial seizures are commonly encountered due to opportunistic infections, such as toxoplasmosis, cytomegalovirus, tuberculosis, and Cryptococcus infections (**Figs. 3** and **4**).

Parasites have the propensity to invade the brain and its vasculature, giving rise to seizures. Parasites can be broadly classified into single-celled organisms, called protozoa, or multicelled helminths (worms). Helminths are further classified into nematodes, trematodes, and cestodes. It is beyond the scope of this article to discuss all epileptogenic CNS infections worldwide in great detail, but **Table 3** lists a few commonly encountered parasitic infections that cause characteristic clinical syndromes. *T solium* is probably the commonest of these helminthic infestations but *Toxocara canis* could be a major culprit of the higher prevalence of epilepsy in low-income economies besides cerebral hydatidosis in sheep-raising areas, mainly from eating food contaminated with dog feces, and paragonimiasis in some endemic areas in the Far East, from eating undercooked or raw crab or crayfish.

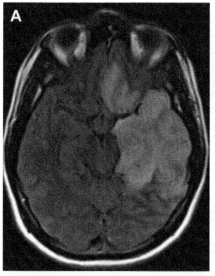

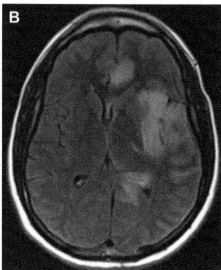

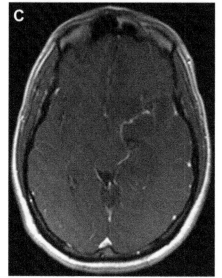

Fig. 1. MRI brain axial fluid-attenuated inversion recovery (FLAIR) images in herpetic encephalitis show (A) abnormal hyperintense signal in the left temporal lobe and left orbitofrontal cortex and (B) left cingulate, left insular cortex, and splenium of the corpus callosum on the left. (C) T_1-weighted image with gadolinium showing minimal contrast enhancement.

Echinococcus granulosus occurs worldwide with the exception of a few countries, such as Iceland and Greenland. Hydatid disease is more common in sheep-raising areas of the Mediterranean, Middle East, Australia, New Zealand, South Africa, and South America and tend to affect liver and lung leading to cerebral hydatidosis and seizures. The cysts develop slowly (usually over many years) into large (up to 1 L), fluid-filled (hydatid) cysts, which contain numerous infective protoscolices. *E multilocularis* does not produce large cysts but invades and destroys surrounding normal hepatic tissue and can result in liver failure and death. It can rarely involves the lungs and brain.

Table 2	
Common regional viral infections associated with epilepsy	
Colorado tick fever	Western United States and Canada
Crimean-Congo hemorrhagic fever	Africa and India
Dengue	Tropical regions of Americas, Africa, Asia, and Oceania
Japanese encephalitis	South and Southeast Asia
Kunjin virus	Oceania
Louping ill viruses	Northern Britain
Murray valley encephalitis	Australia and Papua New Guinea
Powassan encephalitis	Northeast USA and Canada
Rabies	Global, sparing central Europe and Australia
Tick borne	Northern Eurasia (primarily central Europe and across Siberia)
West Nile	Africa, Europe, the Middle East, West and Central Asia, Oceania, North Africa

TREATMENT GAPS IN EPILEPSY CARE

Quality epilepsy care requires expertise and availability of both monitoring equipment and medications. Unfortunately, these can all be resource-heavy requirements. Financial limitations interfere with this care at both intranational and international levels. A recent review demonstrated a "treatment gap," that is, the proportion of epileptic individuals not receiving care, of 75% in low-income countries.[11] Even in high-income countries, however, where the treatment gaps were under 10%, this treatment gap was twice as high as in rural versus urban settings. The causes of this lack of care are multifaceted and complex, involving financial, educational, and social factors.

A lack of physicians care is among the main causes of these disparities; 43% of surveyed African countries and 56.5% of Western Pacific countries reported no access to epilepsy specialists. Overall, African countries have 6 neurologists per 10 million people working predominantly in epilepsy, representing nearly all the neurologists in those countries, whereas European countries had 33 per 10 million people, representing only 6.8% of their neurologists. The higher proportion on psychiatrists and neurosurgeons in these countries who provide epilepsy care fills some of this gap. Similarly, the median number of hospital beds for epilepsy care was more than 8 times greater in high-income versus low-income countries (1.46 vs 0.18 per 100,000 people).[12]

In South Africa, there are 2 separate health care systems, 1 public and 1 private. Although the private care system serves only 15% of the population, it accounts for 57% of health care expenditure; 65% of physicians overall are employed under the private system, including 75% of South Africa's neurologists.[13] These sorts of concentrations of care contribute to situations, such as in India, where a treatment gap is seen of 22% to 50% in urban and suburban settings but 40% to 90% rurally.

Detailed economic analysis has demonstrated a drastically greater benefit of using older anti-epileptic drugs in resource-poor areas.[14] Approximately 93.1% and 95.4% of countries define phenobarbital and carbamazepine as essential drugs, followed by 86.1% and 86.7% that include phenytoin and valproic acid. Although phenobarbital and phenytoin are inexpensive throughout the world, carbamazepine and valproate cost approximately $2.35 to $4.50 for daily dosing, which is prohibitive in many parts of the world. These costs are actually significantly cheaper in high-income countries, where they are $0.69 to $1.

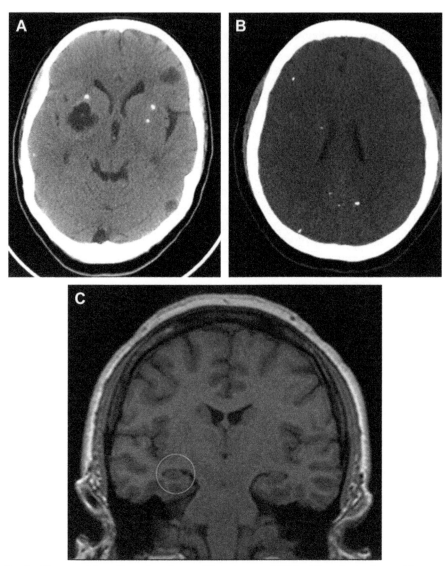

Fig. 2. CT scan axial sections showing multiple stages of NCC—(A) vesicular (cyst with a dot sign) and calcified and (B) healed calcified lesions after albendazole therapy. (C) MRI coronal T1-weighted image showing right hippocampal atrophy (*white circle*) in the same patient.

Social factors also contribute to treatment gaps. Many of the beliefs and taboos surrounding epilepsy (discussed later) can interrupt care. Traditional healers and folk medicine providers can direct patients away from necessary medical interventions for many years.[15] The fear of contagion also interrupts care. Similarly, poor understanding of medication regimens and the cognitive limitations often associated with epilepsy interfere with good medication and follow-up compliance.[16]

To best assess the burden of an illness on a population and the impact of specific interventions, the disability-adjusted life year (DALY) may be calculated as the simple sum of total years of life lost to disability and death. Therefore, interventions in health

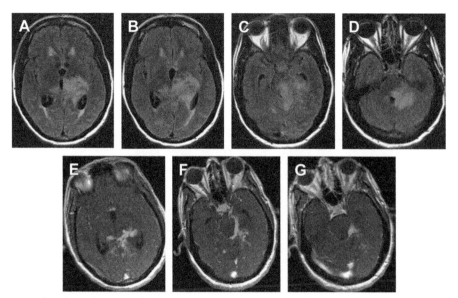

Fig. 3. (A–D) MRI brain axial T2-weighted image fluid-attenuated inversion recovery images show extensive hyperintense signal in bilateral thalami (left much more than right) with surrounding mass effect and vasogenic edema, which extends to basilar cisterns infratentorially. (E–G) Axial T1WI postgadolinium images showing diffuse or nodular enhancement of all cisterns in a patient with HIV and CNS tuberculosis.

care may be compared in overall impact per unit expenditure in dollars/DALY. Recent studies have demonstrated high levels of efficacy in epilepsy care with few simple interventions, which represent 0.8% of all DALYs lost to disease in the world, or 20.6 million DALYs per year.[17] Interventions explored in Nigeria with projected increases in coverage to 50% or 80% with older antiepileptics, including personnel training and distribution, projected $104/DALY and $108/DALY saved (2000 USD).[18] There have been numerous high-benefit and low-cost programs developed in low-income countries involving task-sharing models, in which community members, such as religious leaders and traditional medicine healers, are trained to decrease stigma and improve referral to appropriate medical care as well as training primary care physicians on basic epilepsy treatment.[19] Overall, improved epilepsy treatment infrastructure in underserved communities and nations has the best possibility of decreasing the treatment gap. Improvement in basic sanitation is likely to be crucial to decrease the global burden of epilepsy. Much remains to be done in this area. More basic and clinical research is needed to elucidate the whole spectrum of attributable risk factors for epilepsy.

Drug-resistant epilepsy (DRE) is defined as "failure of adequate trials of two tolerated, appropriately chosen and used automatic external defibrillators schedules (whether as monotherapies or in combination) to achieve sustained seizure freedom." Epilepsy surgery is safe and effective in DRE. Its effects are durable and it is a cost-effective therapy. It is vastly underutilized worldwide, however, despite the emergence of class I evidence.[20] Studies from University of California, Los Angeles,[21] and the State University of New York (SUNY) at Downstate Medical Center in New York City[22] reflect the exaggerated perception of the risks and an instinctive aversion to epilepsy surgery that are widespread and cross-cultural phenomena. Uninsured patients

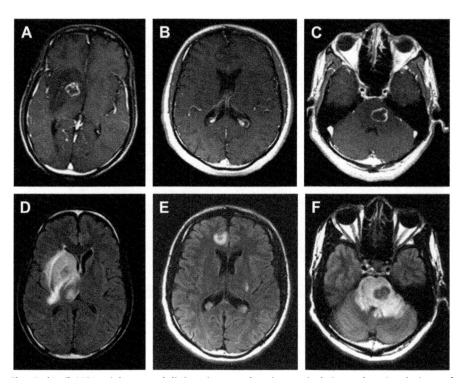

Fig. 4. (*A–C*) MRI axial postgadolinium images showing typical ring-enhancing lesions of toxoplasmosis in the (*A*) right basal ganglia, (*B*) right medial frontal, and (*C*) left pons; (*D–F*) corresponding lesions in the same locations are seen with extensive vasogenic edema on MRI axial T2-weighted image fluid-attenuated inversion recovery images.

with epilepsy and those with Medicaid/Medicare had gaps in access to epilepsy care. There are more than 200 level 3 and level 4 epilepsy centers, representing the majority of epilepsy centers in the United States, according to the National Association of Epilepsy Centers Web page. Schiltz and colleagues[23] looked at the 6 counties that had level 3 or level 4 epilepsy centers in the State of California and concluded that uninsured patients with epilepsy and those with Medicaid/Medicare had gaps in epilepsy care and availability of epilepsy centers had some influence access to care compared with privately insured patients. Epilepsy surgery centers in resource-poor countries lack sophisticated technology to perform comprehensive presurgical evaluations with ancillary tests like magnetoencephalogram, single-photon CT, positron CT, functional MRI, and so forth. The direct costs of presurgical evaluation and surgery amount to a small fraction of the cost incurred in resource-poor countries compared with developed countries. The surgical approaches are modified to single-stage epilepsy surgeries, such as standard temporal lobectomies in straightforward cases and corpus callosotomy in complex cases.

CULTURAL BELIEFS AND TABOOS

Seizures, by their nature, remove a person's consciousness from the control of the body and are both common and unpredictable. Given the dramatic nature of a generalized seizure, which can be shocking even to those with a sound medical understanding of its cause, it is unsurprising that epilepsy has evoked a wide variety of beliefs and

Table 3
Common parasitic infections associated with epilepsy

Protozoa	
Plasmodium falciparum	Malaria
Trypanosoma rhodesiense *Trypanosoma gambiense*	African sleeping sickness
Toxoplasmosis gondii	Toxoplasmosis
Trypanosoma cruzi	Chagas disease
Naegleria fowleri	Primary amebic encephalitis
Acanthamoeba spp	Granulomatous amebic encephalitis
Nematode	
Stronglyloides stercoralis	Disseminated strongyloidiasis
Toxocara canis	Visceral larval migrans (meningoencephalitis, myelitis, cerebral vasculitis, optic neuritis, cognitive and behavioral disorders)
Trichinella	Trichinosis (myositis, myocarditis, pneumonitis, conjunctivitis, and CNS infections
Trematode	
Schistosoma mansoni *Schistosoma haematobium* *Schistosoma japonicum*	Schistosomiasis
Cestode	
T solium	Cysticercosis
T multiceps	Coernurosis
E granulosus	Hydatid disease
Spirometra	Sparganosis

explanations throughout human culture and history. When interacting with patients and family members of patients with epilepsy, it is of vital importance to explore what beliefs they may already hold. As with all matters of cultural sensitivity, these beliefs are not universally held in any specific groups, and individual and family understandings must be explored on a case-by-case basis. Some common and important misunderstandings are discussed.

In many African countries, epilepsy is seen as a demonic curse or the result of witchcraft.[24] This affliction may be communicated through hexes, poisoning, or spiritual possession. Seizures are commonly seen as contagious, which can interrupt the delivery of first aid and care, in addition to furthering social stigma.[25] Many of these beliefs are echoed in European culture. In classical Greece, seizures were attributed to a variety of gods, notably Apollo and Selene. The classic witch hunter's guide, *Malleus Maleficarum*, described seizures as related to curses, and epileptics at the time were excused from communion due to fear of infecting or despoiling the Eucharist.[26] In modern Judaism and Christianity, seizures are often seen as punishment for sins.[27]

Frequently, seizures are seen as the negative consequences of malevolent forces. Exceptions, however, do exist. The Hmong, a group from the mountains between China and Southeast Asia, see epilepsy as a gift and connected to shamanistic divination. As famously discussed in *The Spirit Catches You and You Fall Down*,[28] this can actually encourage families to avoid treatment of seizure disorders as interruptions to these sacred experiences. Elsewhere in Asia, the reactions to seizures can be significantly more negative. In the neighboring countries of Eastern and Southeast Asia, the loss of control inherent in seizures can directly oppose Confucian values. The words for epilepsy in these languages (including Chinese, Japanese, and Thai) are often related to the words for madness or insanity.[29] "Courtesy stigma" can extend throughout the family and limit marriage and employment.[30]

There are situations in which understanding of specific cultural norms can be helpful, and quality language interpretation is vital. Reliance on understanding of specific cultures can lead, however, to further misunderstandings and stereotyping.[31] Every member does not share a bias found within a specific culture, and often there are cultural divisions of which we are unaware. Patients' experience of their culture and their own family cultures are highly idiosyncratic. Therefore, it is obligatory for a provider to explore patients' individual understanding of epilepsy. Open-ended questions exploring a variety of aspects epilepsy are most effective, such as "Where do you believe your symptoms come from?" and "What do you think can help treat them?" Improved understanding on both the part of the physician and the patient can often help soothe any difficulties between religious or cultural beliefs and medical management. When conflicts persist, a shared problem-solving model or involvement of community leaders can lead to improved care.

SUMMARY

Epilepsy is a complex and highly impactful illness with an array of causes. Many aspects of the disease and its treatment are universal; however, there are important regional differences in etiologies, social impact, and treatment. As one of the most common, and most treatable, neurologic illnesses, proper management and closure of the treatment gap are of vital importance. Although advanced management modalities and specialized care are available, which are broadening the contingent of patients whose disease can be controlled, even very basic care can change the lives of many people suffering from epilepsy around the globe.

REFERENCES

1. Sander JW. The epidemiology of epilepsy revisited. Curr Opin Neurol 2003;16: 165–70.
2. Kinnear Wilson JV, Reynolds EH. Texts and documents: translation and analysis of a cuneiform text forming part of a Babylonian treatise on epilepsy. Med Hist 1990;34:185–98.
3. Mishra SK. Concept of neurologic disorders in "Ayurveda" ancient Indian medical treatise [abstract]. Neurology 1987;37(Suppl 1):240.
4. Ngugi AK, Bottomley C, Kleinschmidt I, et al. Estimation of the burden of active and life-time epilepsy: a meta-analytic approach. Epilepsia 2010;51:883–90.
5. Newton CR, Garcia HH. Epilepsy in poor regions of the world. Lancet 2012; 380(9848):1193–201.
6. Bell GS, Sander JW. CPD—Education and self-assessment. The epidemiology of epilepsy: the size of the problem. Seizure 2001;10(4):306–16.
7. Burneo JG, Tellez-Zenteno J, Wiebe S. Understanding the burden of epilepsy in Latin America: a systematic review of its prevalence and incidence. Epilepsy Res 2005;66(1–3):63–74.
8. Carpio A, Hauser WA. Epilepsy in the developing world. Curr Neurol Neurosci Rep 2009;9(4):319–26.
9. Ndimubanzi P, Carabin H, Budke C, et al. A systemic review of the frequency neurocysticercosis with a focus on people with epilepsy. PLoS Negl Trop Dis 2010;4:1–17.

10. Bianchin MM, Velasco TR, Sakamoto AC. Characteristics of mesial temporal lobe epilepsy associated with hippocampal sclerosis plus neurocysticercosis. Epilepsy Res 2014;108(10):1889–95.
11. Meyer AC, Dua T, Ma J, et al. Global disparities in the epilepsy treatment gap: a systematic review. Bull World Health Organ 2010;88(4):260–6.
12. Atlas: epilepsy care in the world 2005. WHO; IBE; ILAE.
13. Benatar SR. Medicine and social responsibility–a role for South African doctors. S Afr Med J 1997;87(3):281–3.
14. Chisholm D. Cost-effectiveness of first-line antiepileptic drug treatments in the developing world: a population-level analysis. Epilepsia 2005;46(5):751–9.
15. Diop AG, Ndiaye M, Diagne M, et al. Filières des soins anti-épileptiques en Afrique [Channels of epilepsy care in Africa]. Epilepsia 1998;10:115–21.
16. Asawavichienjinda T, Sitthi-Amorn C, Tanyanont W. Compliance with treatment of adult epileptics in a Rural District of Thailand. J Med Assoc Thai 2003;86(1): 46–51.
17. (5) WHO methods and data sources for global causes of death 2000-2012. Global Health Estimates Technical Paper WHO/HIS/HSI/GHE/2014.7.
18. Gureje O, Chisholm D, Kola L, et al. Cost-effectiveness of an essential mental health intervention package in Nigeria. World Psychiatry 2007;6(1):42–8.
19. Caraballo R, Fejerman N. Management of epilepsy in resource-limited settings. Epileptic Disord 2015;17(1):13–8.
20. Wiebe S, Blume WT, Girvin JP, et al. A randomized, controlled trial of surgery for temporal-lobe epilepsy. N Engl J Med 2001;345:311–8.
21. Swarztrauber S, Dewar J, Engel J Jr. Patient attitudes about treatments for intractable epilepsy. Epilepsy Behav 2003;4:19–25.
22. Pruss N, Grant AC. Patient beliefs about epilepsy and brain surgery in a multicultural urban population. Epilepsy Behav 2010;17:46–9.
23. Schiltz NK, Koroukian SM, Singer ME, et al. Disparities in access to specialized epilepsy care. Epilepsy Res 2013;107(1–2):172–80.
24. Jilek-aall L. Morbus sacer in Africa: some religious aspects of epilepsy in traditional cultures. Epilepsia 1999;40(3):382–6.
25. Dekker PA. Epilepsy: a manual for medical and clinical officers in Africa. World Health Organization; 2002.
26. Magiorkinis E, Sidiropoulou K, Diamantis A. Hallmarks in the history of epilepsy: from antiquity till the twentieth century, novel aspects on epilepsy. InTech; 2011.
27. Rechard L. Psychological issues of epilepsy. N Engl J Med 1990;1323:18–20.
28. Fadiman A. The spirit catches you and you fall down, a hmong child, her American Doctors, and the collision of two cultures. Macmillan; 2012.
29. Lim KS, Li SC, Casanova-Gutierrez J, et al. Name of epilepsy, does it matter? Neurol Asia 2012;17:87–91.
30. Kheng-Seang L, Chong-Tin T. Epilepsy stigma in Asia: the meaning and impact of stigma. Neurol Asia 2014;19(1):1–10.
31. Carrillo JE, Green AR, Betancourt JR. Cross-cultural primary care: a patient-based approach. Ann Intern Med 1999;130(10):829–34.

Epidemiology of Migraine

Mia T. Minen, MD, MPH[a], David S. Younger, MD, MPH, MS[a,b],*

KEYWORDS

- Migraine • Headache • Public health • Epidemiology

KEY POINTS

- Migraine is a recurrent headache disorder typified by painful attacks lasting 4 to 72 hours. The classification criteria recognize 2 types, migraine with and without aura.
- Migraine affects 12% of the Caucasian population and has a major impact on the well-being and quality of life of sufferers and their families.
- The Global Burden of Disease Study 2013 has provided useful insights into the global burden of migraine.
- Disability-adjusted life years, years of life lost, and years lived with disability are useful summary disability measures for the study of migraine headache.
- A wealth of data provided by genome-wide association studies and metaanalyses have identified new susceptibility loci for migraine.

INTRODUCTION

Epidemiology is an essential starting point in understanding the burden of a disease in the population whether in the United States or worldwide. The epidemiology of migraine has been the most extensively studied of the headache disorders. The most widely used case definitions for migraine were established more than 2 decades age by the International Headache Society,[1] and reiterated in the World Health Organization's *International Classification of Disease and Related Health Conditions, 10th edition*. The original International Headache Society classification defined common and classical migraine respectively as idiopathic, recurring hemicranial pain lasting 4 to 72 hours with moderate to severe pulsatile quality, with the latter preceded by symptoms unequivocally localized to the cerebral cortex or brainstem 5 to 20 minutes, followed as in the former by nausea, photophobia, and phonophobia. Since then, the criteria have been revised multiple times and at the time of publication, we are in the International Classification of Headache Disorders-3-beta edition that no longer uses

The authors have nothing to disclose. Each author provided equal effort in the preparation of the article.
[a] Division of Neuroepidemiology, Department of Neurology, New York University School of Medicine, New York, NY, USA; [b] College of Global Public Health, New York University, New York, NY, USA
* Corresponding author. 333 East 34th Street, 1J, New York, NY 10016.
E-mail address: david.younger@nyumc.org

Neurol Clin 34 (2016) 849–861
http://dx.doi.org/10.1016/j.ncl.2016.06.011
0733-8619/16/$ – see front matter © 2016 Elsevier Inc. All rights reserved.
neurologic.theclinics.com

the terms "common" and "classical" migraine.[2] The newer classification uses the terms migraine with aura (MA) and migraine without aura (MO). Over time, there has been increasing awareness of the disability-related impact of migraine.[3] In addition, there has been work done to determine new metrics of disability, such as the Migraine Disability Index,[4] and measures that incorporate disability-adjusted life years (DALYs), years lived with disability (YLDs), or life lost owing to premature mortality.[5,6] There has been a greater understanding of the pathophysiology of migraine.[7] Importantly, there have been close collaborative efforts among health economists, epidemiologists, public health administrators, physicians, and lay organizations to develop domestic and global campaigns to reduce the burden of migraine headache. One such success was exemplified in the launch of the Global Campaign to reduce the burden of headache worldwide known as "Lifting the Burden" in 2004. It is a joint effort by the World Health Organization, the International Headache Society, the World Headache Alliance and the European Headache Federation.

OVERVIEW

The diagnosis of migraine is established by clinical history. There are no biochemical markers or imaging studies used to make the diagnosis. Any potential relevant secondary headache disorders should be excluded. Nonetheless, it is well-accepted that patients with migraine present a compelling genetic predisposition. For example, people with earlier onset and more severe pain scores report a higher rate of family history compared with those who develop it later on and/or report lower pain intensity scores. In a study of 532 patients with migraine, Stewart and colleagues[8] noted an increased relative risk (RR) of migraine in first-degree relatives (RR, 1.88) compared with controls that was even greater for relatives of probands with onset before age 16 years (RR, 2.5) and more severe pain (RR, 2.38). Based on different rates of comorbidities for MA and MO, there has been some suggestion that MA and MO may be separate disease entities. Those with MA were more likely to develop idiopathic generalized epilepsy and unprovoked seizures.[9] A recent review of migraine and psychiatric comorbidities reported that patients with MA were also more likely to have depression, bipolar disorder, and panic disorder compared with those with MO.[10] However, some studies evaluating the underlying pathophysiology suggest that they may be the same entity.[11]

Epidemiologic studies show an increased risk of ischemic stroke (IS) in migraine patients. Etminan and colleagues[12] analyzed 11 case control studies and 3 cohort studies and found that the risk of stroke was increased in those with migraine (RR, 2.16). The RR for stroke in MA was a RR of 2.27 and in MO was a RR of 1.83. In those taking oral contraceptives, the RR was 8.72. Spector and colleagues[13] conducted a metaanalysis of 35 studies, including 622,381 participants, evaluating stoke risk. They then conducted pooled analysis using data from 21 (60%) of the 35 studies and found using a random effects model that a pooled adjusted OR of IS was 2.30 (95% confidence interval [CI], 1.91–2.76) for migraineurs compared with nonmigraineurs. The pooled adjusted effect estimates for studies that reported RR and hazard ratios, respectively, were 2.41 (95% CI, 1.81–3.20) and 1.52 (95% CI, 0.99–2.35). The overall pooled effect estimate was 2.04 (95% CI, 1.72–2.43). Results were robust to sensitivity analyses excluding lower quality studies.

PUBLIC HEALTH MEASUREMENTS
Incidence

Although cross-sectional data can be used to derive incidence rate estimates, they are better obtained from longitudinal studies.[14] Stewart and colleagues[15] estimated migraine incidence rates using reported age at onset data from a prevalence study admitting its inherent limitations. Noting that migraine both began earlier in males than females with aura than without, the investigators noted that the incidence of MA in males peaked at the age of 5 years with an estimated incidence rate of 6.6 per 1000 person-years. Those without aura peaked at 10 to 11 years with in an estimated 10 per 1000 person-years. New cases were uncommon in men in their 20s. In females, the incidence rate of MA peaked at 12 to 13 years, with an estimated incidence rate of 14.1 per 1000 person-years, and at age 14 and 17 years with in an estimated 18.9 per 1000 person-years. In Olmstead County, Minnesota, Stang and coworkers[16,17] used linked medical records to identify those who sought medical care for migraine noting incidence rates for men and women under the age of 30 of 1.5 to 2 and 3 to 6 per 1000 person-years, respectively.

Prevalence

In the decade before the Global Burden of Disease (GBD) study in 2000, several epidemiologic studies noted varying estimates of migraine prevalence in the United States.[15,18] Stewart and colleagues[15] conducted a population-based study in which a self-administered questionnaire sent to 15,000 households noted that 17.6% of females and 5.7% of males had 1 or more migraines per year. The prevalence of migraine varied considerably by age and was greatest in both men and women between the ages of 35 and 45 years. Migraine prevalence was strongly associated with household income; prevalence in the lowest income group (<$10,000) was more than 60% higher than in the 2 highest income groups (≥$30,000). The proportion of migraine sufferers who experienced moderate to severe disability were not related to gender, age, income, urban versus rural residence, or region of the country. In contrast, the frequency of headaches was lower in higher income groups. Attack frequency was inversely related to disability. A projection to the US population suggested that 8.7 million females and 2.6 million males suffer from migraine headache with moderate to severe disability. Of these, 3.4 million females and 1.1 million males experience 1 or more attacks per month. Females between the ages of 30 and 49 years from lower income households were at especially high risk of having migraines and were more likely than other groups to use emergency care services for their acute condition.

Stewart and coworkers[18] who conducted a metaanalysis of 24 population-based studies predicted 70% of the variance in the prevalence estimates of migraine headache explained by gender and age, noting estimates of migraine varied from 13% to 17% for females and 7.6% to 10% for males. The factors that were significant in predicting the variation in migraine prevalence included the case definitions, method of selecting the study population, the source of the population, the response rate, and whether the diagnoses were confirmed by a clinical assessment; however, none of these factors substantially increased the explained variance. They concluded that after taking sociodemographic factors and case definition into account, estimates of migraine prevalence were remarkably stable among studies. Prevalence rates of migraine were relatively consistent in Western countries, varying from 4% to 9.5% in males and 11.2% to 25% in females, with a lifetime prevalence of 8% in males and 25% in females in the greater Copenhagen study.[19] The authors further noted similar 1-year prevalence estimates of 16% and 6%, respectively, for females and males in American households from about 20,000 respondents.[15] A follow-up study a decade later using identical methodology[20] found migraine prevalence rates of 18.2% among females and 6.5% among males.

Years Lived with Disability

Migraine ranked 19th as a leading cause of YLDs, representing 1.4% of the total causes of YLDs in the 2001 World Health Organization annual report.[6,21] A special edition of *The Lancet* that published the principal findings of the GBD 2010 ranked migraine seventh in global YLDs.[22] The GBD Study 2013 Collaborators[6] reported 28,898.1 YLDs owing to migraine (range, 17,585.8–42,420.1) in 2013, representing a 46.1% change in YLDs from 1990 to 2013 (range, 41.4–50.5), and a percentage change in age-standardized YLDs from 1990 to 2013 of 35.1% (range, 29–41.1).

INHERITANCE

Historically, inheritance studies have shown a genetic predisposition to migraine. In the 1920s, Allan[23] favored autosomal-dominant inheritance because 91% of patients had at least 1 parent affected (n = 500). Among offspring of affected matings, 83.3% had migraine. Goodell and colleagues[24] found 70% penetrance in progeny of affected matings. Dalsgaard-Nielsen[25] found that 90 of 100 women with migraine had affected first-degree relatives. Lateef and colleagues[26] proposed that migraine assessed by family member report alone largely underestimated migraine in relatives. Lucas[27] found that the concordance rate for migraine in monozygotic (MZ) twins was 26% and 13% in dizygotic (DZ) twins, a significant difference ($P<.05$). The concordance rates for migraine in male and female twins were not significantly different. Concordance rates for individual symptoms such as unilaterality and vomiting did not reveal particular features with a markedly higher genetic loading. In 9 MZ and 5 DZ twin pairs, where both twins had common migraine (now known as MO), there was no shared pattern within a twin pair for precipitants or characteristics of attacks. With regard to family history of migraine, there was a common trend in the scores. In MZ twins, there was a family history in 31%, if neither twin had migraine. However, if 1 twin had migraine, the percentage with a family history increased to 45%, and if both twins were affected, the number increased to 60%. Vilatela and coworkers[28] found familial occurrence in migraine in 52.7% of urban Mexican patients and 38.7% of rural patients. Because of a deficiency of affected siblings, they considered autosomal-dominant inheritance very unlikely unless the penetrance of the gene was low. Russell and coworkers[29] studied 121 patients with MO and 72 probands with MA selected from 35 general practices in Denmark noting that, compared with the general population, first-degree relatives of probands with MO had a 3-fold increase of MO, and only 1 first-degree relative of 1 proband with MO had MA. First-degree relatives of probands with MA had a 2-fold increase of both MA and MO. Russell and colleagues[30] analyzed the mode of inheritance in 126 probands with MO and 127 probands with MA from the general population noting multifactorial inheritance with generational differences. In a study of 77 MZ and 134 DZ twin pairs in which at least 1 of the twins had MA, Ulrich and coworkers[31] found a concordance of migraine in 34% of MZ twins and 12% of DZ twins. There was a 50% recurrence risk of migraine in MZ twins, and a 21% recurrent risk of migraine in DZ twins, leading these investigators to conclude that both genetic and environmental factors were important in MA. Gervil and colleagues,[32] who surveyed 2680 Danish twin pairs for MO, noted a pairwise concordance rate of 28% in MZ twin pairs and 18% in DZ twin pairs.

GENETIC SUSCEPTIBILITY LOCI

Wessman and colleagues[33] reported the first genome-wide association study (GWAS) of 50 multigenerational, clinically well-defined Finnish families with MA screened with

350 polymorphic microsatellite markers noting significant evidence of linkage between the MA phenotype and marker D4S1647 at the 4q24 chromosomal locus; statistically significant linkage was not observed in any other chromosomal region. One year later, Bjornsson and colleagues[34] reported the results of a GWAS of 289 patients from 103 Icelandic families with MO noting linkage to a locus on chromosome 4q21 and overlap with the region described by Wessman and colleagues[33] for MA, suggesting that the MGR1 locus could contribute to MA and MO. Chromosomal loci for migraine were identified at 6p21.1-p12.2[35] for MA and MO in migraine type 3 (MGR3); at 14q21.2-q22.3 for MO[36] in MGR4; at 19p13 for MA and MO[37] in MGR5; at 1q31 for MA and MO[38] in MGR6; at 15q11-q13 for MA[39] in MGR7; at 5q21 for MA and MO[40] in MGR8; at 11q24 for MA[41] in MGR9; at 17p13[42] in MGR10; at 18q12 in MA and MO[42] in MGR11; at 10q22-q23[43] in MGR12; and at Xq27 and Xq28 for familial hemiplegia migraine[44] in MGR2. Autosomal-dominant MA (MGR13) is caused by heterozygous mutation in the KCNK18 gene at 10q25 encoding the TWIK-related spinal cord K+ (TRESK) channel.[44] Polymorphisms in the estrogen receptor gene (ESR1) and a polymorphism in tumor necrosis factor may confer susceptibility to migraine.

Arepalli and colleagues[45] reported the results of a meta-analysis across 29 GWAS including a total of 23,285 migraine cases and 95,425 population-matched controls, identifying 142 single nucleotide polymorphisms (SNPs) at a total of 12 loci significantly associated with migraine susceptibility ($P<5 \times 10^{-8}$). Five new loci were near AJAP1 on 1p36, near TSPAN2 on 1p13, within FHL5 on 6q16, within c7orf10 on 7p14, and near MMP16 on 8q21. Four chromosomal loci were suggested to be potential functional candidate genes with significant association to migraine: the APOA1BP gene linked to cholesterol efflux from cells at SNP rs12136718 on chromosome 1; in the TBC1D7 gene that downregulates the tuberous sclerosis gene at rs9349379 on chromosome 6; in the FUT9 gene implicated in neurite outgrowth in brain neuronal cells at rs35128104 on chromosome 6; in STAT6 that transduces activation signals to transcription factors in macrophages at SNP rs4559 on chromosome 12; and in the ATP5B gene and b subunit of mitochondrial ATP synthase, that catalyzes ATP formation using the energy of proton flux through the inner membrane during oxidative phosphorylation, in SNP rs113953523 on chromosome 12.

Freilinger and colleagues[46] analyzed GWAS data of 2326 clinic-based German and Dutch patients and 4580 population-matched controls and selected SNPs from 12 loci with 2 or more SNPs with P-values of less than 1×10^{-5} for follow-up in 2508 patients and 2652 controls. Two loci at 1q22 in the MEF2D gene (rs1050316 and rs3790455) encoding monocyte enhancer factor 2D and 3p24 near the TGFBR2 gene (rs7640543) encoding transforming growth factor beta receptor 2 replicated convincingly ($P = 4.9 \times 10^{-4}$ and $P = 1.0 \times 10^{-4}$, respectively). Meta-analysis of the discovery and replication data yielded 2 additional genome-wide significant loci ($P<5 \times 10^{-8}$) in PHACTR1 at 6p24 (rs9349379) encoding phosphatase and actin regulator 1, and ASTN2 at 9p33 (rs6478241) with a role in glial-guided migration important for development of the laminar architecture of cortical regions in the brain. In addition, SNPs in 2 loci at or near TRPM8 at 3p24 (rs1786920 and rs10166942) with a role in various forms of migraine, and LRP1 at 12q13 (rs11172113) encoding the low-density lipoprotein receptor-related protein 1 expressed in neurons and vasculature was significantly replicated.

Although prior studies on 4 SNPs forming a 22 kb haplotype block in ADARB2 were associated positively with migraine susceptibility in a pedigree-based GWAS of the population of Norfolk Island,[47] Gasparini and coworkers[48] found no association of SNPs in either the adenosine deaminase, RNA-specific, B1 (ADARB1) or B2 (ADARB2) genes in an Australian case-control Caucasian population.

Zhao and colleagues[49] studied the significance of the proportion of shared genes associated with MA and MO in GWAS statistical analyses of the International Headache Genetics Consortium study comparing 4505 MA cases with 34,813 controls and 4038 MO cases with 40,294 controls. The proportion of overlapping genes was almost double the empirically derived null expectation, producing significant evidence of gene-based overlap or pleiotropy. Combining results across MA and MO, 6 genes produced genome-wide significant gene-based P values. Four of these genes (TRPM8, UFL1, FHL5, and LRP1) were located in close proximity to previously reported genome-wide significant SNPs for migraine, whereas 2 genes, TARBP2 and NPFF, were separated by just 259 bp on chromosome 12q13.13, representing a novel risk locus.

Malik and colleagues[50] studied 23,285 migraine cases and 95,425 controls and 12,389 cases of IS and 62,004 controls using 4 different approaches to large-scale GWAS noting a substantial overlap between migraine and IS. MO showed a much stronger overlap with IS and its subtypes than MA. The strongest overlap was between MO and large artery stroke, and between MO and cardioembolic stroke, suggesting shared mechanisms between MO and both large artery stroke and cardioembolic.

One last association addressed by GWAS has been gene set analyses of migraine and sets of synaptic genes predominantly expressed in 3 glial cell types: astrocytes, microglia, and oligodendrocytes, which are involved in various neurotransmitter pathways. Eising and colleagues[51] who analyzed GWAS data of 4954 patients with migraine as well as 13,390 controls noted that gene sets containing astrocyte- and oligodendrocyte-related genes were associated with migraine especially true for gene sets involved in protein modification and signal transduction.

GLOBAL ASPECTS
Global Burden of Disease Study 2013

The GBD Study 2013 Collaborators[5] reported 581,025 × 1000 cases of recurrent migraine (range, 569,050–594,688 × 1000) in 1990 compared with 848,366 (range, 831,035–864,852 × 1000) in 2013, accounting for a 46.06% change (range, 41.44–50.08). The age-standardized rate of migraine in 1990 was 11,690 cases per 100,000 (range, 11,460.6–11,957.8 per 100,000) and 11,714.4 cases per 100,000 in 2013 (range, 11,480–11,939.2 per 100,000) accounting for a 0.33% change. The GBD Study 2013 Collaborators[5] reported 848,366.5 prevalent cases per 1000 of migraine (range, 831,034–864,852.1 per 1000) in 2013, representing a percentage change in prevalence from 1990 to 2013 of 46.1% (range, 41.4%–50.1%) or a 0.3 age-standardized prevalence from 1990 to 2013 of 0.3 (range, −2.8 to 3.0).

Ethiopia

Similar to occidental countries, migraine is highly prevalent among Ethiopians, and issues related to sleep quality and quality of life are reported in the Ethiopian population. A cross-sectional study using a standardized questionnaire that evaluated adults attending outpatient clinics in Ethiopia[52] noted that 14% of participants met criteria for migraine, and 60.5% had poor sleep quality. After adjustments, migraineurs had more than a 2-fold increased OR (OR, 2.4; 95% CI, 1.49–3.38) of overall poor sleep quality as compared with nonmigraineurs, including short sleep duration, long sleep latency, daytime dysfunction owing to sleepiness, poor sleep efficiency, and reduced quality of life. Migraineurs were also more likely to experience poor physical (OR, 1.56; 95% CI, 1.08–2.25) and psychological health (OR, 1.75; 95% CI, 1.20–2.56) as well as poor social relationships (OR, 1.56; 95% CI, 1.08–2.25) and living environments (OR, 1.41; 95% CI, 0.97–2.05) compared with those without migraine.

Nepal

Headache disorders in Nepal have been a burden at the individual and population levels, where structured services are desperately needed. Migraine was a cause of total lost productive time owing to reduced functional capacity. The burden of migraine in Nepal was estimated using a nationwide population-based cross-sectional survey[53] (n = 2100) and 1794 Nepalese (85.4%) reported headache during the preceding year. Those with migraine comprised approximately 4% of the participants in time spent in an ictal state had poorer quality of life than those without (P < .001) migraine. At a population level, migraine was responsible for reduced functional capabilities. Men lost more paid work time than women (P<.001) and women lost more household work time (P<.001).

Italy

The Eurolight project, a partnership activity within the Global Campaign against Headache, assessed the impact of headache disorders in 10 countries in Europe using a structured questionnaire coupled with various sampling methods. Allena and colleagues[54] reported their findings in a stratified sample of 3500 adult inhabitants of the Pavia province representing 1.05% of the general Italian population. The gender-adjusted lifetime prevalence of headache was 82.5%; higher in females than in males (91.2% vs 72.4%; P < .0001) and the 1-year prevalence was 74.2% (females 87.7%, males 61.1%; P < .0001). The most prevalent headache type was migraine (gender-adjusted 1-year prevalence 42.9%; females 54.6%, males 32.5%; P < .0001). Only 16.6% of responders reporting headache had received a diagnosis from a doctor, and very few (2.4%) were taking preventative medications. Headache had negative impacts on different aspects of life: education, career and earnings, and family and social life. In the preceding 3 months, each person with headache had lost, on average, 2.3 days from paid work and 2.4 days from household work, and missed social occasions on 1.2 days.

India

In the Karnataka State of southern India, where migraine has a heavy disease burdens owing to limited access to health care, there were deficient structured headache services in primary care facilities. In a door-to-door survey, Rao and colleagues[55] randomly sampled 2329 participants (nonparticipation rate 7.4%) of whom 1488 (63.9%; 621 male, 867 female) reported headache in the preceding year with a 1-year migraine prevalence of 25.2%. Lost productivity time was 5.8% (equating to 1.5% from the adult population) with lost paid work time accounting for 40%. The population-level disability attributable to migraine for the ictal state was 0.433, and the mean disability per person with migraine was 1.8%, reducing the functional capacity of the entire adult population by 0.46%. Fewer than one-quarter of participants with headache had engaged with health care services for headache in the last year. There was an expressed willingness to pay for effective treatment for headache, signaling dissatisfaction with current treatments.

China

Liu and colleagues[56] conducted a nationwide population-based survey in China studying 5041 respondents noting significantly higher proportions of respondents with migraine (239/452; 52.9%). Multivariate analysis showed associations between disability and probability of consultation in those with migraine (mild vs minimal: adjusted OR, 3.4 [95% CI, 1.6–7.4]; moderate vs minimal: adjusted OR, 2.5 [95% CI, 1.2–5.4]; severe vs minimal: adjusted OR, 3.9 [95% CI, 1.9–8.1]). Consultations in level 3 hospitals were relatively few for migraine (5.9%). Underdiagnosis and misdiagnosis were common in consulters. More than one-half with migraine (52.7%) reported no previous diagnosis. Those with migraine were as likely (13.8%) to be diagnosed with "nervous headache" as migraine. The authors concluded that migraine headache services in China were limited and that there were excessively high rates of underdiagnosis and misdiagnosis in those who sought to access services, characterizing the services as inefficient or cost ineffective.

Zambia

Mbewe and colleagues[57] conducted a cross-sectional population-based survey of 1085 unrelated adults from 1134 households selected by cluster-randomized sampling in the mostly urban Lusaka Province and mostly rural Southern Province with a gender- and habitation-adjusted 1-year prevalence of migraine of 22.9%. Reported mean intensity of migraine attacks was 2.7, representing severe pain. People with migraine spent 10.0% of their time in the ictal state and 4.3% were disabled overall. Average lost productive time in the preceding 3 months for migraine was 4.1 days from work (6.3% loss) and 4.2 days (4.7% loss) from household work. In the population aged 18 to 65 years (effectively the working population), the estimated disability from migraine was 0.98%, with 1.4% of workdays lost.

Spain

Matias-Guiu and colleagues[58] ascertained a 1-year prevalence of migraine of Spain in a population-based sample of adults. The authors[57] contacted 5668 respondents by phone to complete a survey, of whom 476 subjects (8.4%; 95% CI, 7.7%–9.1%) had definite migraine and 236 with probable migraine (4.2%; 95% CI, 3.7%–4.7%). The 1-year prevalence of total migraine (n = 712) was 12.6% (95% CI, 11.6–13.6; 17.2% in females and 8.0% in males). The prevalence rates showed significant geographic variations, from 7.6% in Navarra to 18% in the Canary Islands. One-half of the subjects had MA. One-third of subjects had not been previously diagnosed with migraine. Lara and colleagues[59] reported on the burden of neuropsychiatric disorders in Spain expressing it in DALYs, life lost owing to premature mortality, and YLDs. The burden of neuropsychiatric disorders accounted for 18.4% of total all-cause DALYs generated in Spain for 2010. Within this group, the top 5 leading causes of DALYs were depressive disorders, Alzheimer disease, migraine, substance use disorders, and anxiety disorder, which accounted for 70.9% of all DALYs owing to neuropsychiatric disorders.

Russia

Ayzenberg and colleagues[60] evaluated the prevalence and impact of headache on the preceding day termed headache yesterday nationwide in a cross-sectional survey of the working-age population of 44 settlements of 6 of the 7 Federal Districts of Russia. Among 2025 unrelated adults who were interviewed, approximately 1 in 7 participants (14.5%; men 9.1% and women 19.3%) reported headache yesterday. The overall 1-year prevalence of headache was 62.9%, 20.3% of whom fulfilled standard criteria for definite or probable episodic migraine. In 88.3%, headache intensity was moderate or severe (mean 2.1 on a scale of 1–3) and in 73.9%, headache yesterday impaired daily activity. Loss of productivity at work owing to headache was 2.6 million person-years, or 4.0% of workforce capacity.

Tanzania

Winkler and colleagues[61] studied the 1-year prevalence of migraine headache in a rural population within the catchment area of the Haydom Lutheran Hospital in northern Tanzania. Using a community-based door-to-door survey of 1192 households of 7412 individuals selected by multistage cluster-random sampling, the overall 1-year prevalence of migraine was 4.3% (316/7412; 95% CI, 3.8–4.7) with an age-adjusted rate of 6.0% and a male:female ratio of 1:2.94 (P<.001). One hundred thirty-two individuals did not fulfill all criteria for migraine headache and classified as migraine with a crude prevalence rate of 1.8% (132/7412; 95% CI, 1.5–2.1). The remaining 184 patients met all criteria for migraine resulting in a 1-year prevalence of 2.5% (184/7412; 95% CI, 2.1– 2.9) and a male:female ratio of 1:2.51 (P<.001).

Dent and colleagues[62] conducted a door-to-door survey in northern Tanzania using multistage cluster sampling enrolling 7412 individuals. The migraine patients' average annual attack frequency was 18.4 (n = 308; standard deviation [SD] ± 47.4) with a mean duration of 16.4 hours (SD ± 20.6). The average headache intensity per patient was 2.65 (SD ± 0.59) with a calculated loss of 6.59 (SD ± 26.7) working days per year. Extrapolation of data to the investigated population resulted in annual migraine burden of 281.0 migraine days per 1000 inhabitants.

Germany

Khil and coworkers[63] analyzed data from the Deutsche Migräne und Kopfschmerz Gesellschaft (DMKG) headache study of the German Migraine and Headache Society, assessing the incidence of migraine in Germany via standardized headache questions in a population drawn from a 5-year age-group–stratified and gender-stratified random sample from the population register. Of the 1122 participants, the total sample incidence of migraine ranged between 0% and 3.3%. Straube and colleagues[64] analyzed the data of the DMKG, estimating of the prevalence chronic migraine in 0.2% of the population. The distribution of migraine attacks per subject was highly skewed, with only 14% of all migraine patients having more than 6 migraine attacks per month. Fendrich and coworkers[65] studied the 3-month prevalence of headache, migraine and tension-type headache among adolescents aged 12 to 15 years in Germany in the DMKG study. Students (n = 3324) from 20 schools completed a questionnaire on general and headache-specific pain, which included a sociodemographic module. The overall 3-month prevalence of headache was 69.4% (boys 59.5%, girls 78.9%), with 4.4% of the adolescents suffering from frequent (≥14 days in 3 months) and severe (grade 8–10 on a 10-point visual analog scale) headache and 1.4% (boys 0.9%, girls 1.9%) from headache 15 or more days per month. The 3-month prevalence of migraine was 2.6% (boys 1.6%, girls 3.5%) applying strict criteria, and 6.9% (boys 4.4%, girls 9.3%) with modified criteria; of the 12.6% (boys 8.3%, girls 16.7%) who suffered from probable migraine, 0.07% fulfilled the criteria for chronic migraine. Headache and migraine were more common in girls than in boys and in teenagers, especially in girls, increasing with higher education levels.

Turkey

Demirkirkan and colleagues[66] conducted a cross-sectional 2-stage study of the prevalence of migraine and assessed the disability in the Turkish city of Afyon. The first stage identified students with migraine by using a standardized questionnaire. In this questionnaire, the students were asked about medical consultations and medicines used during attacks. Standard questionnaires applied to 1029 students noted migraine in 128 students (12.4%). The second stage, which examined the impact of migraine on daily life using a disability assessment scale questionnaire, demonstrated minimal disability in 8.6% of students, mild disability in 23.4%, moderate disability in 26.6%, and severe disability in 41.4%. Migraine attacks were associated with a considerable degree of handicap in activities of daily living. Many university students with migraine did not consult a physician and treated their disease symptomatically with simple analgesics.

SUMMARY

Progress in understanding the epidemiologic and clinical aspects of migraine holds the promise of increased understanding and detection of individual and population at risk, and the implementation of effective preventative and therapeutic measures. Such strides if mainstreamed into health care practices may be effective in reducing burden of migraine and the YLDs in the United States and worldwide.

REFERENCES

1. Headache Classification Committee of the International Headache Society. Classification and diagnostic criteria for headache disorders, cranial neuralgias, and facial pain. Cephalalgia 1988;8(Suppl 7):19–28.
2. Headache Classification Committee of the International Headache Society (HIS). The International Classification of Headache Disorders, 3rd edition (beta version). Cephalalgia 2013;33:629–808.
3. Stewart WF, Lipton RB, Simon D. Work-related disability: results from the American migraine study. Cephalalgia 1996;16:231–8.
4. Emeads J, Lainez JM, Brandes JL, et al. Potential of the Migraine Disability Assessment (MIDAS) questionnaire as a public health initiative and in clinical practice. Neurology 2001;56(Suppl 1):S29–34.
5. Global Burden of Disease Study 2013 Collaborators. Global, regional, and national incidence, prevalence, and years lived with disability for 301 acute and chronic diseases and injuries in 188 countries, 1990-2013: a systematic analysis for the Global Burden of Disease Study 2013. Lancet 2015;386:743–800.
6. Leonardi M, Steiner TJ, Scher AT, et al. The global burden of migraine: measuring disability in headache disorders with WHO's Classification of Functioning, Disability and Health (ICF). J Headache Pain 2005;6:429–40.
7. Burtein R, Noseda R, Borsook D. Migraine: multiple processes, complex pathophysiology. J Neurosci 2015;35:6619–29.
8. Stewart WF, Bigal ME, Kolodner K, et al. Familial risk of migraine: variation by proband age at onset and headache severity. Neurology 2006;66:344–8.
9. Ludvigsson P, Hesdorffer D, Olafsson E, et al. Migraine with aura is a risk factor for unprovoked seizures in children. Ann Neurol 2006;59:210–3.
10. Minen MT, Begasse De Dhaem O, Kroon Van Diest A, et al. Migraine and its psychiatric comorbidities. J Neurol Neurosurg Psychiatry 2016;87:741–9.
11. Purdy RA. Migraine with and without aura share the same pathogenic mechanisms. Neurol Sci 2008;29(Suppl 1):S44–6.
12. Etminan M, Takkouche B, Isorna FC, et al. Risk of ischaemic stroke in people with migraine: systematic review and meta-analysis of observational studies. BMJ 2005;330:63.
13. Spector JT, Kahn SR, Jones MR, et al. Migraine headache and ischemic stroke risk: an updated meta-analysis. Am J Med 2010;123:612–24.
14. Lipton RB, Bigal ME, Scher AI, et al. The global burden of migraine. J Headache Pain 2003;4(Suppl 1). S3–S1.

15. Stewart WF, Lipton RB, Celentano DD, et al. Prevalence of migraine headache in the United States. JAMA 1992;267:64–9.
16. Stang PE, Osterhaus JT, Celentano DD. Migraine: patterns of health care use. Neurology 1994;44(Suppl 4):47–55.
17. Stang PE, Yanagihara T, Swanson JW, et al. Incidence of migraine headaches: a population-based study in Olmsted County, Minnesota. Neurology 1992;42:1657–62.
18. Stewart WF, Simon D, Schechter A, et al. Population variation in migraine prevalence: a meta-analysis. J Clin Epidemiol 1995;48:269–80.
19. Rasmussen BK. Epidemiology of headache. Cephalalgia 2001;12:774–7.
20. Lipton RB, Stewart WF, Diamond S, et al. Prevalence and burden of migraine in the United States: data from the American Migraine Study II. Headache 2001;41:646–57.
21. World Health Organization (WHO). World Health report 2001: mental health, new understanding new hope. Geneva (Switzerland): World Health Organization. Available at: http://www.who.int/whr/2001/main/en/overview/outline.htm. Accessed September 1, 2015.
22. Vos T, Flaxman AD, Naghavi M, et al. Years lived with disability (YLDs) for 1160 sequelae of 289 diseases and injuries 1990-2010: a systematic analysis for the Global Burden of Disease Study 2010. Lancet 2012;380:2163–96.
23. Allan W. Inheritance of migraine. Arch Intern Med 1928;42:590–9.
24. Goodell H, Lewontin R, Wolff HG. The familial occurrence of migraine headache: a study of heredity. AMA Arch Neurol Psychiatry 1954;72:325–34.
25. Dalsgaard-Nielsen T. Migraine and heredity. Acta Neurol Scand 1965;41:287–300.
26. Lateef TM, Cui L, Nakamura E, et al. Accuracy of family history reports of migraine in a community-based family study of migraine. Headache 2015;55:407–12.
27. Lucas RN. Migraine in twins. J Psychosom Res 1977;21:147–56.
28. Vilatela EA, Pedroza FG, Ziegler DK, et al. Familial migraine in a Mexican population. Neuroepidemiology 1992;11:46–9.
29. Russell MB, Hilden J, Sorensen SA, et al. Familial occurrence of migraine without aura and migraine with aura. Neurology 1993;43:1369–73.
30. Russell MB, Iselius L, Olsen J. Inheritance of migraine investigated by complex segregation analysis. Hum Genet 1995;96:726–30.
31. Ulrich V, Gervil M, Kyvik KO, et al. Evidence of a genetic factor in migraine with aura: a population-based Danish twin study. Ann Neurol 1999;45:242–6.
32. Gervil M, Ulrich V, Kyvik KO, et al. Migraine without aura: a population-based twin study. Ann Neurol 1999;46:606–11.
33. Wessman M, Kallela M, Kaunisto MA, et al. A susceptibility locus for migraine with aura, on chromosome 4q24. Am J Hum Genet 2002;70:652–62.
34. Bjornsson A, Gudmundsson G, Gudfinnsson E, et al. Localization of a gene for migraine without aura to chromosome 4q21. Am J Hum Genet 2003;73(5):986–93.
35. Carlsson A, Forsgren L, Nylander PO, et al. Identification of a susceptibility locus for migraine with and without aura on 6p12.2-p21.1. Neurology 2002;59:1804–7.
36. Soragna D, Vettori A, Carraro G, et al. A locus for migraine without aura maps on chromosome 14q21.2-q22.3. Am J Hum Genet 2003;72:161–7.
37. Jones KW, Ehm MG, Pericak-Vance MA, et al. Migraine with aura susceptibility locus on chromosome 19p13 is distinct from the familial hemiplegic migraine locus. Genomics 2001;78:150–4.

38. Lea RA, Shepherd AG, Curtain RP, et al. A typical migraine susceptibility region localizes to chromosome 1q31. Neurogenetics 2002;4:17–22.
39. Russo L, Mariotti P, Sangiorgi E, et al. A new susceptibility locus for migraine with aura in the 15q11-q13 genomic region containing three GABA-A receptor genes. Am J Hum Genet 2005;76:327–33.
40. Nyholt DR, Morley KI, Ferreira MAR, et al. Genomewide significant linkage to migrainous headache on chromosome 5q21. Am J Hum Genet 2005;77:500–12.
41. Cader ZM, Noble-Topham S, Dyment DA, et al. Significant linkage to migraine with aura on chromosome 11q24. Hum Mol Genet 2003;12:2511–7.
42. Anttila V, Kallela M, Oswell G, et al. Trait components provide tools to dissect the genetic susceptibility of migraine. Am J Hum Genet 2006;79:85–99.
43. Anttila V, Nyholt DR, Kallela M, et al. Consistently replicating locus linked to migraine on 10q22-q23. Am J Hum Genet 2008;82:1051–63.
44. Lafreniere RG, Cader MZ, Poulin J-F, et al. A dominant-negative mutation in the TRESK potassium channel is linked to familial migraine with aura. Nat Med 2010;16:1157–60.
45. Arepalli S, Cookson MR, Dillman A, et al. Genome-wide meta-analysis identifies new susceptibility loci for migraine. Nat Genet 2013;45:912–7.
46. Freilinger T, Antitila V, de Vries B, et al, The International Headache Genetics Consortium. Genome-wide association analysis identifies susceptibility loci for migraine with aura. Nat Genet 2013;44:777–82.
47. Cox HC, Lea RA, Bellis C, et al. A genome-wide analysis of "bounty" descendants implicates several novel variants in migraine susceptibility. Neurogenetics 2012; 13:261–6.
48. Gasparini CF, Sutherland HG, Maher G, et al. Case-control study of ADARB1 and ADARB2 gene variants in migraine. J Headache Pain 2015;16:31.
49. Zhao H, Eising E, de Vries B, et al. Gene-based pleiotropy across migraine with aura and migraine without aura patients groups. Cephalalgia 2016;36(7):648–57.
50. Malik R, Freilinger T, Winsvold BS, et al. Shared genetic basis for migraine and ischemic stroke. A genome-wide analysis of common variants. Neurology 2015; 84:2132–45.
51. Eising E, de Leeuw C, Min JL, et al. Involvement of astrocytes and oligodendrocyte gene sets in migraine. Cephalalgia 2016;36(7):640–7.
52. Morgan I, Eguia F, Gelaye B, et al. Sleep disturbances and quality of life in Sub-Saharan African migraineurs. J Headache Pain 2015;16:18.
53. Manandhar K, Risal A, Linde M, et al. The burden of headache disorders in Nepal: estimates from a population-based survey. J Headache Pain 2015; 17(1):3.
54. Allena M, Steiner TJ, Sances G, et al. Impact of headache disorders in Italy and the public-health and policy implications: a population based study within the Eurolight Project. J Headache Pain 2015;16:100.
55. Rao GN, Kulbarni GB, Gururaj G, et al. The burden attributable to headache disorders in India: estimates from a community-based study in Karnataka State. J Headache Pain 2015;16:94.
56. Liu R, Yu S, He M, et al. Health-care utilization for primary headache disorders in China: a population-based door-to-door survey. J Headache Pain 2013;14:47.
57. Mbewe E, Zairemthiama P, Paul R, et al. The burden of primary headache disorders in Zambia: national estimates from a population based door-to-door survey. J Headache Pain 2015;16:513.
58. Matias-Guiu J, Porta-Etessam J, Mateos V, et al. One-year prevalence of migraine in Spain: a nationwide population based survey. Cephalalgia 2011;31(4):463–70.

59. Lara E, Garin N, Ferrai AJ, et al. The Spanish Burden of Disease 2010: neurological, mental and substance use disorders. Rev Psiquiatr Salud Ment 2015;8(4): 207–17.
60. Ayzenberg I, Katsarava Z, Sborowski A, et al. Headache-attributed burden and its impact on productivity and quality of life in Russia: structured healthcare for headache is urgently needed. Eur J Neurol 2014;21:758–65.
61. Winkler AS, Dent W, Stalzhammer B, et al. Prevalence of migraine headache in a rural area of northern Tanzania: a community-based door-to-door survey. Cephalalgia 2010;30:582–92.
62. Dent W, Stelzhammer B, Meindi M, et al. Migraine attack frequency, duration, and pain intensity: disease burden derived from a community-based survey in northern Tanzania. Headache 2011;51:1483–92.
63. Khil L, Pfaffenrath V, Straube A, et al. Incidence of migraine and tension-type headache in three different populations at risk within the German DMKG headache study. Cephalalgia 2012;32:326–36.
64. Straube A, Pfaffenrath V, Ladwig KH, et al. Prevalence of chronic migraine and medication overuse headache in Germany-the German DMKG headache study. Cephalalgia 2010;30:207–13.
65. Fendrich K, Vennemann M, Pfaffenrath V, et al. Headache prevalence among adolescents-the German DMKG headache study. Cephalalgia 2007;27:347–54.
66. Demirkirkan MK, Ellidokuz H, Boluk A. Prevalence and clinical characteristics of migraine in university students in Turkey. Tohoku J Exp Med 2006;208:87–92.

I-Cubed (Infection, Immunity, and Inflammation) and the Human Microbiome

David S. Younger, MD, MPH, MS[a,b],*

KEYWORDS

- Infection • Immunity • Inflammation • I-Cubed • Human microbiome • Neurology
- Public health

KEY POINTS

- It has been learned that human beings are superorganisms integrating the identity, function, and immunity of resident micro-oganisms.
- Low-cost high-throughput sequencing of microbial communities comprising the human microbiome is unveiling the identity and function of unculturable microbes.
- Our own innate and adaptive immune systems have evolved to deal with invading organisms.
- Public health officials and neuroepidemiology researchers will be called on to guide the understanding of I-Cubed illnesses and the implications of the human microbiome.

INTRODUCTION

The human microbiome, defined as the collection of micro-organisms that reside within our body, have coevolved over the history of mankind and have been over-looked as determinants of health and disease. Given the appearance of new microbial agents and the everyday occurrence of unexplained lethal neurologic syndromes of suspected infectious cause, scientists have begun to identify a plethora of microbial agents in our body and in the human genome. The true capability of such microbes residing in our body to cause human disease has become the focus of medical science. Postinfectious autoimmune illness is increasingly recognized because of resident and invasive microbial agents that have the capacity to trigger our immune system, turning it on and off at will. With differences in resident microbial niches,

The author has nothing to disclose.
[a] Division of Neuroepidemiology, Department of Neurology, New York University School of Medicine, New York, NY, USA; [b] College of Global Public Health, New York University, New York, NY, USA
* Corresponding author. 333 East 34th Street, 1J, New York, NY 10016.
E-mail address: youngd01@nyu.edu

imperfect host defenses, and susceptibility to epidemic and endemic diseases in the environment, there are ever-increasing opportunities for infectious bacterial, virus, parasitic, and fungal exposures. The triumvirate of infection, immunity, and inflammation, termed I-Cubed, which posits that there are complex and often self-sustaining host adaptive immune responses to acute and chronic infection, forms the etiopathologic basis for diverse medical and neurologic disorders. Public health officials and neuroepidemiology researchers will be called on to guide the understanding of I-Cubed illnesses and the implications of the human microbiome for communicable and noncommunicable diseases, at times one leading to the other, as the natural history is appreciated and the responsiveness of given medical and neurologic disorder to a variety of medical approaches including strong antibiotics and immune-modulatory is established.

BACKGROUND

Imagine the excitement of a scientist at a medical conference claiming to have discovered a new human organ which, like the immune system, contains collections of cells and 100 times more genes than the host. Not only is it tailored to the individual host, but it is modifiable by stress, diet, medications, exercise, and antibiotics. When lost, nearly all aspects of the host's normal physiologic function are altered. Although it has been known for some time that the human body is inhabited by resident flora in a factor greater than 10:1, most researchers have focused instead on a minority of disease-causing or "pathogenic" organisms with far fewer examining the benefits of the resident bacterial flora. The completion of the human genome sequence in 2001, which was the crowning achievement in biology, was incomplete because it did not look at the synergistic activities of humans and microbes living together. With many well-recognized neurologic diseases of likely infectious trigger yet unassigned to infectious microbes, such as most cases of aseptic meningitis, encephalitis, and cerebral vasculitis, there was a need for a second human genome project to provide a comprehensive inventory of microbial genes and genomes at major sites of microbial colonization in the human body. Many investigators envisioned that understanding the microbial contributions to inflammatory disease could be addressed effectively through a thoughtful integration of modern technologies and clinical insight.

The concept of the human microbiome or microbiota originated with the Rockefeller University scientist Joshua Lederberg,[1] as an ecological community of commensal, symbiotic, and pathogenic micro-organisms sharing our body space. It is estimated that 20% to 60% of the human-associated microbiome, depending on body site, is still resistant to conventional culture techniques, making it difficult to accurately estimate its true diversity. More recently, the human microbiome has been studied in different biological states using gene sequencing techniques. Scientists have used molecular tools to extract and compare bits of a particular kind of RNA, the products of DNA transcription and translation, to determine if previously known or new microbes were present in a particular human tissue such as blood. This technique, which is widely used as a biomarker for microbial disease, uses a particular kind of RNA known as 16S ribosomal RNA (rRNA).

Because the genes for rRNA have changed little over millions of years as organisms have evolved, slight changes in their composition provide valuable clues to the very nature of microbial organisms located in the human body. The 16S rRNA gene is very short, just 1542 nucleotide bases, making it quickly and cheaply copied, sequenced, and then compared with libraries of stored 16S rRNA genes from numerous known bacteria. The ones that match up perfectly are microbes that have been previously identified, whereas others that show differences may be previously unknown microbes. Such studies of gastrointestinal microbes at the 16S rRNA gene level have revealed significant diversity in the flora of individuals. An international meeting held in Paris in November 2005, hosted by the French National Institute for Agricultural Research, led to the recommendation of an initiative to precisely define the human intestinal microbiome in health and disease. Directly following the Paris meeting, the National Institutes of Health held discussions about the merits of a Human Microbiome Project, which soon became a roadmap for later biomedical research. Fast-forward to the present: we are presently at a public health crossroads, in a position to make gigantic gains in our knowledge to better understand how microbes impact on human health, transitioning from description to causality and microbial engineering. Underscoring this, 2 papers published simultaneously in the journals *Science*[2] and *Nature*[3] called for the establishment of a Unified [domestic] Microbiome Initiative and International Microbiome Initiative.

With more than 90% of cells in the human microbiome understood to be bacterial, viral, fungal, or otherwise nonhuman in nature, and human metabolism and immunity attributed to the molecular genetic contribution of microbial and human interaction, human beings are being referred to as superorganisms. In the last decade the United States, the Human Microbiome Project and European MetaHit, 2 large-scale genomic projects, along with several private efforts, have investigated the microbiota in a variety of human body niches using new molecular genetic tools. Although many sites such as the skin, oral and nasal cavities, and vagina are all relatively easy to access, most of the research in this area has focused on the gastrointestinal tract, in particular, the colon. The colon is where the greatest density and numbers of bacteria are found. Most of the data regarding the bacterial microbiota comes from fecal samples and tissue specimens lining of the lower intestine. Although the function of colonic microbiota is to efficiently degrade complex indigestible carbohydrates, the small intestine microbiome is shaped by its capacity for fast import and conversion of relatively small carbohydrates, and rapid adaptation to overall nutrient availability. The gut microbiota ferments carbohydrates in the upper colon, whereas other gut flora digest protein and amino acids, liberating short-chain fatty acids. The fermentation of short-chain fatty acids can lead to a range of potentially harmful compounds, some of which play a role in gut diseases such as colorectal cancer and inflammatory bowel disease. Studies in animals show that some compounds, like ammonia, phenols, p-cresol, certain amines, and hydrogen sulfide, play important roles in the initiation or progression of a leaky gut, inflammation, DNA damage, and cancer progression. High dietary fiber or intake of plant-based foods appears to inhibit this, highlighting the importance of maintaining vegetarian gut microbiome carbohydrate fermentation. The newly recognized axis of communication between the gut and brain has led to the recognition of a mind-gut connection, seeking to explain a spectrum of functional symptoms from anxiety and depression to irritable bowel syndrome. So recognized, customized food diets have emerged aimed at improving the gut by impacting on microbiota activities linked to systemic host physiology.

With 5 phyla representing most of the bacteria that comprise the gut microbiota, there are about 160 species in the large intestine alone of any individual, and very few of these are shared between individuals. The functions contributed by these species appear to be found in everybody's gastrointestinal tract, an observation that suggests that microbial function is more important than the identity of the species providing it. The understanding of human microbial biology first derived from pure cultures and genomic sequencing, has been limited by sampling bias toward 4 bacterial phyla, *Proteobacteria*, *Firmicutes*, *Actinobacteria*, and *Bacteroides*, of the 35 bacterial and 18 known archaeal phylum-level lineages. With roughly two-thirds of published microbiological research dedicated to only 8 bacterial genera, all of which grow well on agar culture plates, it is unlikely that they are representative of the 5000 or more species known to us. Phylogenetic molecular genetic methodologies using next generation sequencing have not only revolutionized our understanding of the origin and evolution of microbial organisms, but also have provided scientists with the means for identifying the types of organisms that occur in the environment and in the human microbiome. Molecular biologists using rRNA sequence have revealed a microbial taxonomy based on 1 of 3 aboriginal lines of descent separating bacterial organisms into 3 major kingdoms. The Eubacteria or modern *Eukaryotes* contain all of the typical bacteria-sharing 16S rRNA present in moderately large and varied collections of organisms and organelles of prokaryotic cells. The *Urkaryotes* sharing 18S rRNA comprise major ancestors of eukaryotic cells, including plant, fungal, and slime molds. The *Archaebacteria* possess anaerobic metabolism based on reduction of carbon dioxide to methane, making them well suited for the type of environment presumed to exist on earth 3 to 4 billion years ago.

INFECTION ACTIVATES IMMUNITY

Immunity was originally separated into 2 types based on the purported effects of immunization or vaccine against a given pathogen. The first type was the effect of immunization that resulted in definable changes in the cell-free bodily fluid or serum or humor, whereas another was the observed protective effect associated with multiplication of specific cells. Two primordial types of immune cells are now recognized, one lineage termed B cells that matures in the bone marrow and further differentiates into plasma cells and memory cells. Mature plasma cells are capable of producing antibodies capable of latching onto their target in a lock-and-key specific fashion when their surface antibody receptors recognize other cells displacing foreign antigens. Other B cells mature into memory B cells that circulate in the bloodstream. The other cell lineage of T cells, also derived in the bone marrow, instead passes though the thymus gland, where it achieves final immunoreactivity and is thought to be most protective in recognizing virus-infected cells. These cells participate in the defense against intracellular bacterial, fungal, and protozoan infections; cancers; and transplant rejection. Other aspects of enhanced cellular immunity includes the secretion of cell-signaling molecules termed cytokines that promote cell-to-cell communication in immune responses and stimulate the movement of cells toward sites of inflammation and infection.

Not surprisingly, major understandings of the pathophysiology of autoimmune diseases have been achieved through an appreciation of infectious triggers of the humoral and cell-mediated immune system. When Whipple disease was first identified as the causative agent of the neurologic disorder almost 25 years ago by Relman and coworkers,[4] it was unclear whether the uncultured bacillus *Tropheryma (T) whippelii* was a rare member of the normal human microbial flora and whether it might be associated with other human diseases. Whipple disease causes a systemic inflammatory disorder involving the gastrointestinal tract, heart, and brain. According to phylogenetic analysis, the isolated bacterium was a gram-positive actinomycetes not closely related to any known genus. A molecular genetic approach amplifying a 16S rRNA sequence directly from tissues of 5 unrelated patients determined its nucleotide sequence. A decade later, the same authors[5] performed ultrastructural studies of intestinal biopsy specimens from affected patients. These studies showed the location of *T whippelii* rRNA to be most prevalent near the tips of the intestinal villi in the lamina propria just basal to the epithelial cells, located between cells and not intracellular, indicating that the bacillus grew outside cells and that it was not an obligate intracellular pathogen. Such studies ushered in a generation of molecular genetic technology used today in the study of resident human microbes.

Relman[6] later observed that molecular, cultivation-independent methods revealed that the distribution and diversity of micro-organisms in the world was far greater than previously appreciated. One particular molecular genetic technique compared human tissue–derived DNA sequences with those of known pathogenic and commensal bacterial, viral, fungal, and protozoan genomes in established expressed-sequence tag libraries. However, inefficient and cost-ineffective for screening large numbers of specimens in most laboratories, it revealed surprising findings of nonhuman genetic sequences that appeared to be an inherent feature of the human genome. It appears that all humans have human endogenous retrovirus sequences as an integral part of their genome.[7] At some time during the course of human evolution, exogenous progenitors of the human endogenous retrovirus inserted themselves into the human germ-line reproductive cells where they were replicated along with the host cellular genes. However, intact disease-producing retroviruses differ in the presence of at least one additional coding region, the envelope (*env*) gene that encodes viral membrane proteins that mediate the budding of virus particles to the cellular receptors enabling virus entry as the first step in the pathway to a new replication cycle and disease pathogenicity.

Hajjeh and coworkers[8] observed that unexplained deaths and critical illness possibly due to infectious causes in previously healthy persons occurred at an incidence rate of 0.5 per 100,000 per year from 1995 to 1998 among 7.7 million persons in 4 US Emergency Infectious Programs. However, only two-thirds were diagnosed by reference serologic tests, and the remaining one-third was diagnosed by polymer chain reaction (PCR)-based methods. These findings suggested the need for molecular genetic surveillance approaches to detect present and emerging infectious diseases. New molecular biological techniques have led to the identification of several previously unculturable infectious agents, such as non-A and non-B hepatitis, and hantavirus.[9] Real-time PCR methods with primers and a probe targeting conserved regions of the bacterial 16S rRNA revealed rRNA in blood specimens from healthy individuals, raising the possibility that there were normal populations of bacterial DNA sequences in the blood compartments previously considered sterile at least most of the time. Although persistent infection is a potential source of nonhuman sequences in normally sterile human anatomic sites, not all bona fide pathogens have been associated with abnormality.

The immunologic mechanisms and interactions between resident microbial agents and the human host have been studied at various body sites. The interaction between resident oral bacteria and human gingival epithelial cells in culture demonstrates their potential for virulence. The microbial agents frequently associated with periodontal diseases include *Bacteroides forsythus*, *Campylobacter curvus*, *Eikenella corrodens*, *Fusobacterium (F) nucleatum*, *Porphyromonas gingivalis*, and *Prevotella intermedia*. The effects of these bacteria on the production of interleukin-8, a proinflammatory chemokine, were also measured. *F nucleatum* adheres to and invades human gingival epithelial cells accompanied by high levels of interleukin 8 secretion from the epithelial cells.[10] By electron microscopy, this invasion occurs via a "zipping" mechanism that requires the active involvement of actins, microtubules, signal transduction, protein synthesis, and energy metabolism of the human gingival epithelial cells, as well as protein synthesis by *F nucleatum*.

Other investigators[11] noted a heightened risk of inflammatory bowel disease and colorectal cancer between diffusely adherent *Escherichia coli* and areas of dysplastic mucosa of the colon that made it easier for the bacterial pathogens to gain direct contact with the mucosal surface, a location that is relatively sterile in the normal colon. Such interactions between bacterial components and intrinsic T-cell receptors of the human mucosa with subsequent downstream protein signaling as the mechanism for early oncogenesis illustrating yet another molecular genetic property of the resident bacteria in their putative role in genotoxicity and human disease. If epithelial-associated bacteria play a causative role in inflammatory bowel disease and colorectal cancer, then dietary consumption of soluble plant fibers that prevent mucosal recruitment of bacteria may be protective against both conditions.

Postinfectious autoimmunity is a recognized phenomenon with several theories to explain its occurrence, including molecular mimicry, bystander activation, and viral persistence.[12] Alone or in combination, these mechanisms have been used to account for the immunopathology observed at the site of infection and in distant areas of the body. Molecular mimicry occurs when there are shared immunologic identities or epitopes between the microbe and host. One well-recognized example is rheumatic fever, a systemic autoimmune disease that occurs after group A β-hemolytic streptococci (GABHS) infection wherein affected patients develop and manifest circulating reactive antibodies to the bacterial organism reactive to the heart, joint, and brain, leading to the cardinal manifestations of rheumatic fever. Pediatric autoimmune neuropsychiatric disease associated with GABHS infection or PANDAS, is another example of bacterial-based molecular mimicry.

Viruses with cross-reactive epitopes to hepatitis B virus and myelin basic protein, a constituent of myelin, develop autoimmune experimental allergic encephalomyelitis (EAE) due to circulating T cells that preserve the memory of the virus and cross-react with myelin present in brain white matter of experimental mice. There is a form of postinfectious encephalitis named acute disseminated encephalomyelitis, an inflammatory demyelinating disorder of the brain in children that follows seemingly minor viral infection with a 2- to 30-day latency period that is thought to be postinfectious and autoimmune. It is thought that naissance of autoimmunity in such disorders originates when novel disease-inducing autoantigens are presented by specialized elements of the immune system in a trimolecular complex comprising antigen-presenting cells, major histocompatibility complex class II molecules, and autoreactive CD4$^+$ T cells.

Bystander activation and killing, a second mechanism that can also lead to autoimmune disease, has gained support through the use of experimental animal models mirroring some of the features of autoimmune disease, such as the nonobese diabetic mouse for type 1 diabetes (T1D) and EAE. It states that virus infections lead to significant activation of antigen-presenting cells that potentially activate preprimed autoreactive virus-specific T cells that migrate to areas of virus infection/antigen, such as the pancreas or brain. There, they encounter virus-infected cells presenting certain molecular tags, in turn releasing cytotoxic granules resulting in the killing or death of the infected cells. The dying cells, CD8$^+$ T cells, and inflammatory cells within such inflammatory foci release cytokines that lead to the demise of uninfected neighboring cells and additional immunopathology at sites of infection.

Persistent viral infection is a third mechanism of immune-mediated injury due to the constant presence of viral antigens that in turn drive the immune response. Yet unproven in humans, an example of this occurs in experimental mice who develop a condition termed Theiler murine encephalomyelitis,[13] in which persistent infection leads to a T-cell-mediated immunopathology in genetically susceptible animals. Susceptible strains develop virus-specific delayed-type hypersensitivity responses, whereas resistant strains do not. This response has been proposed as the basis for flaccid paralysis that spreads rapidly to all 4 limbs after an incubation period of 7 to 30 days because of inflammation and demyelination in the brain and spinal cord.

I-CUBED DISORDERS

With the preceding concepts in mind, this section considers 2 exemplary disorders, human leukocyte antigen (HLA) B27-related spondyloarthropathy and T1D and neuropathy, both of public health concern because of its pervasive occurrence in the population.

Spondyloarthropathy

The relationship between microbial infection and the gut, which has been known for decades as the basis for the spondyloarthritides (SpA)[14] has only recently been incorporated into the I-Cubed paradigm. SpA consists of diverse disorders of inflammatory arthritis. The reported incidence of 0.48 to 63/100,000 and prevalence of 0.01% to 2.5% for SpA diseases in the population[15] vary depending on the methodology and case definitions used for case ascertainment, and frequency of HLA-B27 in the population studied. Affected patients with symptoms referable to the vertebral column and limb joints may be seen by a variety of specialists including rheumatologists, neurologists, and general practitioners before the disorder is correctly diagnosed. Documentation of HLA B27 haplotype is a frequent associated feature.

Experimentally induced SpA occurs in mice with a striking resemblance to humans when HLA B27 components are introduced into genetically susceptible animals, establishing its central role in the human sickness.[16] Certain genetically prone mice develop colitis and later SpA when they are colonized with *Bacterioides* flora along with increased colonic cytokine expression compared with germ-free uncolonized animals.[17] The story, however, became more interesting when it was found that such animals also showed activation of Th17 helper cells[18] with HLA-B27 misfolding and a further heightened immune response to the unfolded protein associated with interleukin-23 production.[19]

Taken together, these findings suggested that genetically predisposed animals react to a microbial imbalance by altering their immune system in the intestinal compartment toward a more inflammatory state. The process is mediated by T-cell and interleukin production, which ultimately leads to local and systemic clinical disease manifested as aSpA-like human illness.[20] Such insights of the microbiomes have been used to advance therapy of SpA and other autoimmune arthritides. Empiric broad-spectrum antibiotics do not appear to have a therapeutic role and may select species with even more pathogenic potential. Bacterial modulation using alternative methods drawing from innate benefits of the microbiota,[21] such as fecal microbial transplantation, diet, and probiotics, have instead been used to restore a healthier intestinal microbiome.

Diabetes Mellitus and Neuropathy

Type 1 diabetes

T1D and type 2 diabetes (T2D) are both associated with diverse metabolic diseases that share the common feature of elevated blood glucose levels due to deficient insulin secretion or defective secretion or action, respectively. Both classes of patients are at perpetual risk for the development of nerve, kidney, and retinal disease. T1D usually develops before age 30 years, and such individuals need insulin injections for the rest of their life. Their disease is caused by the gradual loss of insulin-producing β cells in the pancreas.[22] Patients with T2D are typically older, often obese, and at high risk for hypercholesterolemia and heart disease, with relative insulin resistance that perpetuates hyperglycemia. The epidemiology of diabetes is well known. In the United States alone, more than one million people are living with T1D and approximately 80 people per day, or 30,000 individuals per year, are newly diagnosed. The global incidence of T1D is increasing at a rate of approximately 3% to 4% per year, notably among younger children. These statistics highlight the need for both better TID therapies and the continued push toward the prevention of T1D.

In the past several years, several lines of investigations have suggested the importance of environmental factors, including infectious diseases, making T1D an important candidate for an I-Cubed framework of understanding.

First, T1D appears to be caused by autoimmune mechanisms directed against the insulin-producing β cells of the pancreas,[23] with up to 90% of T1D patients harboring one or more autoantibodies.

Second, the pancreas of newly diagnosed T1D patients shows inflammation in the region of the insulin-producing β cells.[24]

Third, the possibility that the onset of T1D might be triggered in genetically predisposed individuals by a preceding infection inducing attack on islets by molecular mimicry was investigated in children with T1D who died prematurely. Their autopsy showed pancreatic islet cell, membrane-bound, superantigens, indicating integrated bacterial or viral genes. The genetic risk of T1D is strongly linked to HLA class II DR3 and DR4 haplotypes, with the highest risk in those with the DR3/DR4 genotype. The importance of HLA genes to T1D risk highlights the role of the adaptive immune system in the development of autoimmunity.

Fourth, T1D occurs with increased frequency in association with several other autoimmune disorders, including Grave disease, pernicious anemia, Hashimoto thyroiditis, myasthenia gravis, anti-phospholipid antibody syndrome, and Addison disease.

Fifth, there is an animal model of autoimmune diabetes in which T cells are strongly implicated in β-cell destruction, similar in nature to studies in humans in which primed autoreactive T cells recognize peptides common to both insulin and microbial antigens, suggesting that molecular mimicry may be the priming event in the destruction of β-islet cells in animals and humans.[25] Moreover, the response of T cells to homologous peptides derived from microbial antigens suggests that their initial priming could occur via molecular mimicry.

Sixth, it is hypothesized that perturbations in normal early microbiome development might predispose to disease whether through direct modulation of innate immunity or via alteration of intestinal permeability, with a downstream effect on adaptive immunity. The gut microbiome is both less diverse and protective in individuals with islet cell autoimmunity or recent onset T1D.[26-28] Whether this difference is causal to T1D in such patients is not known because multiple factors could affect the early intestinal microbiome, some of which also have been shown to correlate with risk of islet autoimmunity and T1D.[29] Nevertheless, increased intestinal permeability as a consequence of prolonged enteric intestinal infections could lead to increased susceptibility to T1D.[22] Viruses, with their potential to induce innate and adaptive immune responses and local inflammation in the pancreas and other organs, have been suspected of initiating these autoimmune processes. The etiologic link between T1D and viruses is based on epidemiologic, serologic, and histologic findings, as well as experimental in vivo and in vitro studies in DNA Herpesviruses and Parvoviruses, and RNA Togaviruses, Paramyxoviruses, Retroviruses, and Picornaviruses. A mechanism of molecular mimicry has been suggested on the observation that some microbial/viral proteins and host proteins have sequence or structural homology and therefore go unrecognized as self-proteins stimulating immune response against the viral antigen, which becomes cross-reactive against the homologous sequence of the host β-cell proteins.[12] Another possible mechanism of infection-induced autoimmunity is bystander activation whereby the infection of neighboring β cells stimulates local inflammation with the appearance of T cells and other inflammatory cells that release inflammatory proteins that lead to bystander killing of β cells.[30]

Diabetic neuropathy

Peripheral neuropathy occurring in association with T1D and T2D affecting large somatic and small pain-sensitive and autonomic fibers may be similarly influenced by inflammatory autoimmune factors. Historically, early investigations of diabetic neuropathy used nerve trunks obtained from diseased limbs obtained at surgical amputation and postmortem examination; such patients had longstanding diabetes that tended to increase the likelihood of arteriosclerosis. However, one early case showed clinicopathologic features of mononeuritis multiplex and vascular thrombosis of arteriae nervorum, suggesting a vascular inflammatory pathogenesis of neuropathy.[31] Decades later, investigations of peripheral nerve microvessels using vital stains to examine endoneurial blood vessels showed thickening of their walls[32] that was subsequently found to be reduplication of the basal lamina, a change also common to retinopathy and nephropathy. Unable to validate the correlation between so-called microangiopathy and neuropathy, attention focused on metabolic alterations in nerve elements, but attempts to correlate chronic hyperglycemia with metabolic derangements and alterations of intrinsic nerve lipids, alcoholic sugars, and a series of biochemical consequences leading to altered protein synthesis, abnormal glycosylation, slowed axon transport, axoglia dysjunction, osmotic swelling, or thickening of axolemmal and endoneurial basement membranes was often inconsistent.

In a series of 2 articles spanning a decade in 107 patients with diabetic neuropathy, Younger and colleagues[33,34] noted a more pervasive contribution of inflammatory and immune-mediated damage to the pathogenesis of diabetic neuropathy than had ever been previously imagined. Inflammatory lesions in diabetic nerves stained by immunoperoxidase comprised primarily CD8+ and CD4+ T cells of varying severity situated around endoneurial and small epineurial arteries or veins measuring 70 μm, leading to perivasculitis so noted in 23% of cases, and transmural inflammation of the vessel wall termed microvasculitis or frank vasculitis each in 3%. Associated immunologic alterations included complement deposition along vessel walls, not simply at sites of vascular inflammation, with expression of various interleukins and tumor necrosis factorα.

Two disorders of known autoimmune etiopathogenesis, chronic inflammatory demyelinating polyneuropathy (CIDP) and lumbosacral radiculoplexus neuropathy (LSRPN), were described in patients with T1D and T2D. Stewart and colleagues[35] and Haq and coworkers[36] described the clinical, electrophysiological, and histopathologic findings of a small series of diabetic patients meeting formal criteria for CIDP, the associated features of which did not discriminate diabetics from nondiabetics. Dyck and colleagues[37] compared 57 patients with LSRPN alone or associated with diabetes in 33 other patients, with regard to natural history variables, electrophysiological features, quantitative sensory and autonomic analysis, histopathology, and outcome, noting no differences in the indices between diabetic and nondiabetic patients.

More recently, Younger[38] described a living patient with diabetic LRPN in whom nerve biopsy showed necrotizing arteritis prompting combination immunosuppressive therapy, who at postmortem examination had perivascular epineurial and endoneurial inflammation in the extradural lumbar plexus, sciatic, and femoral nerve tissue without evidence of systemic vasculitis. Painful small-fiber neuropathy confirmed by intraepidermal nerve fiber analysis also occurs in patients with T1D and T2D as well as in association with diverse connective tissue and infectious and autoimmune neurologic disorders.[39]

REFERENCES

1. Lederberg J, McCray AT. 'Ome Sweet 'Omics—a genealogical treasury of words. New Scientist 2001;15:8.
2. Alivisator AP, Blaser MJ, Brodie EL, et al. MICROBIOME. A unified initiative to harness Earth's microbiomes. Science 2015;350:507–8.
3. Dubilier N, McFall-Ngai M, Zhao L. Create a global microbiome effort. Nature 2015;526:631–4.
4. Relman DA, Schmidt TM, MacDermott RP, et al. Identification of the uncultured bacillus of Whipple's disease. N Engl J Med 1992;327:293–301.
5. Fredericks DN, Relman DA. Localization of Tropheryma whippelii rRNA in tissues from patients with Whipple's disease. J Infect Dis 2001;183:1229–37.
6. Relman DA. The search for unrecognized pathogens. Science 1999;284: 1308–10.
7. Lower R, Lower J, Kurth R. The viruses in all of us: characteristics and biological significance of human endogenous retrovirus sequences. Proc Natl Acad Sci U S A 1996;93:5177–84.
8. Hajjeh RA, Relman D, Cieslak PR, et al. Surveillance for unexplained deaths and critical illnesses due to possibily infectious causes, United States, 1995-1998. Emerg Infect Dis 2002;8:145–53.
9. Gao SJ, Moore PS. Molecular approaches to the identification of unculturable infectious agent. Emerg Infect Dis 1996;2:159–67.
10. Han YW, Shi W, Huang GT, et al. Interactions between periodontal bacteria and human oral epithelial cells: Fusobacterium nucleatum adheres to and invades epithelial cells. Infect Immun 2000;68:3140–6.
11. Prorok-Hamon M, Friswell MK, Alswied A, et al. Colonic mucosa-associated diffusely adherent afaC+ Escherichia coli expressing lpfA and pks are increased in inflammatory bowel disease and colon cancer. Gut 2014;63:761–70.
12. Fujinami RS, von Herrath MG, Christen U, et al. Molecular mimicry, bystander activation, or viral persistence: infections and autoimmune disease. Clin Microbiol Rev 2006;19:80–94.
13. Theiler M. Spontaneous encephalomyelitis of mice, a new virus disease. J Exp Med 1937;65:705–19.
14. Yurkovetskiy LA, Pickard JM, Chervonsky AV. Microbiota and autoimmunity: exploring new avenues. Cell Host Microbe 2015;17:548–52.
15. Stolwijk C, Boonen A, van Tubergen A, et al. Epidemiology of spondyloarthritis. Rheum Dis Clin North Am 2012;38:441–76.
16. Hammer RE, Maila SD, Richardson JA, et al. Spontaneous inflammatory disease in transgenic rates expressing HLA-B27 and human beta 2m: an animal model of HLA-B27-associated human disorders. Cell 1990;63:1099–112.
17. Rath HC, Herfarth HH, Ikeda JS, et al. Normal luminal bacteria, especially Bacteroides species, mediated chronic colitis, gastritis, and arthritis in HLA-B27/human beta2 microglobulin transgenic rats. J Clin Invest 1996;98:945–53.

18. Glatigny S, Fert I, Blaton MA, et al. Proinflammatory Th17 cells are expanded and induced by dendritic cells in spondyloarthritis-prone HLA-B27-transgenic rats. Arthritis Rheum 2012;64:110–20.
19. DeLay ML, Turner MJ, Klenk EI, et al. HLA-B27 misfolding and the unfolded protein response augment interleukin-23 production and are associated with Th17 activation in transgenic rats. Arthritis Rheum 2009;60:2633–43.
20. Scher JU, Littman DR, Abramson SB. Microbiome in inflammatory arthritis and human rheumatic diseases. Arthritis Rheumatol 2016;68(1):35–45.
21. Olle B. Medicines from microbiota. Nat Biotechnol 2013;31:309–15.
22. Precechtelova J, Borsanyiova M, Sarmirova S, et al. Type I diabetes mellitus: genetic factors and presumptive enteroviral etiology or protection. J Pathog 2014; 2014:738512.
23. Atkinson MA, Caclaren NK. The pathogenesis of insulin-dependent diabetes mellitus. N Engl J Med 1994;331:1428–36.
24. Hanninen A, Jolkanen S, Salmi M, et al. Macrophages, T cell receptor usage, and endothelial cell activation in the pancreas at the onset of insulin-dependent diabetes mellitus. J Clin Invest 1992;90:1901–10.
25. Yang J, Chow IT, Sosinowski T, et al. Autoreactive T cells specific for insulin B:11-23 recognize a low-affinity peptide register in human subjects with autoimmune diabetes. Proc Natl Acad Sci U S A 2014;111:14840–5.
26. Giongo A, Gano KA, Crabb DB, et al. Toward defining the autoimmune microbiome for type 1 diabetes. ISME J 2011;5:82–91.
27. Brown CT, Davis-Richardson AG, Giongo A, et al. Gut microbiome metagenomics analysis suggests a functional model for the development of autoimmunity for type 1 diabetes. PLoS One 2011;6:e25792.
28. de Goffau MC, Luopajarvi K, Knip M, et al. Fecal microbiota composition differs between children with beta-cell autoimmunity and those without. Diabetes 2013; 62:1238–44.
29. VanBuecken D, Lord S, Greenbaum CJ. Changing the course of disease in type 1 diabetes. In: De Groot LJ, Beck-Peccoz P, Chrousos G, et al, editors. Endotext. South Dartmouth (MA): MDText.com, Inc.; 2000 [Updated 2015 Jun 29].
30. Roep BO, Hiemstra S, Schloot NC, et al. Molecular mimicry in type 1 diabetes: immune cross reactivity between islet autoantigen and human cytomegalovirus but not Coxsackie virus. Ann N Y Acad Sci 2002;958:163–5.
31. Raff MC, Sangalang V, Asbury AK. Ischemic mononeuropathy multiplex associated with diabetic mellitus. Arch Neurol 1968;18:487–99.
32. Fagerberg SE. Diabetic neuropathy-a clinical and histological study on the significance of vascular affections. Acta Med Scand 1959;164(Suppl 345):1–97.
33. Younger DS, Rosoklija G, Hays AP, et al. Diabetic peripheral neuropathy: a clinical and immunohistochemical analysis of sural nerve biopsies. Muscle Nerve 1996;19:722–7.
34. Younger DS. Diabetic neuropathy: a clinical and neuropathological study of 107 patients. Neurol Res Int 2010;2010:140379.
35. Stewart JD, McKelvey R, Durcan L, et al. Chronic inflammatory demyelinating polyneuropathy (CIDP). J Neurol Sci 1996;142:59–64.
36. Haq RU, Pendlebury WW, Fries TJ, et al. Chronic inflammatory demyelinating polyradiculoneuropathy in diabetic patients. Muscle Nerve 2003;27:465–70.
37. Dyck PJ, Norell JE, Dyck PJ. Non-diabetic lumbosacral radiculoplexus neuropathy: natural history, outcome and comparison with the diabetic variety. Brain 2001;124:1197–207.

38. Younger DS. Diabetic lumbosacral radiculoplexus neuropathy: a postmortem studied patient and review of the literature. J Neurol 2011;258:1364–7.
39. Younger DS. HTLV-1-associated myelopathy/tropical spastic paraparesis and peripheral neuropathy following live-donor renal transplantation. Muscle Nerve 2015;51:455–6.

Epidemiology of Lyme Neuroborreliosis

David S. Younger, MD, MPH, MS[a,b],*

KEYWORDS

- Lyme disease • *Borrelia burgdorferi* • Neurology • Public health • Epidemiology

KEY POINTS

- According to the Centers for Disease Control and Prevention, Lyme disease is the most commonly reported vector-borne illness and the fifth most common disease in the National Notifiable Diseases Surveillance System, making it an important public health concern.
- Lyme disease is caused by the bacterium *Borrelia burgdorferi* and is transmitted to humans through the bite of infected blacklegged *Ixodes* ticks.
- Typical symptoms include fever, headache, fatigue, and a characteristic skin rash called *erythema migrans*.
- Undiagnosed and therefore untreated, infection disseminates to the nervous system.
- The nonhuman primate model of Lyme neuroborreliosis accurately mimicked the microbiological, clinical, immunologic, and neuropathologic aspects of human Lyme neuroborreliosis.

INTRODUCTION

Lyme disease in humans is caused by the transmission of *Borrelia (B) burgdorferi* in the bite of infected blacklegged *Ixodes* ticks. Typical symptoms include fever, headache, fatigue, and a characteristic skin rash called *erythema migrans* (EM). If left undiagnosed and therefore untreated, infection disseminates to the nervous system causing Lyme neuroborreliosis (LNB). The clinical diagnosis is based on symptoms, physical findings, and the probability of exposure to infected ticks in endemic geographic areas and confirmed by serologic and cerebrospinal fluid (CSF) testing with the demonstration of intrathecal production of *Borrelia*-specific antibodies. There is general recognition for the potential of infectious-related autoimmune processes contributing to nervous system disease progression.

The author has nothing to disclose.
a Division of Neuroepidemiology, Department of Neurology, New York University School of Medicine, New York, NY, USA; b College of Global Public Health, New York University, New York, NY, USA
* Corresponding author. 333 East 34th Street, 1J, New York, NY 10016.
E-mail address: david.younger@nyumc.org

Neurol Clin 34 (2016) 875–886
http://dx.doi.org/10.1016/j.ncl.2016.05.005
0733-8619/16/© 2016 Elsevier Inc. All rights reserved.

neurologic.theclinics.com

HISTORY

Originally named for Lyme and Old Lyme, Connecticut, wherein a tight clustering of recurrent attacks of childhood and adult asymmetric oligoarticular arthralgia occurred beginning in 1972, Lyme disease showed a peak incidence of new cases in the summer and early fall.[1,2] Epidemiologic analysis of the clustering suggested transmission of a causative agent by an arthropod vector to humans, in whom 25% describe an expanding annular EM rash before onset of the arthritis. Cultures of the synovium and synovial fluid did not suggest infection with agents known to cause other forms of arthritis. Those in whom arthritis developed seemed to have significantly elevated ESR, lower third and fourth components of complement (C3, C4), higher serum IgM levels, and serum cryoprecipitates at the time of the skin lesions, suggesting an active immunologic response. Five years later, Burgdorfer and colleagues[3] isolated a spirochete from the tick Ixodes (I) dammini that bound immunoglobulins of patients convalescing from Lyme disease and recorded the development of lesions resembling EM in New Zealand white rabbits 10 to 12 weeks after being bitten by the ticks. One year later in the same volume of The New England Journal of Medicine, Steere and co-workers[4] and Benach and colleagues[5] described the spirochetal etiology of Lyme disease. Benach and colleagues[4] isolated spirochetes from the blood of 2 of 36 patients in Long Island and Westchester County, New York with signs and symptoms suggestive of Lyme disease that were morphologically similar and serologically identical to organisms known to infect I dammini ticks, endemic to the area and epidemiologically implicated as vectors of Lyme disease.

CLINICAL INVOLVEMENT

By 1989 Steere[6] summarized the causation, vector and animal hosts, clinical manifestations, pathogenesis, and treatment of human Lyme disease. Three stages of infection were recognized, each with different clinical manifestations. Stage 1 followed the bite by the tick with spread of bacteria locally in the skin in 60% to 80% of patients, resulting in EM rash that faded in 3 to 4 weeks but often accompanied by fever, minor constitutional symptoms, or regional adenopathy. At this time, the patient's mononuclear cells responded minimally to spirochete antigens, and even specific antibody might be lacking. Stage 2 of early infection followed days or weeks after the bite with bloodstream or lymphatic spread to many organ sites. More common in the United States than in Europe, widespread dissemination resulted in recovery of spirochete from tissue specimens of meninges, brain, myocardium, retina, muscle, bone, synovium, spleen, and liver.[7]

NONHUMAN PRIMATE STUDIES

Between 1998 and 1993 two animal models, a murine[8] and nonhuman primate (NHP)[9,10] accurately mimicked the microbiological, clinical, immunologic, and neuropathologic aspects of LNB. Two methods of spirochete inoculation, by needle injection of 1 million N40Br strain spirochetes and feeding of infected ticks were found to be comparable in establishing infection. Transient immunosuppression maximized the yield of infection in some of the NHPs. The central nervous system (CNS) was a major reservoir of spirochetal infection and showed that a strong, well-developed anti-Borrelia humoral immune response did not clear spirochetes from NHP during the months of infection. Accordingly, spirochetal presence was a necessary but not sufficient condition for inflammation.

PUBLIC HEALTH SURVEILLANCE

The public health surveillance of Lyme disease is reviewed elsewhere.[11] Lyme disease is the most commonly reported vector-borne illness and the fifth most common disease in the National Notifiable Diseases Surveillance System. The Centers for Disease Control and Prevention (CDC) reported 22,014 confirmed and 8817 probable incident US cases of Lyme disease reported during 2012. These data were similar to those of 2010 and 2011 but substantially lower than the number reported in 2008 and 2009. One important development, however, was an increase in the geographic distribution. In 2012, a total of 356 counties had a reported incidence of ≥10 confirmed cases per 100,000 persons compared with 324 counties in 2008. In 2013, 95% of confirmed incident cases were reported from 14 northeast and midwestern states including Connecticut, Delaware, Maine, Maryland, Massachusetts, Minnesota, New Hampshire, New Jersey, New York, Pennsylvania, Rhode Island, Vermont, Virginia, and Wisconsin. The seasonal occurrence of Lyme disease follows the life cycle of *Ixodes* ticks. Children age 5 to 14 years and adults age greater than 65 years are most susceptible when they engage in activities that heighten exposure to tick bites infected with *B burgdorferi*. Most cases occur from late spring to early fall when larval ticks mature into nymphs. Nymphs are infected by primary mammalian hosts transmitting the disease to secondary human hosts. Biodiverse habitats have reduced risk of Lyme disease. Forest clearings favor more efficient mammalian hosts such as mice spreading infection to people.

Surveillance methods to ascertain cases of Lyme disease use rigorous clinical and laboratory criteria to verify the diagnosis for reporting purposes, the results of which are verified and tabulated in final numbers in the *Morbidity and Mortality Weekly Report* in early August of the following year and summarized in the annual *Morbidity and Mortality Weekly Report Summary of Notifiable Diseases* (www.cdc.gov/mmwr/mmwr_nd/). A CDC public use dataset provides the number of confirmed cases by county in 5-year intervals, enabling investigators to access and download the information into compatible research-driven computer software for epidemiologic analysis. It should be emphasized that the methodology and specific criteria used in case ascertainment for epidemiologic and public health activities are not intended to be applicable to routine clinical diagnosis or the selection of antibiotic regimens, as a sizable population would be excluded from consideration of the diagnosis and treatment, specifically those with less-compelling, incomplete, or atypical presentations.

For surveillance purposes, the clinical description of Lyme disease is a systemic tick-borne disease with protean manifestations including dermatologic, rheumatologic, neurologic, and cardiac manifestations. The most common clinical marker for the disease is the EM rash, the initial skin lesion so noted in up to three-quarters of confirmed cases. Late manifestations include musculoskeletal (joint swelling, monoarthritis and oligoarthritis), nervous system (lymphocytic meningitis, cranial neuritis, radiculoneuropathy, and encephalomyelitis), and cardiovascular (high-grade heart block and atrioventricular conduction defects). Arthralgia, myalgia, and fibromyalgia; headache, fatigue, paresthesia, stiff neck; and palpitation, bradycardia, bundle branch heart block, and myocarditis, which may be highly suggestive of an index case of Lyme disease–related musculoskeletal, neurologic, and cardiac disease, are not specific criteria for case designation.

The specific laboratory criteria for case ascertainment according to the CDC[12–15] include a positive *B burgdorferi* culture or one of the following: (1) a positive result of 2-tier testing interpreted using established criteria in which a positive IgM titer is used for symptom onset ≤30 days and a positive IgG titer for any point during the infectious illness; (2) single-tier IgG immunoblot or Western blot seropositivity; and (3) CSF positivity for *B burgdorferi* by enzyme-linked immunoassay or immunofluorescence assay notably when the titer is higher in CSF than in serum referred to an intrathecal production of *Borrelia*-specific antibody. The terminology of Lyme exposure often used in clinical notes is defined as having been in wooded, brushy, or grassy areas, all potential tick habitats, in a county in which Lyme disease is endemic. The term *endemic* refers to a county in which at least 2 confirmed cases have been acquired or a county with a population of known tick vectors infected with *B burgdorferi*. A confirmed case of Lyme disease for surveillance meets the criteria of an EM rash with known exposure, or an EM rash with laboratory evidence of infection without known exposure, or one with at least a late clinical manifestation with laboratory evidence of infection. Suspected or probable cases are those with an EM rash or laboratory evidence of infection, respectively. A history of tick bite is not required for case ascertainment. Tokarz and colleagues[16] determined the prevalence of polymicrobial co-infection with *B burgdorferi*, *Anaplasma phagocytophilum*, *Babesia microti*, *Borrelia miyamotoi*, and Powassan virus in 286 adult tick–endemic areas of Lyme disease in New York State using a MassTag multiplex polymerase chain reaction assay.[17] The investigators noted 2 or more co-infections in 30% of ticks and some having up to 3 and 4 organisms.

To improve public health, the CDC has been conducting 3 complementary projects. The first project is to achieve an estimate of the number of people with Lyme disease diagnosed based on medical claims information from a large insurance database. The second study is to estimate the number of people who test positive for Lyme disease based on data obtained from a survey of clinical laboratories. A third study aims to estimate the number of people who report that they have had Lyme disease diagnosed in the previous year.

INFECTION VERSUS IMMUNITY

Inherent in the public health debate is the contribution of infectious versus immune-mediated mechanisms to clinical manifestations and disease progression.

Treatment-Resistant Arthritis

Steere and colleagues[18] first called attention to concomitant immune processes of infectious Lyme disease in the investigation of treatment-resistant Lyme arthritis, a complication rarely noted in Europe. With only about 10% of patients presenting with persistent joint inflammation for months to years after standard courses of antibiotic treatment, Steere and colleagues[19] studied the binding of outer surface protein A and human lymphocyte function–associated antigen 1 peptides to 5 major histocompatibility complex molecules noting the outer surface protein A identified the critical epitope in triggering antibiotic treatment–resistant Lyme arthritis. The hypothesis of infection-induced autoimmunity[20] was based on T-cell epitope mimicry between a spirochetal and host protein of bystander activation of a T-cell response to a self-epitope unrelated to spirochetal proteins. Either way, the T-cell response or linked antibody response to the self-protein could stimulate persistent synovial inflammation. Only some major histocompatibility complex molecules bound particular autoantigens, accounting for the human leukocyte antigen (HLA) association with autoimmune diseases, which made more important that most patients with treatment-resistant Lyme arthritis had the HLA-DRB1*0401 or HLA-DRB1*001 alleles, and to a lesser degree, the HLA-DRB1*0404 alleles. These 3 alleles, which have a similar sequence in the third hypervariable region of the HLA-DRB1 chain were are also associated with the severity of adult rheumatoid arthritis. However, in a study of European Lyme disease,[21] there was no association among 283 patients between HLA determinants and any of the various early or late infectious manifestations. There is limited information on postinfectious autoimmune syndromes of the nervous system caused or mediated by the Lyme spirochete. However, early susceptibility and protracted involvement, combined with the presence of serologic markers of altered immunity in affected patients with neurologic involvement[22] should lead to a consideration of concomitant autoimmune processes and treatment with immune modulatory therapy.

Inflammation in the Pathogenesis of Lyme Neuroborreliosis

With the aim of evaluating whether inflammation induced by B burgdorferi was causal in mediating the pathogenesis of acute LNB, hypothesizing that B burgdorferi–induced production of inflammatory mediators in glial and neuronal cells and that this response had a role in potentiating glial and neuronal apoptosis, investigators[23] recently studied the inflammatory changes induced in CNS, spinal nerves, and dorsal root ganglia (DRG) of rhesus macaques inoculated with live B burgdorferi into the cisterna magna. Some animals were left untreated or given the anti-inflammatory drug, dexamethasone, a corticosteroid that inhibited the expression of several immune mediators and studied for either 8 or 14 weeks postinoculation. Enzyme-linked immunosorbant assay (ELISA) of CSF showed significantly elevated levels of interleukin (IL)-6, IL-8, chemokine ligand 2, and CXCL 13 and pleocytosis in all infected animals except dexamethasone-treated animals; however, CSF and CNS tissues of infected animals were culture positive for B burgdorferi regardless of treatment. B burgdorferi antigen was present in DRG and dorsal roots by immunofluorescence staining and confocal microscopy. Histopathology findings showed leptomeningitis, vasculitis, and focal inflammation in the CNS; necrotizing focal myelitis in the cervical spine cord; radiculitis; neuritis and demyelination in spinal roots; and inflammation with neurodegeneration in the DRG that was concomitant with significant neuronal and satellite glial cell apoptosis. There changes were absent in the dexamethasone-treated animals. In accordance with their hypothesis, the investigators[10] noted that the effective suppression of inflammation by dexamethasone treatment resulted in inhibition of glial and neuronal damage, suggesting that host immunity to infection by B burgdorferi with subsequent inflammation, and not infection alone, had a causal role in the pathogenesis of LNB.

Blood–Brain Barrier

General considerations
Central to the question of active or chronic CNS infection is whether B burgdorferi has disseminated to the CNS across the blood–brain barrier (BBB) and if there is intrathecal production of Borrelia-specific antibodies. The BBB is a neurovascular unit comprising capillary vascular endothelial and neural cells, extracellular matrix components, and a variety of immune cells and has been intensely investigated in health and disease.[24–27]

A schematized and electron microscopic appearance of cerebral capillaries in the BBB (**Figs. 1** and **2**) shows layers of pericytes adherent to the abluminal or parenchymal surface of endothelial cells, together surrounded by a layer of basal lamina comprising extracellular matrix protein molecules. The end feet of neighboring astrocyte processes ensheath the blood vessels. Monolayers of adjacent endothelial cells that form tight junction (TJ) strands connect adjacent endothelial cells by adhesions of transmembrane (occluding-, claudin-, and junctional-associated molecules) across the intercellular space. Cytoplasmic scaffolding and regulatory proteins such as

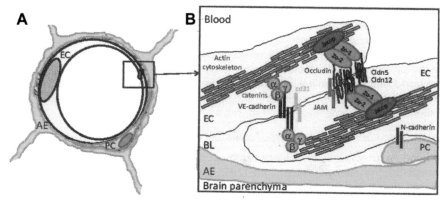

Fig. 1. (*A*) Cross-section schematic representation of a capillary in the human BBB over an endothelial tight junction. (*B*) The insert shows the molecular composition of tight and adherens junctions. (*From* Daneman R. The blood-brain barrier in health and disease. Ann Neurol 2012;72:648–72; with permission.)

zona occludens type 1 and 2 provide linkage to the actin cytoskeleton and initiate several signaling mechanisms via protein-protein interactions. Endothelia BBB cells are also linked by adherens junctions comprising vascular endothelial cadherin, which mediates cell-cell adhesion interactions, linking adherens junctions to the actin

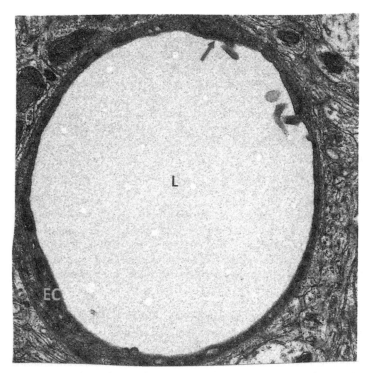

Fig. 2. Electron micrograph of a capillary in the adult murine BBB. Endothelial cells are held together by tight junctions (*red arrow*). (*From* Daneman R. The blood-brain barrier in health and disease. Ann Neurol 2012;72:648–72; with permission.)

cytoskeleton via catenins. The extended neurovascular unit comprises perivascular macrophages that reside between astrocyte end feet and the vessel wall, mast cells associated with specific regions of the CNS, resident microglia that act as antigen-presenting cells, circulating leukocytes that can penetrate the intact BBB via interactions with endothelial adhesion molecules to mediate bidirectional crosstalk between immune cells, and endothelium for normal surveillance. The abnormal entry of plasma components, immune molecules, and cellular elements across the BBB leads to further neural dysfunction and varying degrees of irreversible neural degeneration.

Implications for Lyme neuroborreliosis

Interest in concepts of BBB disruption in LNB started with experimental and clinical observations beginning in the early 1990s focusing on the etiopathogenesis of CNS manifestations, notably encephalopathy in acute and chronic Lyme infection in humans and NHP. The mechanisms by which bacteria breach the BBB have generally been incompletely understood; however, it was proposed that during other forms of bacteremia, microbial factors acted directly or indirectly to trigger production of endogenous inflammatory mediators that altered endothelial TJ to facilitate bacterial entry. There are increasing experimental data in the understanding of the human illness.

In 1990, Szczepanski and colleagues[28] studied the emigration of *B burgdorferi* across cultured human umbilical vein endothelial cells (HUVEC). Low-passage human clinical isolates (HSA1 and HBD1) cultured from skin and blood, respectively, of patients with EM and a tick isolate (T11) from *I dammini* collected in Montauk, NY, adhered 22- to 30-fold greater than the continuously passaged strain B31 to the subendothelial matrix. Spirochete binding and adherence to the subendothelial matrix were inhibited 48% to 63% by pretreatment of the matrix with antiserum to fibronectin, a major component of the matrix produced by cultured endothelial cells and a constituent of the basement membrane of blood vessels in vivo. The inhibition of spirochete adherence to the matrix by antifibronectin indicated that the spirochetes recognized the insoluble matrix form of this glycoprotein. Spirochete migration across endothelial monolayers cultured on amniotic membrane was increased when the monolayers were damaged by chemical or physical means. Electron microscopic examination of spirochete–endothelial interactions demonstrated the presence of spirochetes in the intercellular junctions between endothelial cells and beneath the monolayers. Scanning electron microscopy identified a mechanism of transendothelial migration whereby spirochetes passed between cells into the amniotic membrane at areas where subendothelium was exposed. The adherence of *B burgdorferi* to subendothelial matrix is an important finding, as spirochetes must penetrate the subendothelial basement membrane of the BBB to enter the CNS compartment. Spirochete recognition of endothelial cells or subendothelial matrix seems to be mediated by separate mechanisms, as pretreatment of endothelial cells with antifibronectin antiserum reduced spirochete adherence to the cells slightly, whereas matrix binding was greatly diminished. Moreover, little fibronectin is expressed on the surface of endothelial cells in culture or in vivo. Spirochete transendothelial migration was facilitated by prior damage of the endothelial cell monolayer by physical or chemical injury. Spirochete migration at regions where a small gap in the monolayer exposed the underlying connective tissue on scanning electron microscopy would likewise be expected to occur in vivo in areas where endothelial cell contraction or damage occurred. A similar sequence of events of attachment to the apical surfaces of cultured cells, between cells, and beneath endothelial cell monolayers, and migration via an intercellular route and not by a transcytotic process, was described for the transendothelial migration of *Treponema pallidum* spirochete.[29]

Grab and colleagues[30] studied the traversal of human brain microvascular endo-thelial cells (BMEC) and HUVEC by *B burgdorferi* noting facilitation in the former by proteases. The spirochete organism seemed to bind human BMEC by their tips near or at cell borders, inducing the expression of plasminogen activators, plasmin-ogen activator receptors, and matrix metalloproteinases. Grab and colleagues[30] noted that about a 21-fold more low-passage *Borrelia* crossed HUVEC than BMEC, underscoring the importance of extrapolating data concerning *B burgdorferi* penetra-tion of the BBB from experimental data using nonbrain vascular endothelial cell models. The authors hypothesized that *B burgdorferi* induces the expression of plas-minogen activators and matrix metalloproteinases and that these enzymes, linked by an activation cascade, could lead to the focal and transient degradation of TJ pro-teins. This mechanism allows the spirochete organism to invade the CNS, binding via their tips before crossing the in vitro human BBB model without evidence of loss of BBB integrity. Unlike purulent bacterial meningitis, *B burgdorferi* causes aseptic men-ingitis in which the permeability of the BBB may not be substantially altered.[31] In a later investigation of the traversal of *B burgdorferi* across the human BBB using in vitro model systems constructed of HBMEC, Grab and coinvestigators[32] used cell monolayers pretreated with the intracellular calcium chelator BAPTA-AM (1,2-Bis [2-aminophenoxy]ethane-N,N,N',N'-tetra-acetic acid tetrakis [acetoxymethyl ester]) and the phospholipase C (PLC) inhibitor U-73122 (1-(6-[([17b]-3Methoxyes-tra-1,3,5[10]-trien-17-y1)amino]heyl)1H-pyrrole-2,5-dione). The results were signifi-cant to total inhibition of transmigration of *B burgdorferi* as a result of barrier tightening based on electric cell-substrate impedance sensing. These data suggest a role for calcium in CNS spirochete invasion through the endothelial cell barrier. Nyarko and colleagues[33] noted that *B burgdorferi* and *Anaplasma phagocytophi-lum*–infected neutrophils co-incubated with HUVEC and HBMEC were associated with increased blood and tissue spirochete loads and heightened traversal through endothelial cell barriers.

Garcia-Monco and coworkers[34] found early invasion of the CNS in experimental Lewis rats by *B burgdorferi* accompanied by increased BBB permeability measured as the ratio of Iodine-125-labeled albumin CSF to that in blood. Dose-dependent BBB permeability changes were noted 12 hours after inoculation and reversed within a week. Only live, intravenously inoculated organisms produced disruption of the BBB. More marked BBB charges were noted with inoculation of the more recent low-passage strain termed *J31* acquired from Long Island than with the original isolate of the B31 strain in long-term in vitro culture from Shelter Island, both of which were grown in serum-free media to log phase. Mild pleocytosis and retrievable spirochetes were noted in the CSF of rats with increased BBB permeability. Specific *B burgdorferi* anti-gens were detectable in the CSF of human patients with early Lyme disease with use of murine monoclonal antibodies as probes providing evidence for early CNS invasion.

Garcia-Monco and coworkers[35,36] described the affinity of the Lyme spirochete for cells of primary neonatal rat brain cultures, providing evidence of spirochete binding to cell surfaces and processes of glial fibrillary acidic protein–bearing cells and to the surfaces and processes of myelin basic protein (MBP) and galactocerebroside-bearing cells and their extracellular visible by microscopy. Given that most of the cells in primary rat brain culture were astrocytes and oligodendrocytes, the investigators[35] suggested that affinity and adherence to these cells and their known proximity to brain capillary endothelial cells in the BBB were likely determinants of the initiation of CNS injury and might contribute to the secondary persistence of *B burgdorferi* in the CNS and the development of cross-reactivity between microbial antigens and neural components. Using chromium-51 assays for the detection of damage to cells of neural origin, Garcia-Monco and coworkers[36] showed a higher degree of injury in the primary brain than in astroglial cultures on scanning electron microscopy, revealing marked contraction of the membrane sheets and bleb production of oligo-dendroglia in neonatal rat brain culture after incubation with *B burgdorferi*, whereas the astroglial layers appeared unharmed. The damage to oligodendroglia was evident on the surface of the cells without detection of intracellular *B burgdorferi*, suggesting that the ensuing morphologic changes were not the result of internalization of spirochetes.

The presence of CNS white matter injury and *B burgdorferi*–specific and autoreactive T-cell lines from the CSF have been described in affected patients with Lyme Meningo-radiculo-myelitis,[37,38] as have antibodies to MBP in CSF specimens from patients with chronic meningo-encephalopathy,[39] suggesting a role for antibodies to MBP in the pathogenesis of the disease manifestations. However, a quarter century later, it is still not known with absolute certainty whether autoreactivity causes tissue damage or is a secondary epiphenomenon.[6]

Moriarty and coworkers[40] engineered a fluorescent strain of *B burgdorferi* that expressed green fluorescent protein. Using real-time 3-dimensional and 4-dimensional intravital microscopy with quantitative analysis, the investigators studied fluorescent spirochete dissemination noting it to be a multistage process that included transient tethering-type associations, short-term dragging interactions, and stationary adhesion. The latter in association with extravasating *Borrelia* spirochetes were most commonly observed at endothelial junctions, whereas translational motility of spirochetes seemed to play an integral role in transendothelial migration. Stationary adhesions that projected deep into and sometimes through platelet endothelial cell adhesion molecule 1 (PECAM-1)-stained regions of vessels, a phenomenon termed *embedding*, and that occurred along the length of the spirochete or at one end only, found spirochetes protruding through both sides of the PECAM-1 signal, suggesting migration more deeply into junctions or endothelial cells than partially embedded adhesions. This observation seemed to be consistent with early electron microscopic studies that found that *B burgdorferi* invaded or was taken up by endothelial cells in monolayer cultures.[41] However, the investigators did not study aspects of the BBB.

More recently, Brissette and coworkers[42] analyzed the transcriptional responses to the incubation of *B burgdorferi* in primary cultures with primary human astrocytes and HBMEC over a 72-hour period noting a robust increase in IL-8, CXCL-1, and CXCL-10 chemokines in response to virulent spirochetes. The results were confirmed by ELISA and individual sets of polymerase chain reaction primers. The up-regulation of chemokines receptors from brain microvascular endothelial cells and astrocytes has the potential to facilitate entry of neurotoxic neutrophils into the CNS. NHP astrocytes that expressed the neutrophil chemoattractant IL-8 in response to *B burgdorferi* seemed to contribute to the inflammatory response both in vivo and in vitro in a macaque model of CNS Lyme disease.[43–45]

Future progress in studies of the BBB in humans may yet lead to improved outcome in early and late manifestations of the disease, taking advantage of the selective expression of membrane-bound proteins expressed by brain endothelia cells or circulating leukocytes to target new drugs and improving the effectiveness of conventional oral and parenteral antibiotics.

REFERENCES

1. Steere AC, Malawista SE, Hardin JA, et al. Erythema chronicum migrans and Lyme arthritis. The enlarging spectrum. Ann Intern Med 1977;86:685–98.

2. Steere AC, Malawista SE, Snydman DR, et al. Lyme arthritis: an epidemic of oligoarticular arthritis in children and adults in three Connecticut communities. Arthritis Rheum 1977;20:7–17.
3. Burgdorfer W, Barbour AG, Hayes SF, et al. Lyme disease-a tick-borne spirochetosis? Science 1982;216:1317–9.
4. Steere AC, Grodzicki RI, Kornblatt AN, et al. The spirochetal etiology of Lyme disease. N Engl J Med 1983;308:733–40.
5. Benach JI, Bosler EM, Hanrahan JP, et al. Spirochetes isolated from the blood of two patients with Lyme disease. N Engl J Med 1983;308:740–2.
6. Steere AC. Lyme disease. N Engl J Med 1989;321:586–96.
7. Duray PH, Steere AC. Clinical pathologic correlations of Lyme disease by stage. Ann N Y Acad Sci 1988;539:65–79.
8. Barthold SW, Moody KD, Terwillinger GA, et al. Experimental Lyme arthritis in rats infected with Borrelia burgdorferi. J Infect Dis 1988;157:842–6.
9. Pachner AR, Delaney E, O'Neill T, et al. Inoculation of nonhuman primates with the N40 strain of Borrelia burgdorferi leads to a model of Lyme neuroborreliosis faithful to the human disease. Neurology 1995;45:165–72.
10. Pachner AR, Delaney E, O'Neill T. Neuroborreliosis in the nonhuman primate: Borrelia burgdorferi persists in the central nervous system. Ann Neurol 1995;38:667–9.
11. Younger DS. Epidemiology. Chapter 2. In: Younger DS, editor. Human Lyme neuroborreliosis. New York: Nova Science; 2015. p. 17–24.
12. Centers for Disease Control and Prevention. Recommendations for test performance and interpretation from the Second National Conference on Serologic Diagnosis of Lyme disease. MMWR Morb Mortal Wkly Rep 1995;44:590–1.
13. Dressler F, Whalen JA, Reinhardt BN, et al. Western blotting in the serodiagnosis of Lyme disease. J Infect Dis 1993;167:392–400.
14. Engstrom SM, Shoop E, Johnson RC. Immunoblot interpretation criteria for serodiagnosis of early Lyme disease. J Clin Microbiol 1995;33:419–27.
15. Centers for Disease Control and Prevention. Notice to readers: caution regarding testing for Lyme disease. MMWR Morb Mortal Wkly Rep 2005;54:125–6.
16. Tokarz R, Jain K, Bennett A, et al. Assessment of polymicrobial infections in ticks in New York State. Vector Borne Zoonotic Dis 2010;10:217–21.
17. Tokarz R, Kapoor V, Samuel JE, et al. Detection of tick-borne pathogens by MassTag polymerase chain reaction. Vector Borne Zoonotic Dis 2009;9:147–52.
18. Steere AC, Falk B, Drouin EE, et al. Binding of outer surface protein A and human lymphocytic function-associated antigen 1 peptides to HLA-DR molecules associated with antibiotic-resistant Lyme arthritis. Arthritis Rheum 2003;48:534–40.
19. Steere AC. Treatment of Lyme arthritis. Arthritis Rheum 1994;37:878–88.
20. Steere AC, Glicktein L. Elucidation of Lyme arthritis. Nat Rev Immunol 2004;4:143–52.
21. Reimers CD, Neubert U, Kristoferistch W, et al. Borrelia burgdorferi infection in Europe: an HLA-related disease? Infection 1992;20:197–200.
22. Younger DS, Orsher S. Lyme neuroborreliosis: preliminary results from an Urban Referral Center Employing Strict CDC Criteria for Case Selection. Neurol Res Int 2010;2010:525206.
23. Ramesh G, Didier PJ, England JD, et al. Inflammation in the pathogenesis of Lyme neuroborreliosis. Am J Pathol 2015;185:1344–60.
24. Daneman R. The blood-brain barrier in health and disease. Ann Neurol 2012;72:648–72.

25. Benarroch EE. Blood-brain barrier: recent developments and clinical correlations. Neurology 2012;78:1268–76.

26. Hawkins BR, Davis TP. The blood-brain barrier/neurovascular unit in health and disease. Pharmacol Rev 2005;57:173–85.

27. Weiss N, Miller F, Cazaubon S, et al. The blood-brain barrier in brain homeostasis and neurological diseases. Biochim Biophys Acta 2009;1788:842–57.

28. Szczepanski A, Furie MB, Benach JL, et al. Interaction between Borrelia burgdorferi and endothelium in vitro. J Clin Invest 1990;85:1637–47.

29. Thomas DD, Navab DM, Haake DA, et al. Treponema pallidum invades intercellular junctions of endothelial cell monolayters. Proc Natl Acad Sci U S A 1988;85: 3608–12.

30. Grab DJ, Perides G, Dumler JS, et al. Borrelia burgdorferi, host-derived proteases, and the blood-brain barrier. Infect Immun 2005;73:1014–22.

31. Fikrig E, Coyle PK, Schutzer SE, et al. Preferential presence of decorin-binding protein B (BBA25) and BBA50 antibodies in cerebrospinal fluid of patients with neurologic Lyme disease. J Clin Microbiol 2004;42:1243–6.

32. Grab DJ, Nyarko E, Nikolskaia OV, et al. Human brain microvascular endothelial cell traversal by Borrelia burgdorferi requires calcium signaling. Clin Microbiol Infect 2009;15:422–6.

33. Nyarko E, Grab DJ, Dumler JS. Anaplasma phagocytophilum-infected neutrophils enhance transmigration of Borrelia burgdorferi across the human blood brain barrier in vivo. Int J Parasitol 2006;36:601–5.

34. Garcia-Monco JC, Villar BF, Alen JC, et al. Borrelia burgdorferi in the central nervous system: experimental and clinical evidence for early invasion. J Infect Dis 1990;161:1187–93.

35. Garcia-Monco JC, Fernandez Villar B, Benach JL. Adherence of the Lyme disease spirochete to glial cells and cells of glial origin. J Infect Dis 1989;160: 497–506.

36. Garcia-Monco JC, Fernandez Villar B, Szczepanski A, et al. Cytotoxicity of Borrelia burgdorferi for cultured rat glial cells. J Infect Dis 1991;163:1362–6.

37. Martin R, Ortlauf J, Sticht-Groh V, et al. Borrelia burgdorferi specific and autoreactive T-cell lines from cerebrospinal fluid in Lyme radiculomyelitis. Ann Neurol 1988;24:509–16.

38. R1 Martin, Ortlauf J, Sticht-Groh V, et al. Isolation and characterization of Borrelia burgdorferi-specific and autoreactive T-cell lines from the cerebrospinal fluid of patients with Lyme meningoradiculomyelitis. Ann N Y Acad Sci 1988;540:449–51.

39. Garcia-Monco JC, Coleman JL, Benach JL. Antibodies to myelin basic protein in Lyme disease. J Infect Dis 1988;158:667–8.

40. Moriarty TJ, Norman MU, Colarusso P, et al. Real-time high resolution 3D imaging of the Lyme disease spirochete adhering to and escaping from the vasculature of a living host. PLoS Pathog 2008;4(6):e1000090.

41. Cornstock LE, Thomas DD. Characterizaiton of Borrelia burgdorferi invasion of cultured endothelial cells. Microb Pathog 1991;10:137–48.

42. Brissette CA, Kees ED, Burke MM, et al. The multifaceted responses of primary human astrocytes and brain microvascular endothelial cells to the Lyme disease spirochete, Borrelia burgdorferi. ASN Neuro 2013;5:221–9.

43. Ramesh G, Alvarez AL, Roberts ED, et al. Pathogenesis of Lyme neuroborreliosis: Borrelia burgdorferi lipoproteins induce both proliferation and apoptosis in rhesus monkey astrocytes. Eur J Immunol 2003;33:2539–50.

44. Ramesh G, Borda JT, Dufour J, et al. Interaction of the Lyme disease spirochete Borrelia burgdorferi with brain parenchyma elicits inflammatory mediators from glial cells as well as glial and neuronal apoptosis. Am J Pathol 2008;173:1415–27.
45. Ramesh G, Borda JT, Gill A, et al. Possible role of glial cells in the onset and progression of Lyme neuroborreliosis. J Neuroinflammation 2009;6:23.

Epidemiology of Neurovasculitis

David S. Younger, MD, MPH, MS[a,b],*

KEYWORDS

- Global • Burden • Vasculitis

KEY POINTS

- Vasculitis is defined as inflammation of blood vessel walls for at least some time during the course of the disease and affects arteries and veins of varying calibers.
- The Chapel Hill Consensus Conferences have provided consensus on nosology and definitions for the commonest forms of adult-onset vasculitides.
- The Pediatric Rheumatology European Society and the European League against Rheumatism have proposed specific classification criteria for the commonest childhood vasculitides.
- Although not included in the 2013 Global Burden of Disease Study, adult and childhood vasculitides are a significant source of morbidity and mortality globally.
- Management relies on the use of immunosuppressant and immune modulatory therapy.

CLASSIFICATION AND NOSOLOGY

Vasculitis is defined as inflammation of blood vessel walls for at least some time during the course of the disease and affects arteries and veins of varying calibers. Two Chapel Hill Consensus Conferences (CHCC), one in 1994[1] and the other in 2012,[2] provided consensus on nosology and definitions for the commonest forms of vasculitis. The revised CHCC nomenclature serves as a guide for the categorization of diverse forms of vasculitis based on the vessels involved and provides a scheme for the neurologic aspects thereof (**Box 1**). Large vessel vasculitis (LVV), including giant cell arteritis (GCA) and Takayasu arteritis (TAK), affects the aorta, its major branches, and analogous veins. Medium vessel vasculitis (MVV), inclusive of polyarteritis nodosa (PAN) and Kawasaki disease (KD), involves main visceral arteries and veins and initial branches. The category of small vessel vasculitis (SVV) recognizes involvement of intraparenchymal arteries, arterioles, capillaries, veins, and venules, with a disease mechanism related to antineutrophil cytoplasmic antibody (ANCA) and immune

The author has nothing to disclose.
[a] Division of Neuroepidemiology, Department of Neurology, New York University School of Medicine, New York, NY, USA; [b] College of Global Public Health, New York University, New York, NY, USA
* Corresponding author. 333 East 34th Street, 1J, New York, NY 10016.
E-mail address: david.younger@nyumc.org

neurologic.theclinics.com

Box 1
Classification of primary systemic vasculitides

Large vessel vasculitis

Giant cell arteritis

Takayasu arteritis

Medium vessel vasculitis

Polyarteritis nodosa

Kawasaki disease

Small vessel vasculitis

ANCA-associated vasculitis
  Microscopic polyangiitis
  Granulomatosis with polyangiitis (Wegener)
  Eosinophilic granulomatosis with polyangiitis (Churg-Strauss)

Immune-complex vasculitis
  Cryoglobulinemia
  IgA vasculitis (Henoch-Schönlein)
  Hypocomplementemic urticarial vasculitis (anti-C1q)

Variable vessel vasculitis

Behçet disease

Cogan syndrome

Single-organ vasculitis

Primary CNS vasculitis

Idiopathic aortitis (IgG4)

---

complexes. The category of ANCA-associated vasculitis (AAV) includes granulomatosis with polyangiitis (GPA), Wegener granulomatosis (WG) type, eosinophilic granulomatosis with polyangiitis (EGPA) Churg-Strauss syndrome, and microscopic polyangiitis (MPA) (microscopic polyarteritis), whereas vasculitic disorders associated with immune complexes include immunoglobulin A (IgA) vasculitis (IgAV) (Henoch-Schönlein purpura [HSP]), cryglobulinemic vasculitis (CV), and hypocomplementemia urticarial vasculitis (HUV) associated with C1q antibodies. Vasculitis without a predominant vessel size and caliber, respectively, from small to large, involving arteries, veins, and capillaries, comprises the category of variable vessel vasculitis (VVV), characteristic of Behçet disease (BD) and Cogan syndrome (CS). The category of vasculitis associated with systemic disease includes vasculitis associated with rheumatoid arthritis (RA) and systemic lupus erythematosus (SLE) and other connective tissue disorders, wherein the vasculitic process is secondary to or associated with the underlying systemic disorder. There is a category of vasculitis associated with a probable specific cause, such as substance abuse and infection designated by the specific vasculitic disorder with a prefix to denote the causative agent. The category of single-organ vasculitis (SOV) involves arteries or veins of any size in a single organ without features to indicate that it is a limited expression of a systemic vasculitis characterized by primary central nervous system (CNS) vasculitis, nonsystemic peripheral nerve vasculitis (PNV), and isolated aortitis.

Recognizing that certain forms of vasculitis are more common in childhood and that some vasculitides display different disease courses compared with adult forms,[3] the

Pediatric Rheumatology European Society (PRES) and the European League Against Rheumatism (EULAR) proposed specific classification criteria for the commonest childhood vasculitis syndrome[4] based on vessel size, similar to the CHCC nomenclature.[2] In 2008, the EULAR, PRES, and the Pediatric Rheumatology International Trials Organization reported their methodology and overall clinical, laboratory, and radiographic characteristics for several childhood systemic vasculitides[5] followed by a final validated classification.[6]

HISTORICAL ASPECTS

The early history of vasculitis is debatable, but one fact is clear, the earliest patients with vasculitis appeared to have had neurologic involvement. It is thought that Kussmaul and Maier provided the first complete gross and microscopic description of a patient with leg pains, cramps, and tenderness so prominent that trichinosis was considered in an article entitled, "A hitherto undescribed peculiar disease of the arteries which is accompanied by Bright's disease and a rapidly progressive general paralysis of the muscles." At postmortem examination, there was widespread arteritis that resembled syphilitic periarteritis. The disorder was named periarteritis for the inflammation around blood vessels. The first American patient was described in 1908.[7] This 35-year-old man presented with constitutional symptoms and subacute leg pains. Postmortem examination showed widespread necrotizing arteritis and nodules along small- and medium-sized vessels of the heart, liver, kidney, pancreas, testicles, brain, nerves, and skeletal muscles, sparing the lungs and spleen. The histologic lesions consisted of mononuclear cell infiltration, necrosis of internal and external elastic lamina of the media, fibrin deposition, aneurysmal dilatation, perivascular inflammation of the adventitia, and intimal proliferation resulting in narrowing of arterial lumina. Kernohan and Woltman[8] summarized the clinical and neuropathologic aspects of adult PAN, and Krahulik and colleagues[9] reported the postmortem neurologic findings of fulminant childhood PAN (cPAN). The dominant neurologic picture of both adult and cPAN was a peripheral neuritis that occurred in one-half of patients early in the illness with a predilection for the legs. At postmortem examination, all had arteritic lesions along nutrient arteries of the peripheral nerves, and three-quarters had lesions in arteriae nervorum. The combination of acute and chronic lesions correlated with known exacerbations. Involvement of the CNS was estimated to occur in 8% of cases evident by clinically apparent brain infarcts resulting from occlusion of cerebral vessels, which was often insidious in its progression. In PAN, as in the other systemic necrotizing arteritis, the vasculitic lesion proceeded in a characteristic manner, commencing with invasion of the intima, media, and adventitia by polymorphonuclear, plasma cells, eosinophils, and lymphocytes, leading to swelling of the media, and fibrinoid necrosis that clusters around the vasa vasorum, with fragmentation of the internal elastic lamina. There was focal deposition of perivascular connective tissue, vascular necrosis, and denuding of the endothelium, followed by vascular thrombosis, ischemia, aneurysm formation, rupture, and hemorrhage. Healed lesions coexisted with active lesions. Harry Lee Parker conceptualized nerve and muscle biopsy in a discussion of the paper by Kernohan and Woltman,[8] commenting, "It occurs to me that in any case in which polyarteritis nodosa may be suspected, it is advisable to take a biopsy from a peripheral nerve, muscle or artery." There are no published series confirming the correlation of the extent of systemic necrotizing arteritis that may be predicted by the singular finding of vasculitis in a cutaneous nerve biopsy specimen. Only one reported series[10] reported neither systemic nor isolated PNV found at postmortem after diagnostic cutaneous nerve biopsy evidencing necrotizing vasculitis in life. A variant of PAN was recognized in very young children with mucocu-taneous lymph node syndrome. Although early publications used the term infantile PAN, KD is the preferred term to describe this childhood syndrome with worldwide occurrence, affecting children of all ages and races. Both PAN and KD are prototypical examples of MVV.

Contemporaneously, SVV syndromes were recognized and differentiated from PAN. Early investigators[11–13] described MPA among 34 patients that differed from PAN due to selective involvement of small microscopic arteries, arterioles, capillaries, and ve-nules, including glomerular and pulmonary alveolar capillaries. Fever, arthralgia, pur-pura, hemoptysis, pulmonary hemorrhage, abdominal pain, and gastrointestinal bleeding likewise preceded the explosive phase of systemic necrotizing vasculitis that affected the kidney and lungs, with rapidly progressive glomerulonephritis and pulmonary capillaritis. Two of 5 deaths were attributed to CNS involvement by vascu-litis during periods of disease at 4 and 8 months, respectively; however, that could not be confirmed because postmortem examinations were not performed. The disorder was later reclassified by the CHCC[2] as a necrotizing SVV with little or no immune-complex deposition that primarily affected the kidney and lungs. Medium-sized ar-teries might be involved even though the disease was predominantly considered to affect small-sized arteries, arterioles, capillaries, and venules of the 2 organs most affected, with variable systemic necrotizing vasculitis.

The first patient with EGPA was probably case 1 of Lamb[14] reported in 1914 under the heading of PAN. That patient, a 26-year-old man with 2 years of worsening asthma, developed fever, palpable purpura, nodular skin lesions, hemoptysis, vomit-ing, urinary difficulty, and granular urinary casts. He died 1 month later, and postmor-tem examination showed necrotizing arteritis of small arteries, with dense collections of extravascular eosinophils and tissue eosinophilia in the heart, stomach, and kidney. Decades later, Churg and Strauss[15] described the clinical and postmortem findings of 13 patients with asthma, fever, and hypereosinophilia, accompanied by eosinophilic exudation, fibrinoid change, and granulomatous proliferation that constituted the so-called allergic granuloma that was found within vessel walls and in extravascular connective tissue of major organ systems, leading to cardiac, pulmonary, gastrointes-tinal, skin, peripheral nervous system (PNS), and CNS manifestations. In 1977, Chumbley and coworkers[16] described 30 asthmatic patients from the Mayo Clinic over the period 1950 to 1974 with necrotizing vasculitis of small arteries and veins with extravascular granulomas and infiltration of vessels and perivascular tissue with eosinophilia. The lungs, peripheral nerves, and skin were most frequently involved, and renal failure was encountered in only one patient. Corticosteroids seemed to confer long-term survival. In 1984, Lanham and colleagues[17] emphasized that the combination of necrotizing vasculitis, tissue infiltration by eosinophils, and extravascular granulomas suggested by Churg and Strauss[15] occurred contempora-neously in only a minority of patients. Moreover, such histologic findings could be encountered as well in other granulomatous, vasculitic, and eosinophilic disorders in the absence of clinical asthma, allergic rhinitis, sinusitis, pulmonary infiltrates, and cardiac involvement pathognomonic of EGPA. The investigators described a phasic pattern of EGPA in which allergic disease preceded systemic vasculitis, and eosino-philic tissue infiltrates might occur in the absence of peripheral blood eosinophilia. Pul-monary infiltrates, upper respiratory tract, and gastrointestinal disease often preceded the vasculitic component of the syndrome, leading to cardiac, cutaneous, nervous system, renal, bone, and muscle involvement. In 1990, the American College of Rheu-matology (ACR)[18] developed criteria for the classification of EGPA that included ascer-tainment of 4 or more of the following: asthma, eosinophilia of greater than 10%, mononeuropathy or polyneuropathy, nonfixed pulmonary infiltrates on chest radio-graph, paranasal sinus abnormality, and extravascular eosinophils on tissue biopsy that included an artery, arteriole, or venule. These criteria were inadequate in differen-tiating the various clinicopathologic expressions of SVV, and a patient with asthma and paranasal sinusitis could fit the designation of EGPA. The 1994 CHCC[1] character-ized EGPA as an eosinophil-rich and granulomatous inflammatory process that involved the respiratory tract, with necrotizing vasculitis that affected small- to medium-sized vessels such as capillaries, venules, arterioles, and arteries, with asso-ciated asthma and eosinophilia.

In 1954, Godman and Churg[19] described the syndrome of GPA that included gran-uloma in the nasopharynx, sinuses, and lower respiratory tract with focal segmental glomerulonephritis and disseminated SVV. Nervous system involvement in GPA was found in up to one-half of patients. Fauci and colleagues[20] and Hoffman and col-leagues[21] at the National Institutes of Health (NIH), respectively, reported a prospec-tive series of 85 patients with GPA, and a retrospective assessment of 180 patients followed for 6 months to 24 years, describing nervous system involvement in up to 23% of patients. There was a preponderance of mononeuritis multiplex (MNM) with CNS abnormalities in 8% to 10% of patients. CNS involvement included stroke, cra-nial nerve abnormalities, and diabetes insipidus. Fauci and colleagues[20] established the efficacy of cyclophosphamide and prednisone in achieving complete remissions in 93% of patients as well as the tendency of patients to relapse and accrue additive mortality from both disease and treatment; however, alternative immunosuppressant regimens were not equally effective.[21] The astute conclusion based mainly on patho-logic features was later substantiated by their common association with ANCA, but not so for PAN.

Hypersensitivity vasculitis leading to cutaneous vasculitis was conceptualized as an immunologic response to antigenic material associated with clinically evident purpura, and small vessel inflammation affecting arterioles, capillaries, and postcapillary ve-nules. Between 1948 and 1952, Zeek and colleagues[22,23] separated the hypersensitiv-ity vasculitides from allergic granulomatous angiitis, rheumatic arteritis, PAN, and GCA. Hemorrhage into the skin or palpable purpura was noted in virtually all patients resulting from extravasation of erythrocytes, pronounced endothelial swelling, poly-morphonuclear and later mononuclear cell infiltration, followed by fibrosis, necrosis, fibrinoid deposits, and visible polymorphonuclear debris termed leukocytoclasia. Hy-persensitivity vasculitis was likened to the anaphylactoid Arthus reaction produced by the experimental injection of horse serum into rabbits. Osler[24] first appreciated the relation of purpuric attacks to cerebral manifestations in the report of a patient with transient hemiparesis, and 3 others with potentially fatal cerebral hemorrhages. Gaird-ner[25] described HSP among 12 patients with anaphylactoid purpura, including one child who developed rash, colic, melanotic stools, intussusception, and hematuria fol-lowed by a typical exanthema and convulsion. She died 3 months later, and postmor-tem examination showed scattered cortical hemorrhages associated with cerebral necrotizing arteriolitis. Levitt and Burbank[26] described the clinicopathological findings in 2 previously nonallergic patients with recurrent fatal attacks of HSP after injection of penicillin and ingestion of strawberries, respectively, that included glomerulonephritis alone or with systemic arteriolitis. The finding of IgA deposits in cutaneous blood vessel walls and in glomerular mesangial biopsies of patients with HSP and IgA ne-phropathy[27,28] was circumstantially convincing enough to substitute the term IgAV for HSP.

Wintrobe and Buell[29] described cryoglobulinemia in a patient with progressive fron-tal headache, facial pain, Raynaud symptoms, recurrent nosebleeds, exertional dyspnea, palpitation, and changes in the eyegrounds due to central vein thromboses. Postmortem examination showed infiltrating myeloma of the humerus and lumbar vertebra, and splenic enlargement. A unique plasma protein was detected that spontaneously precipitated with cold temperature and solubilized at high temperature and differed from Bence-Jones proteinuria of other myeloma patients. Lerner and Watson[30] noted the association with purpura, and later Lerner and Watson[31] described its occurrence in 10% of pathologic sera.

Recurrent attacks of erythematous, urticarial, and hemorrhagic skin lesions that lasted 24 hours at a time, associated with recurrent attacks of fever, joint swelling, abdominal distress, and depressed serum complement indicative of HUV, were described by McDuffie and colleagues in 1973[32]; however, small amounts of cryoglobulin were present at one time or another in the serum of each patient. When tested by immunodiffusion against purified preparations of rheumatoid factor and human C1q, 2 patients consistently produced bands against the former, and 2 others reacted strongly with purified C1q. Skin biopsies showed leukocytoclasia characteristic of necrotizing vasculitis in one patient; anaphylactoid purpura in 2 others, and mild nonspecific perivascular infiltration another. Immunofluorescence of skin specimens performed in 3 patients showed fixation of Ig in the patient with necrotizing vasculitis, whereas in 2 others with a pathologic picture of anaphylactoid purpura or nonspecific dermal infiltrate, immunofluorescence was negative. Renal biopsy in 2 patients showed mild to moderate glomerulonephritis indistinguishable for those seen in other forms of chronic membranoproliferative glomerulonephritis. The differences from SLE included more urticarial and purpuric skin lesions, with relatively mild renal or absent and other visceral involvement in the patients with HUV, which was atypical for SLE. Moreover, serum speckled antinuclear and anti-DNA antibodies and basement membrane Ig deposits were absent in those with HUV, also atypical for SLE. An etiopathogenesis related to chronic vascular inflammation resulting from deposits of immune complexes in small vessel walls seemed likely. Zeiss and colleagues[33] characterized C1q IgG precipitins from HUV sera that precipitated C1q in agarose gel among 4 additional patients. Wisnieski and Naff[34] showed C1q binding activity in IgG from HUV sera, which suggested a relation to LE, but that view was later amended.

The historical account of the category of LVV spanned more than a century with notable advances in the past several years. Named for the site of granulomatous giant cell inflammation and vessel involvement, those with biopsy-proven temporal arteritis and associated blindness due to vasculitic involvement of ophthalmic and posterior ciliary vessels were classified as cranial arteritis. The occasional finding of giant cell lesions along the aorta, along its branches, and in other medium- and large-sized arteries at autopsy in other patients warranted the additional diagnosis of generalized GCA. The pathologic heterogeneity of temporal arteritis was further demonstrated by the finding of intracranial lesions in several patients who also qualified for the diagnosis of granulomatous angiitis of the nervous system (GANS).[35] PNS involvement in GCA was exceedingly uncommon in which early lesions of GCA consisted of vacuolization of smooth muscle cells of the media, with enlargement of mitochondria, infiltration of lymphocytes, plasma cells, and histiocytes. With progression, there was extension of inflammation into the intima and adventitia leading to segmental fragmentation and necrosis of the elastic lamina, granuloma formation, and proliferation of connective tissue along the vessel wall eventuating in vascular thrombosis, intimal proliferation, and fibrosis. One other LVV was described in the Japanese literature as unusual changes of the central vessels of the retina in the absence of peripheral arterial pulses in a woman.[36] This pulseless disease and occlusive thromboaortopathy or TAK disease manifested constitutional complaints of malaise, fever, stiffness of the shoulders, nausea, vomiting, night sweats, anorexia, weight loss, and irregularity of menstrual periods weeks to months before the local signs of vasculitis were recognized in up to two-thirds of patients. It is the commonest LVV among Asian women.

One other form of inflammatory aortic disease or aortitis was coming to light in the surgical literature with equally broad and far-reaching implications for concepts of autoimmunity. In 1972, Walker and colleagues[37] noted that 10% of 217 patients presenting with abdominal aneurysms at Manchester Royal Infirmary between 1958 and 1969 for resection showed excessive thickening of aneurysm walls and perianeurysmal adhesions at operation. Subsequent histologic examination of the walls of the aneurysms showed extensive active chronic inflammatory changes, including plasma-cell infiltration. The clinical features of patients with inflammatory aneurysms differed from those with atherosclerotic disease due to generally younger age by a decade, lower incidence of rupture, lack of claudication of intermittent limbs and presence of peripheral pulses, less likelihood of unusual presenting features, elevated erythrocyte sedimentation rate (ESR), and lack of calcification on preoperative abdominal radiographs. In 1985, Pennell and coworkers[38] reported inflammatory aortic or iliac aneurysms in 4.5% of 2816 patients undergoing repair for abdominal aortic aneurysm from 1955 to 1985. Ultrasound and computed tomographic imaging suggested the diagnosis, respectively, in 13.5% and 50% of patients, the former showing a sonolucent halo with clear definition of the aortic wall posterior to the thickened anterior and lateral aortic walls. In 2001, Hamano and colleagues[39] noted a high concentration of IgG4 associated with sclerosing pancreatitis characterized by obstructive jaundice, infrequent attacks of abdominal pain, irregular narrowing of the pancreatic duct, sonolucent swelling of the parenchyma, lymphoplasmacytic infiltration, fibrosis, and a favorable response to corticosteroid treatment. One year later, Hamano and coworkers[40] noted the association of sclerosing pancreatitis with raised concentrations of IgG4 among those with concomitant hydronephrosis that caused ureteral masses later diagnosed as retroperitoneal fibrosis (RPF). Histologic examination of ureteral and pancreatic tissues revealed abundant tissue infiltration by IgG4-bearing plasma cells. In the same year, 2008, 3 important observations were made. First, Sakata and colleagues[41] concluded that inflammatory abdominal aortic aneurysm (IAAA) was related to IgG4 sclerosing disease. Second, Kasashima and colleagues[42] concluded that IAAA was an IgG-related disease (IgG4-RD) together with RPF. Third, Ito and colleagues[43] described a patient with IAAA, hydronephrosis caused by RPF, and high levels of IgG4 I in whom treatment with corticosteroids led to clinical improvement and reduction in IgG4 levels. Histologic inspection of the aortic wall specimen showed lymphocytoplasmacytic infiltration. Immunohistochemical analysis of the tissue showed IgG4-positive plasma cells. The findings suggested that IAAA had an etiopathogenesis similar to autoimmune pancreatitis and that some cases of IAAA and RPF were aortic and periaortic lesions of an IgG4-RD. One year later in 2009, Khosroshahi and colleagues[44] described thoracic aortitis due to IgG4-RD with marked elevation of the serum IgG4 levels with progression to autoimmune pancreatitis, and Stone and coworkers[45] described IgG4-related thoracic aortitis with a media-predominant pattern of aortic wall infiltration and marked elevation of serum IgG4 levels, unequivocally linking IgG4-RD with thoracic lymphoplasmacytic aortitis.

Two forms of VVV, BD and CD, were recognized with very different clinical presentations and systemic involvement. Adamantiades[46] recognized the disorder of relapsing aphthous ulcers of the mouth, eye, and genitalia, the clinicopathological details of which were described in later detail by Behçet and Matteson[47,48] in 2 Turkish patients. Nervous system involvement of a 28-year-old Yemenite with relapsing oral, genital, and oral eruptions over 4 years, was accompanied by severe headache, memory loss, dizziness, lethargy, fatal seizures, and coma. Postmortem examination showed perivascular inflammatory cell infiltration of the meninges, brain, and central retinal artery and optic nerve with necrotic cerebral lesions. The first well-documented American patient with nervous system involvement of BD was described by Wolf and co-workers,[49] a 22-year-old woman with a 5-year history of recurrent oral and genital ulceration, and a 2 year course of progressive visual loss, headache, hemiparesis, ataxia, tremor, dysarthria, cranial nerve palsy, cerebellar and corticospinal tract disease, and mental deterioration, which responded to prednisone therapy.

Mogan and Baumgartner[50] described a 26-year-old man with recurrent pain, spasm, and redness of the left eye with photophobia, excessive tearing, and marked conjunctival injection, followed by a severe attack of dizziness, tinnitus, vertigo, nausea, vomiting, ringing in the ears, profuse perspiration, and deafness. A diagnosis of recurrent interstitial keratitis (IK) and explosive Menière disease was made. In retrospect, he was probably the first reported patient with CS of nonsyphilitic IK. Vestibuloauditory symptoms were later described by Cogan[51] after whom CS was named. In a review of 30 patients seen at the National Eye Institute of the NIH by Cogan,[51] symptoms of IK developed abruptly and gradually resolved, associated with photophobia, lacrimation, and eye pain, which may be unilateral or bilateral. Such symptoms tended to recur periodically for years before becoming quiescent. Vestibuloauditory dysfunction was manifested by sudden onset of Menière-like attacks of nausea, vomiting, tinnitus, vertigo, and frequently progressive hearing loss that characteristically occurred before or after the onset of IK. However, within 1 to 6 months of the onset of eye symptoms, auditory symptoms progressed to deafness over a period of 1 to 3 months, certainly no longer than 2 years.

The histopathologic appearance of vasculitis of the peripheral nerve is similar regardless of whether the process is primary or secondary to underlying systemic vasculitis. Historically, detailed neurovascular anatomy historically arose from the careful dissection of amputated limbs following injection of India ink to opacify peripheral nerve vessels in World War II veterans.[52,53] Such studies indicated that proximal stretches of each of the major nerves were supplied by a single arterial vessel, such as in the axilla-to-elbow and knee-to-elbow segments located peripherally in the nerve trunk, and abundantly along their distal course by a succession of microvessels, which by their repeated division and anastomosis outlined an unbroken vascular net that assured continuous vascular supply. Because there was no evidence for the presence of watershed zones of poor vascular supply along major nerves of the arm or leg, ischemic paralysis of a limb should rarely if ever occur in the absence of widespread arteritis, abrupt occlusion of large named vessels, or focal nerve compression. A quarter-century later, Dyck and coworkers[54] ascribed ischemic centrofascicular nerve fiber degeneration of named upper arm and thigh nerves in a patient with necrotizing angiopathic neuropathy to poor vascular perfusion along presumed watershed zones of the upper arm and thigh regions. However, the clinical details of the patient were not given; the centrofascicular fiber loss was only pronounced in the legs, and extraneural blood vessels of the arms were not studied. Two decades later, Moore and Fauci[55] ascribed progressive weakness and sensory loss in the arms and subsequently in the legs distally from the knees in their patient 8 with extensive MNM due to infarction of specific peripheral nerves, culminating in ambulation with leg braces and good use of the hands. However, that patient was not studied pathologically. Vasculitis of the peripheral nerves leads to specific alterations in the arteriae nervorum with a caliber of 100 μm located in the epineurial compartment as well as in peripheral nerve fascicles ensheathed by perineurium and endoneurium. The key elements of pathologically definite nonsystemic vasculitic neuropathy, generally regarded as a form of SOV, are intramural inflammation accompanied by pathologic evidence of vascular wall damage without evidence of systemic involvement.

Diverse syndromes of adult and childhood primary CNS vasculitis with very different clinical presentation, histopathology, and prognosis have been recognized. Primary CNS vasculitis indicative of granulomatous angiitis of the nervous system (GANS) was first described by Harbitz in 1922[56] in one patient with worsening headaches, mental change, and ataxia culminating in stupor, spastic paraparesis, coma, and death in 2 years. A second patient presented with hallucination and confusion progressing to gait difficulty, stupor, coma, and death in 9 months. At postmortem examination, both had granulomatous vasculitis of the meninges comprising lymphocytes, multinucleate giant cells, and epithelioid cells with vessel necrosis and extension into the brain along involved veins and arteries of varying calibers. Over the ensuing quarter century, additional patients were reported under the rubric of allergic angiitis and granulomatosis, GCA, and sarcoidosis. The identification of angiographic beading and a sausagelike appearance of cerebral vessels at sites of presumed arteritis captured the attention of Cupps and Fauci[57] in other patients with so-called isolated angiitis of the CNS (IACNS). The angiographic features of presumed vasculitis along with the judged efficacy of a combination immunosuppressive regimen of oral cyclophosphamide and alternate day prednisone, including 3 patients with IACNS defined angiographically, and another with biopsy-proven GANS of the filum terminale, led to prospective diagnostic and therapeutic recommendations. At that time, investigators at the NIH regarded IACNS and GANS as equivalent entities, with the former term emphasizing the restricted nature of the vasculitis and the latter term emphasizing the granulomatous histology. Giant cells and epithelioid cells, usually found at autopsy in GANS, were an inconsistent finding in a meningeal and brain biopsy, and therefore, were considered unnecessary for antemortem diagnosis. In the same year of 1988, Calabrese and Mallek[58] proposed criteria for the diagnosis of primary angiitis of the central nervous system vasculitis (PACNS), whereas Younger and colleagues[59] contemporaneously described the limits of granulomatous angiitis of the brain and GANS. The past quarter century has witnessed an expansion in the present understanding of primary CNS vasculitis in children and adults.

EPIDEMIOLOGY

The publication of recent genome-wide association studies (GWAS) has brought awareness to the understanding and susceptibility factors and designated genetic risk loci for many of the vasculitides supporting the interplay of immunologic, environmental, and shared genetic susceptibility in the etiopathogenesis of these disorders. They show a very complex cause in which both environmental and genetic factors contribute to the predisposition and clinical phenotype. With an incidence and prevalence of primary systemic vasculitis that is steadily increasing, and an impact that is being reported worldwide in developed countries, governments, nongovernmental organizations, and other key stakeholders have not developed sufficient programs for the prevention and surveillance of these disorders. This section focuses on the epidemiology of the major large-, medium-, and small-sized vessel vasculitides shown in **Box 1**. There is a recent review of the epidemiology and classification of primary systemic vasculitides.[60]

Large Vessel Vasculitis

Giant cell arteritis
Background GCA is a chronic granulomatous vasculitis of large- and medium-sized vessels that frequently affect the thoracic aorta and its branches. Both GCA and

PMR, a related disorder, are probably polygenic disease in which multiple environmental and genetic factors influence susceptibility and severity. For the purpose of epidemiologic studies and in clinical practice, GCA has been classified by 5 discriminatory features that include age greater than 50 years at onset, new onset of localized headache, temporal artery tenderness or decreased temporal artery pulse, ESR greater than 50 mm/h, and biopsy, including an artery showing necrotizing arteritis, characterized by a predominance of mononuclear cells or a granulomatous process with multinucleated giant cells. Unrecognized and therefore untreated or inadequately treated, there is a high likelihood of large artery complications, including increased morbidity and mortality, especially due to aortic aneurysm and dissection, and large artery stenosis.

Epidemiology The epidemiology of GCA was reviewed by Gonzalez-Gay and colleagues.[61] Since 2000, relatively large cohort studies exemplifying the epidemiologic aspects of GCA in different regions of the world were reported from Australia, Germany, Israel, Japan, New Zealand, Norway, Spain, Sweden, the United Kingdom, and the United States (US).[62–74] Smaller nonepidemiological case series of patients with GCA reported in Brazil, Saudi Arabia, and Mexico exemplifying the incalculably low incidence,[75–77] and similarly, in Japan[66] where a nationwide survey of GCA was untaken despite the relatively low incidence, demonstrated a prevalence of 1.47 cases per 100,000 population. The highest known incidence of GCA was reported without major differences between northern and western Norway compared with those of Southern Norway. By comparison, very low incidence rates of GCA were found in Saudi Arabian, Mexican, and Japanese populations. The global incidence and prevalence of GCA are summarized in **Table 1**.

According to Herlyn and colleagues,[64] who studied inhabitants of the city of Lubeck and the rural region of Segeberg in northern Germany, GCA was the most prevalent systemic vasculitis in 2006 with 171 per million inhabitants followed by GPA with a prevalence rate of 98 per million inhabitants. The prevalence rate of GCA doubled in northern Germany from in those aged 50 years or more from 240 to 440 per million inhabitants between 1994 and 2006, and from 87 to 171 per million population overall. There was a difference in period prevalence and incidence rates between the urban and rural areas, with an incidence of GCA of 27.1/million/y in Lubeck compared

Table 1
Global incidence and prevalence of giant cell arteritis

Authors[a]	Country	Study Period	Incidence per 10^6	Prevalence per 10^6
Kobayashi et al	Japan	1997	1.47	—
Herlyn et al	Germany	2006	2.71	171 per 10^6
Dunstan et al	Australia	1992–2011	3.20	—
Bas-Lando et al	Israel	1980–2004	9.50	—
Gonzalez-Gay et al	Spain	1981–2005	10.13	—
Gonzalez-Gay et al	New Zealand	1996–2005	12.7	—
Mohammad et al	Sweden	1997–2010	13.3	—
Salvarani et al	US	1950–1999	18.8	—
Smeeth et al	UK	1990–2001	22.0	—
Haugeberg et al	Norway	1992–1996	27.50	—
	Norway	1992–1996	36.70	—
	Norway	1992–1996	32.8	—

[a] See text.

with 14.7/million/y in Segeberg ($P = .2$), whereas respective prevalence rates were 237 and 116 per million population overall, and 586 and 311 per million inhabitants aged 50 years or more. Differences in incidence between regional populations of the world may be explained in part by immunogenetic and environmental factors that account for differences in susceptibility and may contribute to severity and outcome. In 1980, Kemp and coworkers[78] performed HLA tissue-type antigen determinations for A-B, C-antigens in the sera of 88 mixed cases of clinical GCA and polymyalgia rheumatica (PMR) with an overwhelming representation of women and only sporadic familial occurrence, demonstrating no significant deviation from a sample compared with 3164 blood donor controls. In 1983, Armstrong and colleagues[79] studied 55 patients with GCA and PMR, typed for HLA A, B, C, and DR loci, noting a significantly increased frequency of DR4, Cw3, and Cw6, with the increase in Cw3 possibly attributed to linkage disequilibrium to DR4. Among 128 DNA samples for 128 patients and 145 ethnically matched controls in a case-control association study to determine whether those with patients with GCA and PMR sample from Lugo in northwestern Spain exhibited identical HLA class II associations, Dababneh and colleagues[80] found that the association of HLA-DRB 1*0401 and GCA reached statistical significance in the total GCA group of patients, less so for DRG1*0101 and *0102. An association was also observed between the RA DRB1 shared epitope (SE) and GCA that was primarily accounted by the presence of a single copy of the SE; moreover, an SE-bearing allele of DRB1 was observed in those with jaw claudication and visual manifestations. The genetic susceptibility to GCA has been supported by the contribution of shared HLA class II gene polymorphisms in mannose-binding lectin variant alleles, in DR4, DR3, Cw3, and MHC class I and HLA-B gene polymorphisms.[81–91]

Takayasu Disease

Background
In contrast to GCA, TAK occurs in those less than 40 years of age and presents with large vessel-sized vasculitis of the aorta and its branches. For the purpose of epidemiologic studies, the case definition has generally followed the ACR 1990 criteria for the classification of TAK.[92] An understanding of the inflammatory lesions in TAK, like that of GCA, has been advanced by immunologic studies, revealing a clearer understanding of the pathophysiology, which may be impacted by the genetic background of different global regions. The inflammatory cell infiltrate in aortic tissue specimens of affected patients is composed of neutrophils, macrophages, CD4$^+$, and CD8$^+$ T cells, natural killer (NK) cells, and macrophages. Infiltrating $\alpha\delta$T cells and NK cells appear to facilitate endothelial cell apoptosis through production of perforin and killer cell lectinlike receptor subfamily K. The latter activating C-type lectin family receptor triggers NK cells and costimulates CD8$^+$ α/β T-cell receptor + T cells, whereas CD4$^+$ Th1 cells that secrete interferon-γ promote giant cell and granulomatous lesion formation. Peripheral T cells, notably Th1 and Th17, contribute to the pathophysiology of GCA and TAK as do major histocompatibility complex class (MHC) I and II molecules and endothelial intracellular adhesion molecules, expressed in tissue lesions of the aorta with TAK.

Epidemiology
Two GWAS conducted in TAK identifying 379 UK cases and 1985 controls and 451 US/Turkish cases and 1115 controls, respectively,[93,94] noted strong associations with *IL12B* located at the 5q33.3 chromosome locus (rs6871626), and susceptibility to the Max-like protein X (*MAX*) gene transcription factor-like 4 positioned at the 17q21.2 chromosome locus (rs665268), whereas those in the United Kingdom alone

exhibited independent associations at the 6p21.32 chromosome locus in *HLA-DQB1/HLA-DRB1* (rs113452171; rs189754752). *HLA-DQB1* specifies the autoimmune response against insulin-producing islet cells that leads to insulin-dependent diabetes mellitus, whereas the function of *HLA-DRB1* is to present processed foreign antigens to T cells. The US/Turkish group reported another susceptibility locus at the Fc fragment of IgG, low affinity IIa and IIIa receptor (*FCGR2A/3A*) at the 1q23.3 chromosome locus (rs10919543), leading to increased mRNA expression of *FCGR2A*, and proteasome-assembling chaperone 1 (*PSMG1*). With receptors present on monocytes, macrophages, neutrophils, NK cells, and T and B lymphocytes, *FCGR2A/3A* play an essential role in the protection of the organism against foreign antigens by removing antigen-antibody complexes from the circulation and participate in diverse functions such as phagocytosis of immune complexes and modulation of antibody production by B cells. Located at the 21q22.2 chromosome locus, *PSMG1* is involved in the maturation of the mammalian 20S proteasomes with a yet clear implication for TAK.

The global incidence and prevalence of TAK is summarized in **Table 2**. Watts and colleagues[95] reviewed the primary care UK General Practice Research Database and the secondary care–based Norfolk Vasculitis Register from 2000 to 2005. With a population of 445,000, 16 cases with a first diagnosis of TAK were identified with an annual incidence of 0.8 per million. The annual prevalence of TAK was 4.7 per million, with an increase during the course of the study period from 3.6 to 6.3 per million. Mohammad and Mandl[96] studied 3 health care districts of southern Sweden with a total population of 983,419 as of 2011 to identify incident cases of TAK among 5 hospitals in the study area and in all private Rheumatology clinics between 1997 and 2011, noting 13 cases fulfilling the ACR 1990 criteria for TAK. Among them, 8 were of Swedish ancestry, 1 Asian, 2 Arabs, 1 African, and 1 northern European descent. The annual incidence rate was estimated at 0.8 per million for the whole population. The point prevalence as of June 2012 was estimated at 13.2 per million for the whole population. The incidence findings were comparable with the reported incidence of 0.8, 0.5, and 0.4 per million, respectively, in previous studies from Sweden, Germany, and eastern Denmark,[97–99] although the prevalence of TAK was somewhat higher than the prevalence of 6.4 per million previously reported in Sweden.

MEDIUM-SIZED VESSEL VASCULITIS
Polyarteritis Nodosa

Background
The ACR 1990[100] and the CHCC[2] criteria for PAN have been used in the case definitions of adult cases in most epidemiologic studies as well as the criteria of the Turkish Pediatric Vasculitis Study Group[4,101] for pediatric cases, stratified into cutaneous and classic PAN. This author was unable to find GWAS for PAN.

Table 2
Global incidence and prevalence of Takayasu arteritis

Authors[a]	Country	Study Period	Incidence per 10^6	Prevalence per 10^6
Watts et al	UK	2000–2005	0.8	4.7
Mohammad et al	Sweden	1997–2011	0.8	—
Waern et al	Sweden	1969–1976	0.8	6.4
Reinhold-Keller et al	Germany	1998–2000	0.5	—
Dreyer et al	Demark	1990–2009	0.4	—

[a] See text.

Epidemiology

The global incidence and prevalence of PAN are shown in **Table 3**. Mahr and colleagues[102] defined PAN as a predominantly medium-sized vessel that occurs alone or in association with hepatitis B virus (HBV) infection, with angiographically documented aneurysms or histologic proof of vessel inflammation, without glomerulonephritis, lung hemorrhage, or ANCA positivity. An analysis of the prevalence of PAN, MPA, GPA, and EGPA in Seine-St. Denis, a northeastern suburb of Paris, included a population of 1,093,515 adults, 28% of were of non-European ancestry. Their capture-recapture study of the entire calendar year of 2000 identified cases by general practitioners, departments of all of the public hospitals, 2 large private clinics, and the National Health Insurance System. The prevalence of PAN was estimated at 30.7 per million adults; however, previous studies based on the most restrictive and biopsy-dependent CHCC[2] criteria estimated PAN to be 9 per million adults, in comparison to 33 per million based on the less specific ACR criteria[100] that fail to discriminate between MPA and PAN. The total prevalence estimate for all disorders was 90.3 per million, which substratified for geographic origin showed a 2-fold higher incidence rate for subjects of European than non-European ancestry, respectively, 104.7 compared with 52.5 per million. Not more than 30% of the PAN cases appeared to be HBV-related with most diagnosed during the 1980s, suggesting that the reported incidence of HBV-associated PAN of 77 per million so noted in a small population of Alaskan Eskimos with high rates of HBV infection[103] was currently decreasing as a consequence of vaccination campaigns and the improved safety of blood products. Mohammad and colleagues[104] studied incident cases of PAN, GPA, MPA, and EGPA in 2 health care districts of South Sweden of central and southwest Skåne containing 14 municipalities with a population of 641,763 for the period 1997 to 2006 from hospital databases identifying 144 cases of primary systemic vasculitis, of which 6 were PAN. The annual incidence rates were 21.8 per million for all patients and 0.9 per million for PAN. Watts and colleagues[105] studied incident cases of PAN, GPA, MPA, and EGPA in 2 regions of Europe, among general medical practices of the Norwich Health Authority (NHA) in Norfolk, UK covering 413,500 patients, and in the referral center of Lugo, Spain at the Hospital Xeral-Calde, with a population of 250,000 people between 1988 and 1998, noting an overall incidence of primary systemic vasculitis that was 18.9 Norwich compared with 18.3 per million in Spain, with a higher incidence of PAN in Norwich than in Spain, 9.7 versus 6.2 per million, respectively. Omerod and Cook[106] studied the prevalence and incidence for primary systemic vasculitides for the two 5-year periods of 1995 to 1999, and 2000 to 2004, in

Table 3
Global incidence and prevalence of polyarteritis nodosa

Authors[a]	Country	Study Period	Incidence per 10⁶	Prevalence per 10⁶
Jennette et al	US	2012	—	30.7
Lightfoot et al	US	1990	—	9.0
Mohammad et al	Sweden	1997–2006	0.9	—
Watts et al	UK[b]	1988–1998	9.7	—
	Spain[c]	1988–1998	6.2	—
Omerod & Cook	UK[a] + Spain[b]	1995–1999	2.3	—
	UK[a] + Spain[b]	2000–2004	1.1	—

[a] See text.
[b] Norwich.
[c] Lugo.

the Australian Capital Territory and the surrounding rural regions. Altogether, 41 cases of primary systemic vasculitides including PAN, GPA, MPA, and EGPA were identified between 1995 and 1999, and 67 between 2000 and 2004. Their study[106] yielded a prevalence of 95 and 148 per million, with a similar annual incidence of 17 per million for Norwich, UK and Lugo, Spain, and disease-specific incidences for PAN of 2.2 and 1.1 for the 2 successive periods.

Kawasaki Disease

Background

KD, or mucocutaneous lymph node syndrome, is an acute, self-limited systemic vasculitis of medium- and small-sized vessels occurring predominantly in children aged 6 months to 5 years. It is the second commonest childhood vasculitis and the leading cause of acquired childhood heart disease in developed countries. The distribution is worldwide with an incidence in Japanese populations 10- to 15-fold greater than in Caucasians. Before revision of the criteria for KD, the classification was based either on Japanese[107] or on the American Heart Association (AHA) classification.[108] The former criteria, used in Japanese epidemiologic studies of KD, required the presence of 5 of the following 6 criteria, including characteristic fever, bilateral conjunctivitis, changes in lips and oral cavity, polymorphous exanthema, changes of peripheral extremities, and cervical lymphadenopathy, whereas those of the latter criteria used in American and Caucasian studies generally required fever plus 4 of the remaining 5 criteria. Two recent modifications to the criteria for KD made by the EULAR/PRES consensus criteria conference,[4] which may alter the carriage of epidemiologic studies in the future, included the addition of perineal desquamation describing changes in the extremities; moreover, fewer than 4 of the remaining 5 criteria were deemed necessary in the presence of fever and coronary arterial involvement demonstrated by echocardiography. To emphasize pediatric vasculitis disease even before retrospective and prospective epidemiologic studies, a half century of 1,335,045 postmortem examinations from the Annual of Pathological Autopsy Cases in Japan from 1958 to 2008 identified 380 cases of vasculitis in children, more than one-half of which were KD and other disease entities, including unclassified vasculitis, PAN, purpuric vasculitis, TAK, and others. Moreover, the postmortem findings for 24 of 125 childhood vasculitides performed before 1976 and diagnosed as non-KD were later consistent with KD.

Epidemiology

The global incidence and prevalence of KD are shown in **Table 4**. Saundankar and colleagues[109] identified hospitalized patients in Western Australia with the diagnosis of KD, noting a steady increase in the mean annual incidence from 7.96 between 1990 and 1999 to 9.34 per 100,000 children aged less than 5 years between 2000 and 2009, with the peak incidence of 15.7 per 100,000 in 2005. Lin and colleagues[110] identified hospitalized discharges with the diagnosis of KD in Ontario, noting a mean annual incidence of 26.2 per 100,000 for less than 5 year olds, and 6.7 per 100,000 for 5- to 9-year-old children, and 0.9 per 100,000 for those 10 to 14 years old, that steadily increased from 14.39 to 26.24 per 100,000 from 1995 to 2006. Ma and colleagues[111] studied all children sent to one of 50 hospitals in Shanghai, noting a mean annual incidence of 46.32 per 100,000 children less than 5 years of age that steadily increased from 36.78 to 53.28 between 2003 and 2007. Li and coworkers[112] identified cases of KD less than 5 years of age among 212 hospitals in the Sichuan Province, noting a steady increase in the incidence in the children from 8.57 to 9.81 per 100,000, with an average incidence throughout the latest 5 years of 7.06 per 100,000. Du and coworkers[113] conducted a hospital-based survey of KD in 45 Beijing

Table 4				
Global incidence and prevalence of Kawasaki disease				
Authors[i]	**Country**	**Study Period**	**Incidence per 10^6**	**Prevalence per 10^6**
Saundankar et al	Australia	1990–1999	7.96 per 10^6	—
	Australia	2000–2009	9.34	—
	Australia	2005	15.7	—
Lin et al	Canada[a]	1995–2006	26.2[b]	—
	Canada[a]	1995–2006	6.8[c]	—
	Canada[a]	1995	14.39[d]	—
	Canada[a]	2006	26.24[d]	—
Ma et al	China[e]	2003–2007	46.32[b]	—
	China[e]	2003	36.78[b]	—
	China[e]	2007	53.28[b]	—
Li et al	China[f]	1997–2001	7.06[b]	—
	China[f]	1997	8.57[b]	—
	China[f]	2001	9.81[b]	—
Du et al	China[g]	2000–2004	49.4[b]	—
	China[g]	2000	40.9[b]	—
	China[g]	2004	55.1[b]	—
Fischer et al	Denmark	1981–2004	4.5–5.0	—
Holman et al	Hawaii	1996–2006	50.4	—
Ng et al	Hong Kong	1994–1997	26.0	—
	Hong Kong	1994–1997	39.0	—
Singh et al	North India	1994	0.51	—
	North India	2007	4.5	—
Nakamura et al	Japan	2009	206.2	—
	Japan	2010	239.6	—
Park et al	Korea	2006–2008	113.1	—
	Korea	2006	108.7	—
	Korea	2008	113.1	—
Schiller et al	Sweden	1990–1992	2.9	—
	Sweden	1990–1992	6.2[b]	—
Lue et al	Taiwan	2006	66.24[b]	—
Huang et al	Taiwan	2003–2006	153.0	—
	Taiwan	2003–2006	69.0[b]	—
Harnden et al	UK	1991	4.8	—
	UK	2000	9.2	—
Holman et al	US	2006	20.8	—

[a] Ontario.
[b] Age less than 5 years.
[c] Age 5 to 9 years.
[d] Age 10 to 14 years.
[e] Shanghai.
[f] Sichuan Province.
[g] Beijing.
[i] See text.

hospitals identifying 1107 KD patients with a mean annual incidence of 49.4 per 100,000 less than 5-year-old children and a steady increase from 2000 to 2004 that varied from 40.9 to 55.1 per 100,000. Fischer and colleagues[114] performed a population-based hospital study of KD children in Denmark from 1981 to 2004 identifying 360 children younger than 15 years and noting a mean annual incidence of 4.5

to 5 per 100,000 person-years with a gradual increase over the study period. Holman and colleagues[115] conducted a retrospective analysis of children aged less than 18 years, notably those less than 5 years, hospitalized in Hawaiian hospitals from 1996 to 2006, noting a mean annual incidence of 50.4 per 100,000 children less than 5 years of age ranging from 45.5 to 56.5. Japanese children who had the highest mean annual incidence of 210.5 per 100,000 exceeded the mean Asian and Pacific children annual incidence of 62.9 per 100,000 children, followed by native Hawaiian children with an incidence of 86.9, other Asian children with an incidence of 84.9, and Chinese children with an incidence of 83.2 per 100,000, exceeding that of whites with an incidence of KD of 13.7 per 100,000 children. Ng and colleagues[116] conducted retrospective and prospective studies of KD in Hong Kong between 1994 and 1997 and from 1997 to 2000, respectively, identifying 696 children less than 15 years of age and noting a higher incidence of KD in the prospective period (39 vs 26 per 100,000 children). Singh and colleagues[117] analyzed the records of children with KD less than 15 years of age in Chandigarh, North India identifying 196 children. There was an increasing incidence of disease from 0.51 cases to 4.5 cases during the period from 1994 to 2007. Nakamura and coworkers[118] conducted the 21st nationwide survey of 23,730 KD children treated between 2009 and 2010 and noted an annual incidence rate of 206.2 and 239.6 per 100,000, establishing the highest rate ever for Japan in 2010. Park and coworkers[119] surveyed Korean hospitals for the period of 20062008 and identified 9039 KD children, noting an outbreak rate of 108.7 in 2006 that increased to 113.1 per 100,000 in 2008, with a mean annual incidence of 113.1 per 100,000 children. Schiller and contributors[120] examined a national prospective study over a 2-year period from 1990 to 1992 of KD children recording an annual incidence rate of 2.9 per 100,000 children younger than 16 years, and a rate of 6.2 per 100,000 children less than 5 years of age. Lue and colleagues[121] conducted nationwide hospital surveys of KD in Taiwan in 2006, noting an incidence of 66.24 per 100,000 children less than 5 years of age representing the highest of any preceding survey. Huang and colleagues[122] investigated the epidemiology of KD using national insurance claims between 2003 and 2006, noting an annual incidence of KD of 153 per 100,000 in less than 1-year-old children with an overall incidence of 69 per 100,000 children aged less than 5 years. Harnden and colleagues[123] analyzed hospital admission data in England for the period 1991–2000 of childhood KD, identifying 2215 emergency admissions representing an incidence that increased from 4.8 to 9.2 per 100,000 in this time period. Holman and coworkers[124] performed a retrospective analysis of emergency childhood admission in the United States using the Kids' Inpatient Database and a Nationwide Inpatient Sample for 2006 noting an incidence of 20.8 per 100,000 children.

Eight GWAS and linkage analysis studies of KD[125–129] have led to susceptibility genetic loci for KD. Onouchi and colleagues[125] performed a nonparametric GWAS of sibling pairs on 75 full sibling pairs, 3 sibling trios, and 1 half-sibling identifying candidate gene locus at 12q24 (maximum logarithm of odds [LOD] score = 2.69), with possible linkage to 4q35, 5q35, 5q34, 6q27, 7p15, 8q24, 18q23, 19q13, Xp22, and Xq27. Moreover, 90 genes were thought to be expressed in organs related to immune function among the 128 genes that mapped within 1 LOD confidence interval of the linkage position on chromosome 12. Burgner and coworkers[126] on behalf of the International Kawasaki Disease Genetics Consortium investigated genetic determinants of KD susceptibility in a GWAS of 119 Caucasian KD patients and 135 matched controls using the AHA criteria. The investigators[126] noted associations with 40 single-nucleotide polymorphisms (SNP) and 6 haplotypes, however, most significantly at *NAALADL2* (rs17531088) and *ZRHX3* (rs7199343). The latter, also known as ATBF1, which encodes a large enhancer-binding transcription factor known to be polymorphic and interactive with several proteins including protein inhibitor of activated signal transducer and activator of transcription-3, is activated by interleukin (IL)-6 involved in innate immune reactivity. The function of the N-acetylated α-linked acidic dipeptidase-like 2 gene, which showed the greatest change in transcript levels between acute and convalescent KD, contributes to Cornelia de Lange syndrome, a multisystem malformation syndrome. Tsai and coworkers[127] conducted a GWAS in a Han Chinese population in 250 KD patients and 446 controls residing in Taiwan. The most strongly associated SNP were detected in 3 novel loci close to the coatomer protein complex β-2 subunits (COPB2) gene (rs1873668, rs4243399, rs16849083) as well as in the intronic region of the endoplasmic reticulum amino peptidase 1 (ERAP1) gene (rs14981). COPB2 coats non-clathrin-coated vesicles and is essential for Golgi budding and vesicular trafficking, whereas ERAP1 plays a role in trimming peptides to the optimal length for HLA class I presentation cleaving cell surface receptors for proinflammatory cytokines. Kim and coworkers[128] on behalf of the Korean Kawasaki Disease Genetics Consortium conducted a GWAS among 186 Korean KD patients and 600 controls noting susceptibility loci for KD at the 1p31 region and 2p13.3 chromosomal loci. A putative KD susceptibility locus (rs5277409) mapped to chromosome 1p31 and the coronary artery lesion (CAL) locus (rs7604693) mapped to the Pellino 1 protein (PELI1) (rs7604693) gene in the 2p13.3 region encoding PEL1, an intermediate component in the signaling cascade initiated by Toll-like receptors and the IL1 receptor (IL1R) gene, that are associated with innate and adaptive immune responses. Khor and colleagues[129] performed a GWAS in 2173 KD patients of European and Asian descent, noting 2 significant loci in the Fc fragment of IgG, low-affinity 2A receptor (FCGR2A) (rs1801274), and for the rs2233152 SNP near the melanoma inhibitory activity (MIA), inositol 1,4,5-trisphosphate 3-kinase C (ITPKC) gene. Whereas the FCGR2A, present on monocytes, macrophages, neutrophils, NK cells, T and B cells, participates in the phagocytosis of immune complexes and modulation of antibody production by B cells, ITPKC acts as a negative regulator of T-cell activation through the Ca^{2+}/NFAT signaling pathway, contributing to immune hyperactivity. Lee and coworkers[130] performed a GWAS in 622 KD patients and 1107 controls in a Han Chinese population residing in Taiwan, noting 2 loci significantly associated with KD, including one at the B-lymphoid tyrosine kinase (BLK) gene and the other at CD40. Whereas the BLK gene appears to play an important role in the expression of B-cell signaling, activation, and antibody secretion, CD40 is instead a member of the tumor necrosis factor receptor superfamily, and its interaction with the CD40 ligand (CD40L) leads to cross-talk integrating strong antigenic signals and microbial stimuli to induce IL-17-producing $CD4^+$ T cells that contribute to inflammation and the development of autoimmune disease. Onouchi and coworkers[131] performed a GWAS in 428 Japanese KD patients and 3379 controls noting significant associations in the FAM167A-BLK region at 8p22-23 (rs2254546) in the HLA region at 6p21.3 (rs2857151), and in the CD40 region at 20q13 (rs48130030), also replicating the association of a function SNP of FCGR2A (rs1801274). Although ubiquitously expressed, the function of FAM167A has not been well characterized. Yan and coworkers[132] analyzed variants of 6 SNP in 358 Japanese KD patients and 815 controls identifying 3, rs1801274, rs2857151, and rs22554546, respectively, corresponding to FCGR2A, HLA, and BLK genes, noting significant effect and stronger association on KD than single-, 2-, and 3-locus combinations; moreover, a significant association to CAL was noted in KD with high-risk genotypes at both rs1801274 and rs2857151.

SMALL-SIZED VESSEL VASCULITIS
Antineutrophil Cytoplasmic Antibody–Associated Vasculitis

Background

Early observations of ANCA differentiated clinicopathological subtypes.[133] Proteinase 3 (PR3) is a serine protease found in the azurophilic granules of neutrophils and peroxidase-positive lysosomes of monocytes. Myeloperoxidase (MPO), which constitutes about 5% of the total protein content of the neutrophilic cell, is localized to the same cellular compartment as PR3. However, PR3 in contrast to MPO is also found on the plasma membrane of resting neutrophils and monocytes in many patients. Autoantibodies directed against PR3 and MPO are directed against multiple epitopes. Although sera from different patients may recognize different epitopes, all ANCA recognized restricted epitopes of PR3 involve its catalytic site.[134] An AAV classification appears to better recognize ANCA disease and predict prognosis than other any existing clinical classification system.[135] However, as with other autoimmune disorders, the cause and pathogenesis appeared multifactorial, involving the interplay of initiating and predisposing environment and genetic factors. Important contributing factors to the mediation of vascular and extravascular inflammation included a loss of regulatory T- and B-cell function, acute neutrophilic cell injury with release of ANCA antigens, cytokine priming of neutrophilic cells, and subsequent complement activation by Fc and Fab2 engagement, and enhancement of complement-dependent cytotoxicity with release of ANCA antigens into the microenvironment. The ANCA lesion typical of GPA includes both vasculitic and granulomatous features in lung, with focal segmental glomerulonephritis typified pathologically by lysis of glomerular tufts, basement membrane disruption, accumulation of fibrinoid material, thrombosis of glomerular capillary loops, acute tubular necrosis, and cant deposition of Ig and complement. There are genetic distinctions between MPO and GPA suggested by the strong association of PR3-ANCA disease with antigenic specificity of HLA-DP and the genes encoding α1-antitrypsin (SERPINA1) and PR3 (PRTN3), and HLA-DQ for MPO-ANCA.[136] An immunofluorescence technique (IFT) has been standard method for routine determination of ANCA in vasculitis using ethanol-fixed human neutrophils as substrate. Two main immunofluorescence patterns are distinguished, a cytoplasmic ANCA and perinuclear ANCA. The 1999 International Consensus Statement on testing and reporting ANCA[137] required laboratories to screen for ANCA by IFT and to confirm the specificity of fluorescent sera by enzyme-linked immunoassay (ELISA) for PR3 and MPO-ANCA. However, conventional ELISA using PR3 immobilized to the surface of the ELISA plate shows great variation in performance and often lacks sensitivity. Capture ELISA is superior in overall diagnostic performance to direct ELISA,[138] but the sensitivity of capture ELISA may be reduced by the capturing antibodies hiding relevant epitopes. High-sensitivity PR3 (hsPR3)-ANCA ELISA, which immobilizes PR3 via a bridging molecule to the plastic plate and preserves nearly all epitopes for the binding of ANCA, was superior to direct and capture techniques in GPA.[139]

Although the clinical classification of the AAV has been controversial, the European Medicines Agency algorithm has provided a standardized method for their application in epidemiologic studies, each with separate deficiencies, especially when applied to unselected patients. These systems were developed as classification criteria and not as diagnostic criteria. As there were no validated diagnostic criteria for AAV, the Diagnostic and Classification Criteria for Vasculitis Study, developed by Watts and colleagues,[140] led to the consensus development and validation of diagnostic criteria by an algorithm to avoid inclusion of patients with other conditions. So defined, Watts and colleagues noted an annual incidence of 11.3 for GPA and 5.9 per million for MPA, with respective prevalence at the end of calendar year 2008 of 145.9 for GPA and 63.1 per million for MPA. Lyons and colleagues[136] conducted a GWAS in a cohort of 1233 UK subjects with AAV and 5884 controls noting both MHC and non-MHC associations with AAV, with the strongest genetic association with the antigenic specificity of ANCA, not with the clinical syndrome. Those with PR3 ANCA were associated with *HLA-DP* (rs3117242) at the 6p21.32 chromosome locus as well as those encoding α1-antitrypsin (*SERPINA1–SERPINA11*) (rs7151526) at the 14q32 chromosome locus and PR3 (*PRTN3*) (rs62132295) at the 19p13.3 chromosome locus, while anti-MPO ANCA was associated with *HLA-DQ* (rs5000634) at the 6p21.32 chromosome locus. These studies confirmed that the pathogenesis of AAV had a genetic component and that the genetic distinction between GPA and MPA was associated with ANCA specificity. Moreover, the response against the PR3 autoantigen was a central pathogenic feature of PR3-AAV, distinct from MPO-AAV.

Epidemiology

The global incidence and prevalence are summarized in **Table 5**. Watts and colleagues,[141] Omerod and Cook,[106] and Mohammad and colleagues[104] evaluated the epidemiologic aspects of AAV globally in adults. In 2 regions of Europe, Norwich, UK and Lugo, Spain, the incidence rate of GPA in Norwich was 10.6 per million compared with that in Lugo of 4.9 per million for 2008 with virtually equal age distribution of 34.1 per million between aged 45 and 74 years, suggesting that environmental factors might be important in the their etiopathogenesis. In a 10-year study of primary

Table 5
Global incidence and prevalence of ANCA-associated vasculitis

Authors[i]	Country	Study Period	Incidence per 10^6	Prevalence per 10^6
Watts et al	UK	1988–1992	8.7[a]	—
	UK	1988–1992	6.8[b]	—
	UK	1988–1992	1.5[c]	—
	UK	1993–1997	10.3[a]	—
	UK	1993–1997	8.9[b]	—
	UK	1993–1997	3.7[c]	—
Ormerod et al	Australia + UK	1995–1999	8.8[a]	64.3[a]
		2000–2004	8.4[a]	95.0[a]
		1995–1999	2.3[b]	17.5[b]
		2000–2004	5.0[b]	39.1[b]
		1995–1999	2.3[c,d,e]	11.7[c]
		2000–2004	2.2[c]	22.3[c]
Mahr et al	Seine-St. Denis County, Paris	2000	—	23.7[a]
	Seine-St. Denis County, Paris	2000	—	25.1[b]
	Seine-St. Denis County, Paris	2000	—	10.7[c]
Mohammad et al	Sweden	1997–2006	9.8[a]	—
	Sweden	1997–2006	10.1[b]	—
	Sweden	1997–2006	0.9[c]	—

[a] GPA.
[b] MPA.
[c] EGPA.
[d] Capital Territory.
[e] New South Wales.
[i] See text.

systemic vasculitis in the United Kingdom[141] in the NHA from 1988 to 1997, the annual incidence of GPA was 9.7, EGPA was 2.7, and MPA was 8.0 per million during the entire study period; however, a comparison of the period from 1988 to 1992 with 1993 to 1997 showed respective annual incidences toward an increase in all conditions (8.7 for GPA, 1.5 for EGPA, and 6.8 for MPA, compared with 10.3 for GPA, 3.7 for EGPA, and 8.9 for MPA). In a comparison of primary systemic vasculitis in the Australian Capital Territory and southeastern New South Wales between 1995 and 1999, and between 2000 and 2004, Omerod and colleagues[106] noted similar disease-specific incidences for each of the 2 periods, with 8.8 and 8.4 per million for GPA, 2.3 and 5.0 per million for MPA, and 2.3 and 2.2 per million for EGPA in the Australian Capital Territory compared with southeastern New South Wales with a trend for higher values in MPA and GPA in rural areas. A similar relation was found in disease-specific prevalence for each of the 2 periods, with 64.3 and 95.0 per million for GPA, 17.5 and 39.1 per million for MPA, and 11.7 and 22.3 per million for EGPA in the Australian Capital Territory compared with southeastern New South Wales. In incident cases of primary systemic vasculitis identified in Seine-St. Denis County, Paris, Mahr and colleagues[102] estimated the prevalence of GPA 23.7, MPA 25.1, and EGPA 10.7 per million adults in a population of 1,093,515, 28% of whom were of non-European ancestry, with an overall prevalence that was 2-fold higher for those of European (104.7 5 per million) compared with others of non-European ancestry (52.5 per million). Mohammad and colleagues[104] estimated incident cases of GPA, MPA, and EGPA in southern Sweden, respectively, of 9.8, 10.1, and 0.9 per million in a total population of 641,000 between 1997 and 2006, with a progressive increase in age-specific incidence rates over the study period.

IMMUNE COMPLEX VASCULITIS
Cryoglobulinemic Vasculitis

Background

CV is a prototypic immune complex vasculitis. Cryoglobulins reversibly precipitate at temperatures less than 37°C. They are composed of IgG and IgM, complement, lipoprotein, and antigenic protein moieties. They are classified into 3 types with implications for clinical and etiologic specificity. Type 1 is composed of a single monoclonal IgM or IgG antibody; type II, mixed, has monoclonal IgM, possessing activity against polyclonal IgG; and type III has mixed polyclonal and nonimmunoglobulin molecules in the form of immunoglobulin–anti-immunoglobulin immune complexes. Types I and II cryoglobulins are associated with lymphoproliferative diseases, particularly multiple myeloma and Waldenström macroglobulinemia. Type III cryoglobulins are associated with infection and collagen vascular diseases. One subgroup, termed essential mixed cryoglobulinemia (EMC), harbors circulating hepatitis C virus (HCV) RNA and corresponding antibodies in the cryoprecipitate. Type I cryoglobulins cause the hyperviscosity syndrome.

Four vascular lesions are noted in cryoglobulinemia: (1) occlusion of small and large vessels in those with high levels of cryoglobulins of type I or II; (2) bland thrombosis of small arteries and arterioles; (3) endothelial swelling, proliferation, and basement membrane thickening; and (4) leukocytoclastic vasculitis. True vasculitis is occasionally seen, mainly in those with associated PAN. Dermatitis is the most conspicuous feature accompanied by palpable purpura that persists for a week to 10 days, heralded by a sharp or burning sensation. Purpura is noted in all types but is more common with type III and in EMC. PNS and CNS manifestations are more common with types II and III. Renal disease is a major feature of EMC. Hepatic disease is far more common with this syndrome by virtue of its association with HCV. The appearance of high levels of cryoglobulins in the blood in patients reporting cold sensitivity and vasomotor symptoms led to the presumption that cryoprecipitation is the cause of ischemia of arterioles and capillaries due to hyperviscosity and the direct plugging of small vessels. However, it is now known that the cryoprecipitate, when present, may be tangential to the pathogenesis of the clinical syndrome and even an artifact for several reasons. First, cryoprecipitation occurs in systemic organs of normal temperature. Second, the temperature at which precipitates occur in vitro is far less than that achieved in the body. Third, symptoms do not correlate with serum cryoglobulin levels, viscosity, or cryoprecipitate concentration. Fourth, in EMC in which levels of cryoglobulins are typically quite low, the abnormality can still be explained on the basis of immune-complex deposition. Several factors that may contribute to the clinical manifestations of cryoglobulinemia include intravascular activation of complement and the clotting cascade by aggregated immunoglobulin and immune complexes; secondary vessel wall damage; cold agglutination of erythrocytes; local tissue reaction to precipitated proteins; and vascular endothelial cell proliferation. Nervous system manifestations in types I and II disease are related to vascular occlusion with or without vasculitis. Cryoglobulinemia should be considered in patients with features of characteristic skin lesions, MNM, hyperviscosity, easily coagulable blood, IgM monoclonal paraproteinemia, and risk factors for HCV infection. If found, the presence of cryoglobulinemia will direct the performance of bone marrow studies, nerve biopsy, and studies for HCV and HIV-1 infection, AIDS, occult cancer, infection, plasma cell dyscrasia, and collagen vascular disease.

Epidemiology

This author did not find reports of the global prevalence and incidence of CV. Recognizing the etiopathogenesis of HCV infection in mixed cryoglobulinemia (MC), it is noteworthy that the Global Burden of Disease, Injuries, and Risk Factors (GBD) 2010 that produced age-standardized prevalence estimates for each of 21 GBD regions using a model-based meta-analysis[142] found that the prevalence and number of people with anti-HCV increased from 2.3% (95% uncertainty interval [UI]: 2.1%–2.5%) to 2.8% (95% UI: 2.6%–3.1%) and greater than 122 million to greater than 185 million between 1990 and 2005. The highest prevalences (>3.5%) were found in Central and East Asia and North Africa/Middle East. Cacoub and coauthors[143] noted that the presence of the DR11 phenotype was associated with a significantly increased risk for the development of type II MC in patients with chronic HCV infection. In contrast, HLA-DR7 protected against the production of type II MC, suggesting that host immune response genes may play a role in the pathogenesis of HCVF-associated MC. One GWAS of HCV and CV was reported by Zignego and colleagues,[144] who compared 899,641 SNP compared between cases and controls, noting the most significant association on chromosome locus 6p21.32 at which an SNP rs2071286, located within an intronic region of *NOTCH4*, conferred 2.15 times the odds of having cryoglobulin-related vasculitis within chronically infected patients for each risk allele. The second most significant association was found nearly 400 kilobases within the MHC between *HLA-DRB1* and *HLA-DQA1* at SNP 9461776 (odds ratio = 2.16, $P = 1.16E-07$).

Behçet Disease

Background

This disorder is a prototypic VVV characterized by relapsing aphthous ulcers of the mouth, eye, and genitalia. The most widely used diagnostic criteria of BD were formulated by the International Study Group (ISG)[145] that included recurrent oral ulcerations plus any 2 of genital ulceration, typical defined eye lesions, typical skin lesions, or a positive pathergy. Recurrent oral ulcerations were categorized as minor aphthous, major aphthous, and herpetiform ulcerations that recurred at least 3 times in a 12-month period. Recurrent genital ulcerations were defined as aphthous ulceration and scarring. Eye lesions were defined as anterior uveitis, posterior uveitis, or cells in the vitreous on slit-lamp examination, and retinal vasculitis. Compatible skin lesions included erythema nodosum, pseudofolliculitis, papulopustular lesions, and aceniform nodules in postadolescent patients not receiving corticosteroids. A positive pathergy test of cutaneous hypersensitivity was defined as positive when a sterile pustule developed after 24 to 48 hours at the site of a needle prick to the skin. Although the usual onset of BD is in the third or fourth decade of life, pediatric onset patients have been described. Uluduz and colleagues[146] studied 2 large Istanbul BD cohorts totaling 728 patients, ascertaining and comparing pediatric-onset (26 patients) and adult adult-onset (702 patients) neurologic Behçet disease (NBD). The mean age of pediatric-onset of BD and NBD onset were 13 and 13.5 years, respectively, compared with adult-onset BD and NBD of 26 and 32 years. The commonest initial neurologic symptom in the pediatric-onset patients was headache in 92% followed by seizures in 11.5%, compared with adult-onset BD that manifested corticospinal tract signs in 59% followed by headache in 58% and dysarthria in 23%. Significant differences in neurologic involvement consisted of a higher frequency of cerebral venous sinus thrombosis so noted in 88.5% of children and 17% of adults, whereas parenchymal involvement was noted in 74.8% of adults compared with 11.6% of children. None of the children had associated cortical venous infarcts. Oral ulcers were noted in 100% of both groups, and there were no significant statistical differences in the occurrence of skin lesion, uveitis, or arthralgia; however, genital ulcers were less common in children compared with adults (54% compared with 84%).

Epidemiology

Although this author was unable to find comparative incidence rates for BD, 2 population-based studies, both fulfilling ISG criteria,[145] studied prevalence data for BD, including one from France[147] and another from the United States.[148] The overall prevalence in France was 7.1 per 100,000, with immigrants of North African and Asian ancestry manifesting significantly higher prevalence rates of BD than those of European ancestry (17.5 per 100,000 compared with 2.4 per 100,000), comparable with those of North Africa and Asia suggesting that BD risk was not related to age at immigration but was a primarily hereditary basis. The point prevalence of BD in the US was 5.2 per 100,000.

Genetic studies that focused on molecules related to innate immune responses[149] identified an association with endothelial nitric oxide (eNOS) gene located on chromosome 7q35-36, a variant of which causes deficient NOS and contributes to the pathogenesis of endothelial abnormalities and increases thrombotic tendency in BD. Dhifallah and colleagues[150] identified a polymorphism of eNOS that was associated with BD susceptibility as well as skin lesions. Park and coworkers[151] identified SNP of the promoter and exons regions in the cytotoxic T lymphocyte antigen 4 genes that predisposed to BD related to the immunologic abnormalities and disease expression associated with BD. Kim and colleagues[152] noted that genital ulceration, eye involvement, and NBD were associated with mannose-binding lectin 2 (MBL2) polymorphisms and production of high levels of MBL or functional MBL.

GWAS data have produced a major step forward by in the genetic of BD,[153] providing insights into the underlying mechanisms in BD with the discovery of a new susceptibility gene that implicates defects in sensing and processing of microbial and endogenous danger signals as well as the regulation of innate and adaptive immune responses. Fei and colleagues[154] conducted a GWAS identifying a genetic association between BD and SNP in KIAA1529, the BD-risk allele (rs2061634) that led to a substitution of serine to cysteine at amino acid position 995 in the KIAA1529 protein. Hou and coworkers[155] conducted a GWAS suggesting that *STAT4* SNP (rs7574070, rs7572482, rs897200) was a novel locus underlying BD in a model in which upregulation of *STAT4* expression and subsequent *STAT4*-driven production of inflammatory cytokines, such as IL-17, constituted a potential etiopathogenic pathway. Lee and colleagues[156] conducted a GWAS suggesting that GIMAP cluster mapped to chromosome 7q36.1 (rs1608157) in a minor dominant model (rs11769828), representing a novel susceptibility locus for BD that is involved in T-cell survival, and that T-cell aberration could contribute to the development of this disease.

REFERENCES

1. Jennette JC, Falk RJ, Andrassay K, et al. Nomenclature of systemic vasculitides. Proposal of an international conference. Arthritis Rheum 1994;37:187–92.
2. Jennette JC, Falk RJ, Bacon PA, et al. 2012 Revised International Chapel Hill Consensus Conference Nomenclature of Vasculitides. Arthritis Rheum 2013; 65:1–11.
3. Yildiz C, Ozen S. The specificities of pediatric vasculitis classification. Presse Med 2013;42:546–50.
4. Ozen S, Ruperto N, Dillon MJ, et al. EULAR/PRES endorsed consensus criteria for the classification of childhood vasculitides. Ann Rheum Dis 2006;65:936–41.
5. Ruperto N, Ozen S, Pistorio A, et al. EULAR/PINTO/PRES criteria for Henoch-Schönlein purpura, childhood polyarteritis nodosa, childhood Wegener granulomatosis and childhood Takayasu arteritis: Ankara 2008. Part I: overall methodology and clinical characterization. Ann Rheum Dis 2010;69:790–7.
6. Ozen S, Pistorio A, Iusan SM, et al. EULAR/PRINTO/PRES criteria for Henoch-Schönlein purpura, childhood polyarteritis nodosa, childhood Wegener granulomatosis and childhood Takayasu arteritis. Ankara 2008. Part II: final classification. Ann Rheum Dis 2010;69:798–806.
7. Longcope WT. Periarteritis nodosa with report of a case with autopsy, vol. 1. Bull Auyer Clin Lab, Pennsylvania Hospital; 1908.
8. Kernohan JW, Woltman HW. Periarteritis nodosa: a clinicopathologic study with special reference to the nervous system. Arch Neurol 1938;39:655–86.
9. Krahulik L, Rosenthal M, Loughlin EH. Periarteritis nodosa (necrotizing panarteritis) in childhood with meningeal involvement. Report of a case with study of pathologic findings. Am J Med Sci 1935;190:308–17.
10. Younger DS. Diabetic neuropathy: a clinical and neuropathological study of 107 patients. Neurol Res Int 2010;2010:140379.
11. Wohlwill F. Uber die mur mikroskopisch erkenbarre form der periarteritis nodosa. Arch Pathol Anat 1923;246:377–411.
12. Davson J, Ball M, Platt R. The kidney in periarteritis nodosa. Q J Med 1948;17: 175–202.
13. Wainwright J, Davson J. The renal appearance in the microscopic form of periarteritis nodosa. J Pathol Bacteriol 1950;62:189–96.
14. Lamb AR. Periarteritis nodosa—a clinical and pathological review of the disease with a report of two cases. Arch Intern Med 1914;14:481–516.

15. Churg J, Strauss L. Allergic granulomatosis, allergic angiitis, and periarteritis nodosa. Am J Pathol 1951;27:277–301.
16. Chumbley LC, Harrison EG, DeRemee RA. Allergic granulomatosis and angiitis (Churg-Strauss syndrome). Report and analysis of 30 cases. Mayo Clin Proc 1977;52:477–84.
17. Lanham JG, Elkon KB, Pussey CD, et al. Systemic vasculitis with asthma and eosinophilia: a clinical approach to the Churg-Strauss syndrome. Medicine (Baltimore) 1984;63:65–81.
18. Masi AT, Hunder GG, Lie JT, et al. The American College of Rheumatology 1990 criteria for the classification of Churg-Strauss syndrome (allergic granulomatosis and angiitis). Arthritis Rheum 1990;33:1094–100.
19. Godman GC, Churg J. Wegener's granulomatosis: pathology and review of the literature. Arch Pathol 1954;58:533–53.
20. Fauci AS, Haynes BF, Katz P, et al. Wegener's granulomatosis: prospective clinical and therapeutic experience with 85 patients over 21 years. Ann Intern Med 1983;98:76–85.
21. Hoffman GS, Kerr GS, Leavitt RY, et al. Wegener granulomatosis: an analysis of 158 patients. Ann Intern Med 1992;116:488–98.
22. Zeek PM, Smith CC, Weeter JC. Studies on periarteritis nodosa. III. The differentiation between the vascular lesions of periarteritis nodosa and of hypersensitivity. Am J Pathol 1948;24:889–917.
23. Zeek PM. Periarteritis nodosa—a critical review. Am J Clin Pathol 1952;22: 777–90.
24. Osler W. The visceral lesions of purpura and allied conditions. BMJ 1914;1: 517–25.
25. Gairdner D. The Schönlein-Henoch syndrome (anaphylactoid purpura). Q J Med 1948;17:95–122.
26. Levitt LM, Burbank B. Glomerulonephritis as a complication of the Schonlein-Henoch syndrome. N Engl J Med 1953;248:530–6.
27. Faille-Kuyber EH, Kater L, Kooiker CJ, et al. IgA-deposits in cutaneous blood-vessel walls and mesangium in Henoch-Schonlein syndrome. Lancet 1973;1: 892–3.
28. Conley ME, Cooper MD, Michael AF. Selective deposition of immunoglobulin A1 in immunoglobulin A nephropathy, anaphylactoid purpura nephritis, and systemic lupus erythematosus. J Clin Invest 1980;66:1432–6.
29. Wintrobe MM, Buell MV. Hyperproteinemia associated with multiple myeloma. With report of a case in which an extraordinary hyperproteinemia was associated with thrombosis of the retinal veins and symptoms suggesting Raynauds disease. Bull Johns Hopkins Hosp 1933;52:156–65.
30. Lerner AB, Watson CJ. Studies of cryoglobulins. I. Unusual purpura associated with the presence of a high concentration of cryoglobulin (cold precipitable serum globulin). Am J Med Sci 1947;214:410–5.
31. Lerner AB, Watson CJ. Studies of cryoglobulins. II. The spontaneous precipitation of protein from serum at 5°C in various disease states. Am J Med Sci 1947; 214:416–21.
32. McDuffie FC, Sams WM, Maldonado JE, et al. Hypocomplementemia with cutaneous vasculitis and arthritis. Possible immune complex syndrome. Mayo Clin Proc 1973;48:340–8.
33. Zeiss CR, Burch FX, Marder RJ, et al. A hypocomplementemic vasculitic urticarial syndrome: report of four new cases and definition of the disease. Am J Med 1980;68:867–75.

34. Wisnieski JJ, Naff GB. Serum IgG antibodies to C1q in hypocomplementemic urticarial vasculitis syndrome. Arthritis Rheum 1989;32:1119–27.
35. Save-Soderbergh J, Malmvall B, Anderson R, et al. Giant cell arteritis as a cause of death. JAMA 1986;255:493–6.
36. Takayasu M. Case with unusual changes of the central vessels in the retina [Japanese]. Acta Soc Ophthal Jap 1908;12:554–5.
37. Walker DI, Bloor K, Williams G, et al. Inflammatory aneurysms of the abdominal aorta. Br J Surg 1972;59:609–14.
38. Pennell RC, Hollier LH, Lie JT, et al. Inflammatory abdominal aortic aneurysms: a thirty-year review. J Vasc Surg 1985;2:859–69.
39. Hamano H, Kawa S, Horiuchi A, et al. High serum IgG4 concentrations in patients with sclerosing pancreatitis. N Engl J Med 2001;344:732–8.
40. Hamano H, Kawa S, Ochi Y, et al. Hydronephrosis associated with retroperitoneal fibrosis and sclerosing pancreatitis. Lancet 2002;359:1403–4.
41. Sakata N, Tashiro T, Uesugi N, et al. IgG4-positive plasma cells in inflammatory abdominal aortic aneurysm: the possibility of an aortic manifestation of IgG4-related sclerosing disease. Am J Surg Pathol 2008;32:553–9.
42. Kasashima S, Zen Y, Kawashima A, et al. Inflammatory abdominal aortic aneurysm: close relationship to IgG4-releated periaortitis. Am J Surg Pathol 2008;32: 197–204.
43. Ito H, Kalzaki Y, Noda Y, et al. IgG4-related inflammatory abdominal aortic aneurysm associated with autoimmune pancreatitis. Pathol Int 2008;58:421–6.
44. Khosroshahi A, Stone JR, Pratt DS, et al. Painless jaundice with serial multiorgan dysfunction. Lancet 2009;373:1494.
45. Stone JH, Khosroshahi A, Hilgenberg A, et al. IgG4-related systemic disease and lymphoplasmacytic aortitis. Arthritis Rheum 2009;60:3139–45.
46. Adamantiades B. Sur un cas d'iritis a hypopion recidivant. Ann D'Ocul 1931; 168:271–8.
47. Behçet H. Ueber rezidivierende, aphthöse, durch ein virus verursachte Geschwüre am Mund, am Auge und an den Genitalien. Dermat Wchnschr 1937;105: 1152–7.
48. Behçet H, Matteson EL. On relapsing, aphthous ulcers of the mouth, eye and genitalia caused by a virus. 1937. Clin Exp Rheumatol 2010;28(Suppl 60):S2–5.
49. Wolf SM, Schotland DL, Phillips LL. Involvement of nervous system in Behçet's syndrome. Arch Neurol 1965;12:315–25.
50. Mogan RF, Baumgarten CJ. Meniere's disease complicated by recurrent interstitial keratitis: excellent results following cervical ganglionectomy. West J Surg 1934;42:628.
51. Cogan DG. Syndrome of nonsyphilitic interstitial keratitis and vestibuloauditory symptoms. Arch Ophthalmol 1945;33:144–9.
52. Sunderland S. Blood supply of the sciatic nerve and its popliteal divisions in man. Arch Neurol 1945;53:283–9.
53. Sunderland S. Blood supply of the nerves of the upper limb in man. Arch Neurol 1945;53:91–115.
54. Dyck PJ, Conn DL, Okazaki H. Necrotizing angiopathic neuropathy. Three-dimensional morphology of fiber degeneration related to sites of occluded vessels. Mayo Clin Proc 1972;47:461–75.
55. Moore PM, Fauci AS. Neurologic manifestations of systemic vasculitis. A retrospective and prospective study of the clinicopathologic features and responses to therapy in 25 patients. Am J Med 1981;71:517–24.

56. Harbitz F. Unknown forms of arteritis with special reference to their relation to syphilitic arteritis and periarteritis nodosa. Am J Med Sci 1922;163:250–72.

57. Cupps T, Fauci A. Central nervous system vasculitis. Major Probl Intern Med 1981;21:123–32.

58. Calabrese HL, Mallek JA. Primary angiitis of the central nervous system: report of 8 new cases, review of the literature, and proposal for diagnostic criteria. Medicine 1988;67:20–39.

59. Younger DS, Hays AP, Brust JC, et al. Granulomatous angiitis of the brain. An inflammatory reaction of diverse etiology. Arch Neurol 1988;45:514–8.

60. Scott DG, Watts RA. Epidemiology and clinical features of systemic vasculitis. Clin Exp Nephrol 2013;17:607–10.

61. Gonzalez-Gay MA, Vazquez-Rodriguez TR, Lopez-Diaz MJ, et al. Epidemiology of giant cell arteritis and polymyalgia rheumatica. Arthritis Rheum 2009;61: 1454–61.

62. Dunstan E, Lester SL, Rischmueller M, et al. Epidemiology of biopsy-proven giant cell arteritis in South Australia. Intern Med J 2014;44:32–9.

63. Ninan J, Nguyen AM, Cole A, et al. Mortality in patients with biopsy-proven giant cell arteritis: a south Australian population-based study. J Rheumatol 2011;38: 2215–7.

64. Herlyn K, Buckert F, Gross WL, et al. Doubled prevalence rates of ANCA-associated vasculitides and giant cell arteritis between 1994 and 2006 in northern Germany. Rheumatology (Oxford) 2014;53(5):882–9.

65. Bas-Lando M, Breuer GS, Berkun Y, et al. The incidence of giant cell arteritis in Jerusalem over a 25-year period: annual and seasonal fluctuations. Clin Exp Rheumatol 2007;25(Suppl 44):S15–7.

66. Kobayashi S, Yano T, Matsumoto Y, et al. Clinical and epidemiologic analysis of giant cell (temporal) arteritis from a nationwide survey in 1998 in Japan: the first government-supported nationwide survey. Arthritis Rheum 2003;49:594–8.

67. Abdul-Rahman AM, Molteno ACB, Bevin TH. The epidemiology of giant cell arteritis in Otago, New Zealand: a 9-year analysis. N Z Med J 2011;124:44–52.

68. Haugeberg G, Irgens KA, Thomsen RS. No major differences in incidence of temporal arteritis in northern and western Norway compared with reports from southern Norway. Scand J Rheumatol 2003;32:318–9.

69. Haugeberg G, Paulsen PQ, Bie RB. Temporal arteritis in Vest Agder County in southern Norway: incidence and clinical findings. J Rheumatol 2000;27:2624–7.

70. Gonzalez-Gay MA, Barros S, Lopez-Diaz MJ, et al. Giant cell arteritis: disease patterns of clinical presentation in a series of 240 patients. Medicine 2005;84: 269–76.

71. Gonzalez-Gay MA, Miranda-Filloy JA, Lopez-Diaz MJ, et al. Giant cell arteritis in northwestern Spain. A 25-year epidemiological study. Medicine 2007;86:61–8.

72. Mohammad AJ, Nilsson JA, Jacobsson LT, et al. Incidence and mortality rates of biopsy-proven giant cell arteritis in southern Sweden. Ann Rheum Dis 2015; 74(6):993–7.

73. Smeeth L, Cook C, Hall AJ. Incidence of diagnosed polymyalgia rheumatica and temporal arteritis in the United Kingdom, 1990-2001. Ann Rheum Dis 2006;65:1093–8.

74. Salvarani C, Crowson CS, O'Fallon M, et al. Reappraisal of the epidemiology of giant cell arteritis in Olmsted County, Minnesota, over a fifty-year period. Arthritis Rheum 2004;51:264–8.

75. De Souza AW, Okamoto KY, Abrantes F, et al. Giant cell arteritis: a multicenter observational study in Brazil. Clinics (Sao Paulo) 2013;68:317–22.

76. Chaudhry IA, Shamsi FA, Elzaridi E, et al. Epidemiology of giant-cell arteritis in an Arab population: a 22-year study. Br J Ophthalmol 2007;91:715–8.

77. Alba MA, Mena-Madrazo JA, Reyes E, et al. Giant cell arteritis in Mexican patients. J Clin Rheumatol 2012;18:1–7.

78. Kemp A, Marner K, Nissen SH, et al. HLA antigens in cases of giant cell arteritis. Acta Ophthalmol (Copenh) 1980;58:1000–4.

79. Armstrong RD, Behn A, Myles A, et al. Histocompatibility antigens in polymyalgia rheumatica and giant cell arteritis. J Rheumatol 1983;10:659–61.

80. Dababneh A, Gonzalez-Gay MA, Garcia-Porrua C, et al. Giant cell arteritis and polymyalgia rheumatica can be differentiated by distinct patterns of HLA class II association. J Rheumatol 1998;25:2140–5.

81. Jacobsen S, Baslund B, Madsen HO, et al. Mannose-binding lectin variant alleles and HLA-DR4 alleles are associated with giant cell arteritis. J Rheumatol 2002;29:2148–53.

82. Bignon JD, Ferec C, Barrier J, et al. HLA class II genes polymorphism in DR4 giant cell arteritis patients. Tissue Antigens 1988;32:254–8.

83. Bignon JD, Barrier J, Soulillou JP, et al. HLA DR4 and giant cell arteritis. Tissue Antigens 1984;24:60–2.

84. Richardson JE, Gladman DD, Fam A, et al. HLA-DR4 in giant cell arteritis: association with polymyalgia rheumatica syndrome. Arthritis Rheum 1987;30: 1293–7.

85. Barrier J, Bignon JD, Soulillou JP, et al. Increased prevalence of HLA-DR4 in giant-cell arteritis. N Engl J Med 1981;305:104–5.

86. Martinez-Taboda VM, Bartolome MJ, Lopez-Hoyos M, et al. HLA-DRB1 allele distribution in polymyalgia rheumatica and giant cell arteritis: influence on clinical subgroups and prognosis. Semin Arthritis Rheum 2004;34:454–64.

87. Weyand CM, Hicok KC, Hunder GG, et al. The HLA-DRB1 locus as a genetic component in giant cell arteritis. Mapping of a disease-linked sequence motif to the antigen binding site of the HLA-DR molecule. J Clin Invest 1992;90: 2355–61.

88. Weyand CM, Hunder NN, Hicok KC, et al. HLA-DRB1 alleles in polymyalgia rheumatica, giant cell arteritis, and rheumatoid arthritis. Arthritis Rheum 1994; 37:514–20.

89. Gonzalez-Gay MA, Garcia-Porrua C, Llorca J, et al. Visual manifestations of giant cell arteritis. Trends and clinical spectrum in 161 patients. Medicine (Baltimore) 2000;79:283–92.

90. Hansen JA, Healey LA, Wilske KR. Association between giant cell (temporal) arteritis and HLA-Cw3. Hum Immunol 1985;13:193–8.

91. Gonzalez-Gay MA, Rueda B, Vilchez JR, et al. Contribution of MHC class I region to genetic susceptibility for giant cell arteritis. Rheumatology (Oxford) 2007;46:431–4.

92. Arend WP, Michel BA, Bloch DA, et al. The American College of Rheumatology 1990 criteria for the classification of Takayasu arteritis. Arthritis Rheum 1990;33: 1129–34.

93. Terao C, Yoshifuji H, Kimura A, et al. Two susceptibility loci to Takayasu arteritis reveal a synergistic role of the IL12B and HLA-B regions in a Japanese population. Am J Hum Genet 2013;93:289–97.

94. Saruhan-Direskeneli G, Hughes T, Aksu K, et al. Identification of multiple genetic susceptibility loci in Takayasu arteritis. Am J Hum Genet 2013;93:298–305.

95. Watts R, Al-Taiar A, Mooney J, et al. The epidemiology of Takayasu arteritis in the UK. Rheumatology 2009;48:1008–11.

96. Mohammad A, Mandl T. Takayasu's arteritis in southern Sweden. Presse Med 2013;42:719.

97. Waern AU, Andersson P, Hemmingsson A. Takayasu's arteritis: a hospital-region based study on occurrence, treatment and prognosis. Angiology 1983;34: 311–20.

98. Reinhold-Keller E, Herlyn K, Wagner-Bastmeyer R, et al. Stable incidence of primary systemic vasculitides over five years: results from the German vasculitis register. Arthritis Rheum 2005;53:93–9.

99. Dreyer L, Faurschou M, Baslund B. A population-based study of Takayasu's arteritis in eastern Denmark. Clin Exp Rheumatol 2011;29(Suppl 64):S40–2.

100. Lightfoot RW Jr, Michel BA, Bloch DA, et al. The American College of Rheumatology 1990 criteria for the classification of polyarteritis nodosa. Arthritis Rheum 1990;33:1088–93.

101. Ozen S, Bakkaloglu A, Dusunsel R, et al. Childhood vasculitides in Turkey: a nationwide survey. Clin Rheumatol 2007;26:196–200.

102. Mahr A, Guillevin L, Poissonnet M, et al. Prevalences of polyarteritis nodosa, microscopic polyangiitis, Wegener's granulomatosis, and Churg-Strauss syndrome in a French urban multiethnic population in 2000:a capture–recapture estimate. Arthritis Rheum 2004;51:92–9.

103. McMahon BJ, Heyward WL, Templin DW, et al. Hepatitis B-associated polyarteritis nodosa in Alaskan Eskimos: clinical and epidemiologic features and long-term follow-up. Hepatology 1989;9:97–101.

104. Mohammad AJ, Jacobsson LT, Westman KW, et al. Incidence and survival rates in Wegener's granulomatosis, microscopic polyangiitis, Churg-Strauss syndrome and polyarteritis nodosa. Rheumatology (Oxford) 2009;48:1560–5.

105. Watts RA, Gonzalez-Gay MA, Lane SE, et al. Geoepidemiology of systemic vasculitis: comparison of the incidence in two regions of Europe. Ann Rheum Dis 2001;60:170–2.

106. Omerod AS, Cook MC. Epidemiology of primary systemic vasculitis in the Australian Capital Territory and south-eastern New South Wales. Intern Med J 2008;38:816–23.

107. Japan Kawasaki Disease Research Committee. Diagnostic guidelines for Kawasaki disease. 5th edition. Tokyo: 2002. Available at: http://www.kawasaki-disease.org/diagnostic/index.html.197.

108. Newburger JW, Takahashi M, Gerber MA, et al. Diagnosis, treatment and long-term management of Kawasaki disease: a statement for health professionals from the Committee on Rheumatic Fever, Endocarditis, and Kawasaki Disease, Council on Cardiovascular Disease in the Young. Pediatrics 2004;114:1708–33.

109. Saundankar J, Yim D, Itotoh B, et al. The epidemiology and clinical features of Kawasaki disease in Australia. Pediatrics 2014;133:e1009–14.

110. Lin YT, Manlhiot C, Ching JC, et al. Repeated systematic surveillance of Kawasaki disease in Ontario from 1995 to 2006. Pediatr Int 2010;52:699–706.

111. Ma XJ, Huang M, Chen SB, et al. Epidemiologic features of Kawasaki disease in Shanghai from 2003 through 2007. Chin Med J 2010;123:2629–34.

112. Li XH, Li HJ, Xu M, et al. Epidemiological survey of Kawasaki disease in Sichuan Province of China. J Trop Pediatr 2008;54:133–6.

113. Du AD, Zhao D, Du J, et al. Epidemiologic study on Kawasaki disease in Beijing from 2000 through 2004. Pediatr Infect Dis J 2007;26:449–51.

114. Fischer TK, Holman RC, Yorita KL, et al. Kawasaki syndrome in Denmark. Pediatr Infect Dis J 2007;26:411–5.

115. Holman RC, Christensen KY, Belay ED, et al. Racial/ethnic differences in the incidence of Kawasaki syndrome among children in Hawaii. Hawaii Med J 2010;69:194–7.
116. Ng YM, Sung RY, So LY, et al. Kawasaki disease in Hong Kong, 1994 to 2000. Hong Kong Med J 2005;11:331–5.
117. Singh S, Aulakh R, Bhalla AK, et al. Is Kawasaki disease incidence rising in Chandigarh, North India? Arch Dis Child 2011;96:137–40.
118. Nakamura Y, Yashiro M, Uehara R, et al. Epidemiologic features of Kawasaki disease in Japan: results of the 2009-2010 nationwide survey. J Epidemiol 2012;22:216–21.
119. Park YW, Han JW, Hong YM, et al. Epidemiologic features of Kawasaki disease in Korea, 2006-2008. Pediatr Int 2011;53:36–9.
120. Schiller B, Fasth A, Bjorkhem G, et al. Kawasaki disease in Sweden: incidence and clinical features. Acta Paediatr 1995;84:769–74.
121. Lue HC, Chen LR, Lin MT, et al. Epidemiologic features of Kawasaki disease in Taiwan, 1976-2007: results of five nationwide questionnaire hospital surveys. Pediatr Neonatol 2014;55(2):92–6.
122. Huang WC, Huang LM, Chang IS, et al. Epidemiologic features of Kawasaki disease in Taiwan, 2003-2006. Pediatrics 2009;123:e401–5.
123. Harnden A, Alves B, Sheikh A. Rising incidence of Kawasaki disease in England: analysis of hospital admission data. BMJ 2002;324:1424–5.
124. Holman RC, Belay ED, Christensen KY, et al. Hospitalizations for Kawasaki syndrome among children in the United States, 1997-2007. Pediatr Infect Dis J 2010;29:483–8.
125. Onouchi Y, Tamari M, Takahashi A, et al. A genomewide linkage analysis of Kawasaki disease: evidence for linkage to chromosome 12. J Hum Genet 2007;52: 179–90.
126. Burgner D, Davila S, Breunis WB, et al. A genome-wide association study identifies novel and functionally related susceptibility Loci for Kawasaki disease. PLoS Genet 2009;5:e1000319.
127. Tsai FJ, Lee YC, Chang JS, et al. Identification of novel susceptibility loci for Kawasaki disease in a Han Chinese population by a genome-wide association study. PLoS One 2011;6:e16853.
128. Kim JJ, Hong YM, Sohn S, et al. A genome-wide association analysis reveals 1p31 and 2p13.3 as susceptibility loci for Kawasaki disease. Hum Genet 2011;129:487–95.
129. Khor CC, Davila S, Breunis WB, et al. Genome-wide association study identifies FCGR2A as a susceptibility locus for Kawasaki disease. Nat Genet 2011;43: 1241–6.
130. Lee YC, Kuo HC, Chang JS, et al. Two new susceptibility loci for Kawasaki disease identified through genome-wide association analysis. Nat Genet 2012;44: 522–5.
131. Onouchi Y, Ozaki K, Burns JC, et al. A genome-wide association study identifies three new risk loci for Kawasaki disease. Nat Genet 2012;44:517–21.
132. Yan Y, Ma Y, Liu Y, et al. Combined analysis of genome-wide-linked susceptibility loci to Kawasaki disease in Han Chinese. Hum Genet 2013;132:669–80.
133. Falk RJ, Jennette JC. Anti-neutrophil cytoplasmic autoantibodies with specificity for myeloperoxidase in patients with systemic vasculitis and idiopathic necrotizing and crescentic glomerulonephritis. N Engl J Med 1988;318:1651–7.
134. Griffith ME, Coulthart A, Pemberton S, et al. Anti-neutrophil cytoplasmic antibodies (ANCA) from patients with systemic vasculitis recognize restricted

epitopes of proteinase-3 involving the catalytic site. Clin Exp Immunol 2001;123: 170–7.

135. Lionaki S, Blyth ER, Hogan SL, et al. Classification of anti-neutrophil cytoplasmic autoantibody vasculitides: the role of anti-neutrophil cytoplasmic autoantibody specificity for myeloperoxidase or proteinase 3 in disease recognition and prognosis. Arthritis Rheum 2012;64:3452–62.

136. Lyons PA, Rayner TF, Trivedi S, et al. Genetically distinct subsets within ANCA-associated vasculitis. N Engl J Med 2012;367:214–23.

137. Savige J, Gillis D, Benson E, et al. International consensus statement on testing and reporting of anti-neutrophil cytoplasmic antibodies (ANCA). Am J Clin Pathol 1999;111:507–13.

138. Csernok E, Holle J, Hellmich B, et al. Evaluation of capture ELISA for detection of antineutrophil cytoplasmic antibodies against proteinase-3 in Wegener's granulomatosis: first results from a multicenter study. Rheumatology 2004;43: 174–80.

139. Hellmich B, Csenok E, Fredenhagen G, et al. A novel high sensitivity ELISA for detection of antineutrophil cytoplasm antibodies against proteinase-3. Clin Exp Rheumatol 2007;25(Suppl 44):S1–5.

140. Watts RA, Lane S, Hanslik T, et al. Development and validation of a consensus methodology for the classification of the ANCA-associated vasculitides and polyarteritis nodosa for epidemiological studies. Ann Rheum Dis 2007;66:222–7.

141. Watts RA, Lane SE, Bentham G, et al. Epidemiology of systemic vasculitis. Arthritis Rheum 2000;43:414–9.

142. Mohd Hanafiah K, Groeger J, Flaxman AD, et al. Global epidemiology of hepatitis C virus infection: new estimates of age-specific antibody to HCV serotypes. Hepatology 2013;57:1333–42.

143. Cacoub P, Renou C, Kerr G, et al. Influence of HLA-DR phenotype on the risk of hepatitis C virus-associated mixed cryoglobulinemia. Arthritis Rheum 2001;44: 2118–24.

144. Zignego AL, Wojclk GL, Cacoub P, et al. Genome-wide association study of hepatitis C virus- and cryoglobulin-related vasculitis. Genes Immun 2014;15: 500–5.

145. International Study Group for Behçet's Disease. Lancet 1990;335:1078–80.

146. Uluduz D, Kürtüncü M, Yapici Z, et al. Clinical characteristics of pediatric-onset neuro-Behçet disease. Neurology 2011;77:1900–5.

147. Mahr A, Belarbi L, Wechsler B, et al. Population-based prevalence study of Behçet disease. Differences by ethnic origin and low variation by age at immigration. Arthritis Rheum 2008;58:3951–9.

148. Calamia KT, Wilson FC, Icen M, et al. Epidemiology and clinical characteristics of Behcet's disease in the US: a population-based study. Arthritis Rheum 2009; 61:600–4.

149. Dursun A, Durakbasi-Dursun HG, Dursun R, et al. Angiotensin-converting enzyme gene and endothelial nitric oxide synthase gene polymorphisms in Behcet disease with or without ocular involvement. Inflamm Res 2009;58:401–5.

150. Dhifallah IB, Houman H, Khanfir M, et al. Endothelial nitric oxide synthase gene polymorphism is associated with Behcet's disease in Tunisian population. Hum Immunol 2008;69:661–5.

151. Park KS, Baek JA, Do JE, et al. CTLA4 gene polymorphisms and soluble CTLA4 protein in Behçet's disease. Tissue Antigens 2009;74:222–7.

152. Kim J, Im CH, Kang EH, et al. Mannose-binding lectin gene-2 polymorphisms and serum mannose-binding lectin levels in Behcet's disease. Clin Exp Rheumatol 2009;27(Suppl 53):S13–7.
153. Gul A. Genetics of Behcet's disease: lessons learned from genomewide association studies. Curr Opin Rheumatol 2014;26:56–63.
154. Fei Y, Webb R, Cobb BL, et al. Identification of novel genetic susceptibility loci for Behcet's disease using a genome-wide association study. Arthritis Res Ther 2009;11:R66.
155. Hou S, Yang A, Du L, et al. Identification of a susceptibility locus in STAT4 for Behçet's disease in Han Chinese in a genome-wide association study. Arthritis Rheum 2012;64:4104–13.
156. Lee YJ, Horie Y, Wallace GR, et al. Genome-wide association study identifies GIMAP as a novel susceptibility locus for Behcet's disease. Ann Rheum Dis 2013; 72:1510–6.

Epidemiology of Multiple Sclerosis

Jonathan Howard, MD[a],*, Stephen Trevick, MD[b], David S. Younger, MD, MPH, MS[c]

KEYWORDS

- Multiple sclerosis • Neuroepidemiology • Public health

KEY POINTS

- Multiple sclerosis (MS) which includes a clinically isolated syndrome, neuromyelitis optica or Devic disease, and acute disseminated encephalomyelitis are common complex neurodegenerative disease of the central nervous system. It manifests as a progressive disease through dissemination in time and space in the brain and spinal cord, due mainly to autoimmune inflammation.
- The disorder engenders an enormous burden of disease and comorbidity, varying with world regions and population ethnicity.
- Genome-wide association studies serve as powerful tools for investigating the genetic substrate of MS.
- There are novel biologic treatments, including fingolimod and natalizumab.
- Supportive treatment includes management of disability, support of generalized symptoms, and psychiatric care.

EPIDEMIOLOGY
Prevalence and Incidence

The Americas

In 2007, Poser and Brinar[1] noted that published prevalence rates of multiple sclerosis (MS) could be misleading with the reliance on clinical information and brain MRI interpretation leading to one-third of incorrect MS diagnoses. This opinion was epitomized by the findings of a clinical questionnaire survey of 30 complete MS clinical histories and examinations, including cerebrospinal fluid (CSF), sent to prominent clinical neurologists around the world.[2] All of the cases were autopsied, 25 patients had clinical MS, 1 had MS plus brain tumor, 1 had MS and stroke, and 3 did not have MS at all. When asked to indicate if the diagnosis was probable, possible, or unlikely MS

[a] Division of Neuroepidemiology, Department of Neurology, Comprehensive Care Center, New York University, New York, NY, USA; [b] New York University Langone Medical Center, New York, NY, USA; [c] Division of Neuroepidemiology, Department of Neurology, New York University School of Medicine, College of Global Public Health, New York University, New York, NY, USA
* Corresponding author.
E-mail address: Jonathan.howard@nyumc.org

Neurol Clin 34 (2016) 919–939
http://dx.doi.org/10.1016/j.ncl.2016.06.016
0733-8619/16/© 2016 Elsevier Inc. All rights reserved.

neurologic.theclinics.com

according to their own diagnostic criteria, 108 neurologists responded, correctly identifying only two-thirds of the cases but not the same ones. Experience, country of training, and practice and specialization in MS were inconsequential. Poser and Brinar[1] noted that common errors in global prevalence studies might be the failure to distinguish between the clinical and MRI characteristics of MS and disseminated encephalomyelitis (DEM) in both their acute and chronic forms, cases with onset before entering the study group or moving to the geographic area, and counting cases of the variant neuromyelitis optica (NMO) as an oriental form of MS, falsely inflating prevalence rates of MS in Far Eastern countries and failing to recognize some cases of NMO as instances of DEM.

Evans and colleagues[3] reviewed the incidence and prevalence of MS in the Americas, noting high heterogeneity among all studies even when stratified by country, making comparisons difficult, and noting variation in the quality of the studies. Among 9 epidemiologic studies that estimated MS prevalence and incidence in the United States reported between 1989 and 2007,[4–12] prevalence was highest in Olmstead County, Minnesota,[7] with age-standardized rate (ASR) of 191.2 per 100,000, and lowest in Lubbock, Texas, and the 19 surrounding counties, with an ASR of 39.9 per 100,000. Incidence of MS was reported in Olmstead County, MN[7] with an ASR of 7.3 per 100,000.

Among 12 epidemiologic studies estimating prevalence and incidence in Canada from 1986 to 2010,[13–24] 1 nationwide study used self-reporting information from a national population-based health survey conducted in 2000 to 2001 from a stratified random sample that estimated the crude prevalence of MS to be 240 per 100,000[19] Crude prevalence in individual regions of Canada ranged from 56.4 per 100,000 in Newfoundland in 1985[13] to 298 per 100,000 in Saskatoon in 2005.[22] The highest reported incidence of MS was in Alberta, with an ASR of 20.6 per 100,000 in 2002[25] and 23.9 per 100,000 for 2004.[23] However, the latter was based on invalidated administrative health claims.

A total of 6 studies from 4 countries in Central and South America examined the prevalence and incidence of MS from 1992 to 2009[26–31] but only 1[31] produced estimates for the entire country, noting a crude prevalence for Panama during 2000 to 2005 of 5.24 per 100,000 and annual incidence from 1990 to 2005 of 0.15 per 100,000.[31] Both prevalence and incidence were highest in the Argentine Patagonia region with a 2002 crude prevalence of 17.2 per 100,000 and annual incidence of 1.4 per 100,000.[29]

A meta-analysis evaluating prevalence estimates from 59 countries found a statistically significant latitudinal gradient for prevalence even after age-standardization and adjustment for prevalence year,[32] whereas a previous review of MS prevalence in Canada found no striking latitudinal or longitudinal gradient[33] similar to another study[29] that found and no south-north gradient in prevalence within the Argentine Patagonia. Prevalence estimates of MS were much lower in South America compared with North America, according to Evans and colleagues,[3] despite the studied regions being similar distances from the equator. This was possibly due to variations in the methodologies used, the quality of medical care, and the differential population susceptibility to MS.[34] Such conflicting findings suggest that geography alone may not predict the prevalence or risk of MS. Although it has been suggested that the prevalence of MS has increased in recent years,[35] it may partly be explained by a longer life expectancy in those with MS, and not necessarily an indicator of an increased risk of the disease, as well as advances in the identification of affected cases as a consequence of increased access to neurologists and improved methods of case ascertainment. Although most studies examine prevalence, incidence may be a better measure of increased disease risk.[34]

Europe

Kingwell and colleagues[36] did a comprehensive literature search of population-based studies of MS prevalence and incidence in European populations published between 1985 and 2011, noting that study estimates were highly heterogeneous also within regions or countries. Together with the Italian peninsula, the British Isles was the most studied. Prevalence estimates in the British Isles ranged from 96 per 100,000 in Guernsey[37] to more than 200 per 100,000, with the highest estimates originating from Scotland and Northern Ireland.[38,39] These 2 countries had the highest annual incidence rates, ranging from 7.2 to 12.2 per 100,000. With rare exceptions, prevalence and incidence estimates were higher in women with ratios of 3 to 1. Epidemiologic data at the national level were uncommon and there were marked geographic disparities in available data, with large areas of Europe unrepresented and other regions well-represented in the literature. Only 37% of the studies provided standardized estimates.

In the Italian peninsula, Sardinia had a higher incidence and prevalence of MS compared with the rest of Italy.[40] Of 6 studies of the Sardinian population,[41–45] 5 found an estimated prevalence of MS greater than 100 per 100,000. The only study with a lower estimate noted 69 per 100,000 in 1985.[46] When considering the incidence of MS, the Sardinian estimates of 3.4 to 6.8 per 100,000 were not unlike those seen across the entire Italian peninsula.

Although prevalence and incidence estimates tended to be higher in the northern regions of the British Isles and in the Nordic countries, implicating the role of latitude, this pattern was not uniform, with higher estimates originating as far south as Greece. There, the crude prevalence rate of definite MS cases increased between 1984 and 2006 from 10.1 per 100,000 recorded in northeastern Greece to 119.61 per 100,000; and mean annual incidence rates that increased between 1984 and 1989 from 2.71 per 100,000 to 10.73 per 100,000.[47]

Asia

Makhani and colleagues[48] examined published studies between 1985 and 2011 of MS incidence and prevalence from Kuwait, Israel, Turkey, Jordan, Iran, India, China, Japan, and Taiwan,[49–69] noting MS incidence and prevalence lowest in Africa and highest in Australia. Prevalence of MS increased over time in many countries, ranging from 0.67 per 100,000 per year in Taiwan to 3.67 per 100,000 in Australia; with the lowest prevalence in South African blacks of 0.22 per 100,000 and highest among Australian-born of 125 per 100,000.

Genetic Aspects

Genes involved in MS have long been sought and several approaches to this problem have been applied with varied success. A candidate gene approach was used for many decades wherein genes potentially associated with MS were chosen based on family aggregation and twin studies but, more recently, on the presumed autoimmune MS etiopathogenesis invoking human leukocyte antigen (HLA) class I and II, particularly the latter, which control immune response genes.[70]

Family aggregation studies

Familial aggregation in MS has not been compelling. Monozygotic twins of afflicted individuals had a 30% risk of the disease, with a similar rate in dizygotic twins to other siblings, demonstrating a significant genetic component to the illness without likely contribution of intrauterine factors.[71,72] Siblings were conferred a 2% to 5% lifetime risk, and parents and children of MS patients had a 1% lifetime risk.[73] The Multiple Sclerosis Genetics Group[74] reported demographic and clinical characteristics of 89 multiplex families, noting a mean difference in age of onset between probands and affected siblings of 8.87 years and a higher concordance rate among sister pairs than among brother pairs but without differences in affection rate among sons or daughters of either affected mothers or affected fathers. In a cohort of 807 MS families with 938 affected aunt or uncle and niece or nephew pairs ascertained from a longitudinal, population-based Canadian database, Herrera and colleagues[75] observed an increased number of avuncular pairs connected through unaffected mothers compared with unaffected fathers ($P = .008$) noting a maternal parent-of-origin effect in susceptibility to MS. Ebers and colleagues[72] (1986) studied familial aggregation of MS in a sample of 5,463 MS cases in Canada, noting an excess of monozygotic twins and a marked excess of concordance among monozygotic twin pairs. They quoted previous studies that indicated a 300-fold increase of risk for monozygotic twins of index cases and 20-fold to 40-fold increase for biological first-degree relatives.[76] Together, these studies suggested that familial aggregation in MS was genetic. However, because most monozygotic twins remained discordant, nongenetic risk factors are clearly important. Baranzini and colleagues[77] reported the genome sequences of 1 MS-discordant monozygotic twin pair, and mRNA transcriptome and epigenome sequences of CD4+ lymphocytes from 3 MS-discordant, monozygotic twin pairs, noting no reproducible differences between cotwins among approximately 3.6 million single nucleotide polymorphisms (SNPs) or in approximately 0.2 million insertion-deletion polymorphisms; nor was there evidence for genetic, epigenetic, or transcriptome differences that explained disease discordance.

Genome-wide association studies

Bashinskaya and colleagues[78] provided an excellent review of genome-wide association studies (GWAS) in MS. Powerful tools for investigating the genetic architecture of MS, GWAS have the potential to identify the genetic factors of disease susceptibility, clinical phenotypes, and treatment response. The GWAS data for MS can be found in the regularly updated National Human Genome Research Institute-European Bioinformatics Institute website: www.ebi.ac.uk/gwas.[79] Established in 2008, it includes data of all published GWAS assaying at least 100,000 SNP.

The role of the GWAS has been led by 3 international consortia possessing individual DNA samples from various clinics worldwide, including the International Multiple Sclerosis Genetic Consortium (IMSGC), Welcome Trust Case Control Consortium 2 (WTCCC2), and Australia and New Zealand Multiple Sclerosis Genetics Consortium (ANZgene). Affymetrix and Illumina genome-wide platforms are used by most GWAS for targeting SNPs regularly distributed throughout the genome, covering arrays with a range of 262 to 600 K. Formed in 2 phases, the first or discovery phase of a GWAS includes detection of associations followed by a second or replication phase.

Of 13 GWAS described by Bashinskaya and colleagues,[78] the most significant signals mapped to HLA-*DRB1* class II gene.[80–83] Their review of GWAS in MS summarized more than a dozen studies, several of which met significance levels of association of $P < 4 \times 10^{-225}$.[80–82] Two chromosomal loci mapping to 6p21.32 in HLA-*DRB1* and *DQB1* gene loci (Online Mendelian Genetics in Man [MIM] 142857 and 604305) and another at 2q37.3 in the *PDCD1* gene (MIM 604305) locus share phenotypic-genetic relationships with either susceptibility (MIM 142857, 604305) or disease progression of MS (MIM 600244).[84] SNPs identified and replicated in GWAS of MS have been located mainly in or near protein-coding genes directly involved in immune-related functions. Because it is well known that the HLA locus is an essential component directing the immune response and immune developments, it is not surprising that the major histocompatibility complex (MHC) region still represents about one-half of the MS genetic risk.

Non-HLA genes associated with MS are associated with T-cell function and may indicate the leading role of T-cell immunity in MS development. Many aspects of the immune system have demonstrated involvement in MS. Circulating T cells bind to blood brain barrier endothelium and then pass into the parenchyma. Microglia stimulate proliferation, leading to the release of a broad range of cytokines; further recruitment of T cells; activation of B cells; and, collectively, the destruction of myelin. Th1-like cytokines levels and other T-cell–related cytokines in the CSF have been correlated with disease progression.[85] Reciprocal upregulation of T-cell migration mediated by T-cell–released cytokines via interaction with MCH class II molecules provides an important avenue for neuroinflammation. A variety of inflammatory mediators are involved, including tumor necrosis factor (TNF), oxygen free radicals, and nitric oxide. The effects of these on neuronal function may contribute to myelin breakdown.[86] Pathogenic B-cell activation is suggested by elevated CSF oligoclonal bands (OCBs), increased levels of CSF immunoglobulin-G (IgG), and anti–myelin-associated glycoprotein (MAG) antibody in affected patients.[87] Viral and other infectious exposures may predispose a host to an autoimmune attack. An association with latent Epstein-Barr virus (EBV) has been implicated; activation of latent EBV has been found in some active MS lesions,[88] although this has been inconsistently replicated.[89,90] Whatever the associating factors, critical exposure seems to occur before the age of 15 years, based on migration studies.[91,92] In keeping with most autoimmune illnesses, female patients are affected 2 to 3 time more frequently than male patients. Individuals of white ancestry have the highest incidence of the disease. Although the disease is less common in African Americans, it tends to have a more severe course in this population. Overall, MS is the third most common cause of disability in United States in individuals 15 to 50 years of age, following only trauma and musculoskeletal disease.[93] The calculation of disability-adjusted life years, a measure of premature morbidity and disability, equivalent to years of healthy life lost due to MS, occurs in the adult population between 25 and 54 years of age, which results in major financial burdens of the patient, family, health system, and society.[94]

PATHOLOGIC FINDINGS

The primary trigger of immune response in MS is unknown. Early in the inflammatory cascade, a response is triggered against myelin antigens, such as myelin basic protein (MBP), proteolipid protein (PLP), myelin/oligodendrocyte glycoprotein, MAG, and gangliosides. Although plaques may occur throughout the CNS, they are most common in the optic nerves, cerebral periventricular white matter, brainstem, and spinal cord white-matter tracts. MS lesions are classified histologically as acute, chronically active, and inactive. Acute lesions have marked perivascular inflammatory cell infiltrates, composed predominantly of mononuclear cells, T cells, and macrophages, with occasional B cells and plasma cells. Over time, demyelination ensues, with phagocytosis of myelin debris by macrophages and microglial cells. Oligodendrocytes, the myelin-producing cells, proliferate but are destroyed by inflammatory infiltration and gliosis. The resulting demyelination leads to slowed conduction or even conduction block, as well as ectopic signal transmission, which leads to symptomatology.[95] Remyelination is activated by oligodendrocyte progenitor cells, not the surviving oligodendrocytes. With severe and longstanding demyelination, axonal loss is often found on histologic examination. This process is likely responsible for the nonremitting, chronic, and progressive symptoms in MS patients. The extent of axonal injury is associated with the inflammation in active MS lesions, although later in the course even clinically silent acute lesions may contribute to axonal injury. Subpial gray matter lesions may contribute to permanent disability even early in the disease.[96]

PATHOPHYSIOLOGY

A variety of motor deficits can result from MS lesions, including spasticity, weakness, tremor, and ataxia. Spasticity, an upper motor neuron (UMN) sign, results from the loss of inhibitory inputs from the corticospinal tracts to γ-motor neurons and interneuron networks. Weakness and impairment of fine motor control are due to interruption of input to α-motor neurons. Although the primary pathologic finding is UMN in nature, chronic disuse will rarely lead to muscle weakness, wasting, and atrophy, resembling lower motor neuron disease. Tremor and ataxia are related to lesions of the cerebellum and related pathways through the brainstem, red nucleus, thalamus, and basal ganglia. Ganglia in the Mollaret triangle, comprising the dentate nucleus of the cerebellum, inferior olive, and red nucleus, are specifically implicated in the development of tremor. In some patients, proprioceptive loss may be the primary cause of tremor, though a wide variety of injuries and circuit involvements may lead to this symptom. Fatigue, defined as a loss of force-generating capacity during sustained motor activity, contributes to disability in patients without other objective signs of motor dysfunction on examination.[97]

CLINICAL AND LABORATORY DIAGNOSIS

MS is typically divided into relapsing-remitting MS (RRMS) noted in about 85% of cases; and a chronic progressive pattern known as primary progressive MS (PPMS) in about 10% of cases. One-half of those with RRMS may evolve into secondary progressive MS.[98] Discrete episodes of neurologic dysfunction develop over hours to days and are called relapses, flares, attacks, or exacerbations. Attacks may be quite devastating, though most patients recover well. Occasionally, however, attacks can be debilitating if left untreated, especially if the brainstem or spinal cord is involved. During a severe exacerbation, inflammatory damage to myelin affects underlying axons, which can lead to poor recovery and permanent disability. Although patients may have residual disability from MS attacks, there is no progression of disability independent of attacks. Some inference on course can be made based on early prognostic features with initial sensory symptoms generally prognostically positive,[99] whereas motor and cerebellar signs, early relapse, and onset after age 40, are typically prognostically negative and associated with a more aggressive and rapid debilitating course.[100–102] Unlike RRMS, PPMS presents equally in men and women, and tends to occur at an older age. Certain presentations, such as optic neuritis, are common in RRMS but rare in PPMS compared with RRMS. The classic presentation is a male patient presenting after age 40 with progressive myelopathy that steadily worsens with eventual paraparesis, variable upper limb involvement and few other deficits, or symptomatic lesions in cerebral subcortical white matter.

The diagnosis of MS is based on 2 discrete episodes of neurologic dysfunction at least 30 days apart in different locations of the CNS, alternatively, in those with 1 relapse who show evidence of dissemination in time (DIT) and dissemination in space (DIS) on MRI. Patients with a single attack that does not meet formal criteria for MS are considered to have a clinically isolated syndrome (CIS), whereas those with imaging consistent with MS but discovered incidentally are considered to have a radiographically isolated syndrome. The diagnosis of MS is, therefore, based on the demonstration of multiple lesion DIT and DIS, while excluding alternative diagnoses through clinical, radiographic, and laboratory methods.

DIS is recognized by the following:

- One or more T_2 lesions in at least 2 out of 4 areas of the CNS: periventricular, juxtacortical, infratentorial, or spinal cord
- Gadolinium enhancement of lesions is not required for DIS.

DIT is recognized by either of the following:

- A new T_2 and/or gadolinium-enhancing lesion on follow-up MRI, with reference to a baseline scan, irrespective of the timing of the baseline MRI
- Simultaneous presence of asymptomatic gadolinium-enhancing and nonenhancing lesions at any time.

Diagnostic criteria for MS suggested by Poser and colleagues[103] were initially defined for the purposes of epidemiologic studies and clinical trials, whereas later criteria by McDonald,[104] and Polman and colleagues,[105] were clinically relevant and applicable to practice. They included the caveat that MRI could aid in diagnosis and even mitigate it as in CIS,[106,107] early conversion to clinically definite MS,[108] as well as in predicting responsiveness to immunotherapy with interferon beta-1a[109] and in documenting the first demyelinating episode.[110] The revised McDonald criteria[111] incorporated MRI criteria for the demonstration of DIS,[112,113] whereas those of Montalban and colleagues[111] demonstrated DIT.[107] Recognizing the special diagnostic needs of spinal PPMS, the 2010 McDonald criteria[104,106] maintained that 2 of 3 MRI or CSF findings for PPMS replaced previous brain imaging criteria for DIS.[112] The final criteria for PPMS included 1 year of retrospective or prospective disease progression, plus 2 of the 3 following: (1) 1 or more T_2 lesions in at least 1 area characteristics for MS, such as periventricular, juxtacortical, or infratentorial; (2) 2 or more T_2 lesions in the cord; or (3) positive CSF by isoelectric focusing evidence of OCB and/or elevated IgG index. Gadolinium enhancement on MRI was not required.

The MRI appearance of MS lesions in the brain and spinal cord is shown in **Figs. 1–9**. Typical MS brain lesions are ovoid foci of T_2/fluid-attenuated inversion

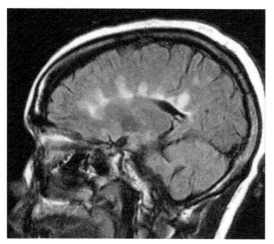

Fig. 1. Sagittal fluid-attenuated inversion recovery (FLAIR) image demonstrates typical periventricular lesions so called, Dawson fingers.

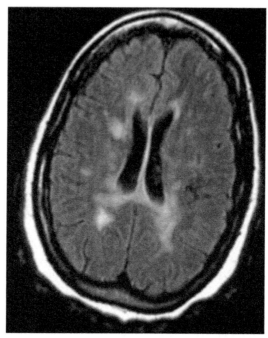

Fig. 2. Axial FLAIR image demonstrates typical periventricular lesions so called, Dawson fingers.

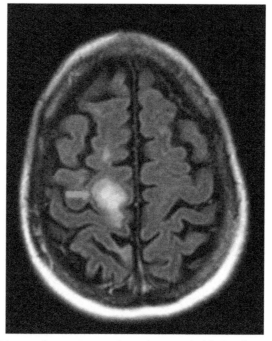

Fig. 3. Axial FLAIR image demonstrates a large juxtacortical lesion (*arrow*).

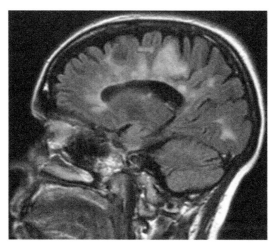

Fig. 4. Sagittal FLAIR image demonstrates a large juxtacortical lesion (*arrow*).

recovery (FLAIR) hyperintensity that radiate away from the ventricles best appreciated on sagittal FLAIR images. For every clinical relapse the patient experiences, the MRI shows 5 to 10 times as many lesions. Actively inflamed lesions demonstrate enhancement after the administration of gadolinium secondary to breakdown of the blood-brain barrier. There is characteristic complete or incomplete ring enhancement, often with the opening of the ring pointing to the cortex. Other times, lesions may enhance homogenously.

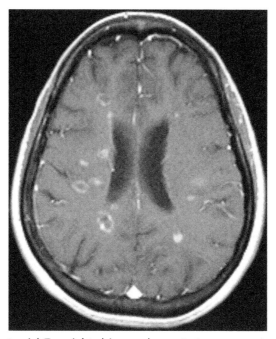

Fig. 5. Postcontrast axial T_1-weighted image demonstrates numerous enhancing lesions. Incomplete ring-enhancing lesions are highly suggestive of MS.

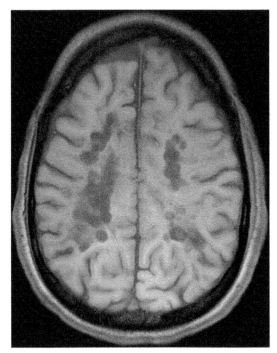

Fig. 6. Axial T₁-weighted image demonstrates hypointense lesions in the white matter. Older lesions appear hypointense on T₁-weighted images. They are called black holes and are evidence of irreversible axonal damage.

Magnetic resonance spectroscopy (MRS) is based on organic molecules in tissue as opposed to water. MRS has been studied with creatine (Cr), N-acetyl aspartate (NAA), choline, and myoinositol. NAA, which localizes to neurons, and Cr, which localizes to neurons and glial cells, relate to neuronal integrity, with deviations from normal levels indicating loss and injury; while correlating with neurologic disability.[114] Lymphocytic CSF pleocytosis of 5 to 50 cells/mm3 present in up to two-thirds of patients with MS; and OCB are found in greater than 90% of cases[115]; however it may not be recognized for several years. The latter is a nonspecific marker for CNS and may be found in encephalitis, meningitis, Guillain-Barré syndrome, and cerebral infarction.[116] Trimodal visual evoked responses, brainstem auditory evoked responses, and somatosensory evoked responses are potentially useful adjunctive studies in selected patients. Transcranial magnetic stimulation can demonstrate significant intraspinal delays in motor conduction.[117]

MULTIPLE SCLEROSIS VARIANTS AND DIFFERENTIAL DIAGNOSIS
Neuromyelitis Optica

Neuromyelitis optica has phenotypic similarities to MS although the underlying pathophysiology is quite different.[118] This disorder presents with inflammation and demyelination, which may relapse similarly to MS but, unlike MS, there is little to no progression independent of relapses. It is an uncommon disease that affects 0.5 to 5 per 100,000 persons. It is 10 times more common in women than in men, compared with MS, which is only 2 to 3 times more common in women. Unlike MS, it is more

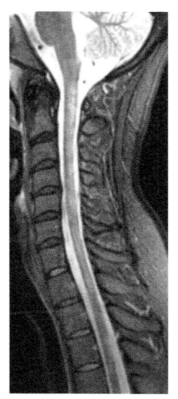

Fig. 7. Sagittal T_2-weighed image demonstrates hyperintense spinal cord lesions typical for MS. These lesions appear as discrete plaques within spinal cord white matter becoming more confluent over time. On axial imaging, the lesions are typically eccentric within the cord and do not occupy the entire cord.

common in African Americans, Asians, and Hispanics than in white persons. It typically presents between the ages of 30 and 40 years, although it may present at any age. It results in optic neuritis and transverse myelitis, both of which are longitudinally extensive. Patients can present with brainstem syndromes manifesting nausea, vomiting, and intractable hiccups, as well as hypothalamic lesions leading to narcolepsy, excessive sleepiness, obesity, and autonomic dysfunction.

The formal criteria for NMO are divided into those with and without NMO-IgG antibodies directed against the aquaporin-4 (AQP4) water channel present on astrocyte foot processes of the blood-brain-barrier. Seropositivity is reported in about 75% of patients with a clinical symptom consistent with NMO, whereas nearly 100% are specific for NMO.[119,120] Guidelines have been developed for the diagnosis and management of NMO.[121]

There are no randomized clinical trials of disease-modifying treatments in NMO, but small case series support the use of immunosuppressive agents, such as mycophenolate mofetil and azathioprine. The monoclonal antibody rituximab, which eliminates circulating B cells, has shown the greatest efficacy. The anti–interleukin-6 receptor antibody, tocilizumab, has shown promise in a small series of patients. Patients are often maintained on oral glucocorticoids as well. The disease-modifying agents in MS do not play a role in NMO, and they may worsen

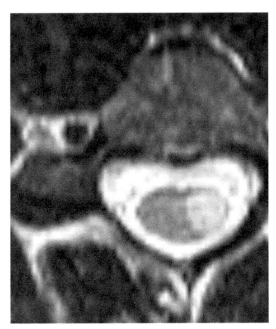

Fig. 8. Axial T$_2$-weighed image demonstrates hyperintense spinal cord lesions typical for MS. These lesions appear as discrete plaques within spinal cord white matter becoming more confluent over time. On axial imaging, the lesions are typically eccentric within the cord and do not occupy the entire cord.

the disease. However, other agents currently under study include aquaporumab, which is a nonpathogenic antibody-blocking AQP4-IgG–binding agent; sivelestat, which inhibits neutrophil elastase; and eculizumab, which inhibits the complement cascade.[122]

Acute Disseminated Encephalomyelitis

This monophasic immune-mediated CNS-demyelinating disorder can initially mimic MS; however, it is a predominantly a disorder of childhood and often postviral due to preceding measles, rubella, and mumps infection or vaccination, especially during the spring and winter months. Onset is characterized by fever, vomiting, headache, gait disturbance, and generalized seizures with signs of altered sensorium, nystagmus, diplopia, isolated or multiple cranial nerve palsies; as well as speech disturbance, dystonia, chorea, bladder disturbances, paraparesis, and quadriparesis.[123] Up to one-third of affected patients experience optic neuritis and CSF pleocytosis can be identified in up to two-thirds of patients. MRI shows multifocal demyelinating lesions through the subcortical white matter, midbrain, pons, corpus callosum, basal ganglia, medulla, and cerebellum. Only about one-third of patients have spinal cord lesion on neuroimaging. About 70% of patients will have remission within a week of commencing treatment with high-dose corticosteroids, although the remainder may experience residual symptoms.

Many other illnesses may initially mimic MS, most frequently other autoimmune, infectious or postinfectious, or genetic diseases. Autoimmune differential diagnosis may include systemic lupus erythematosus, Sjögren syndrome, Behçet syndrome, sarcoidosis, and CNS vasculitis.[124] Commonly considered infectious disorders

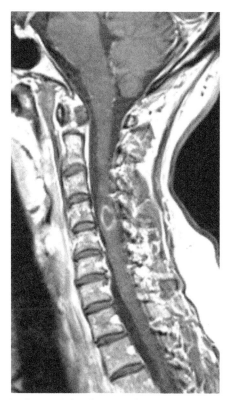

Fig. 9. Postcontrast sagittal T$_1$-weighted image demonstrates an enhancing lesion in the cervical spinal cord in patients with MS. Such lesions can have a ring-like appearance or a more punctate pattern of enhancement. Active lesions in the spinal cord, like active lesions in the brain, enhance with the administration of gadolinium.

include syphilis, tuberculosis, Lyme borreliosis, human T-lymphotropic virus type I, cytomegalovirus, herpes simplex virus, and varicella zoster virus. Hereditary disorders that may mimic MS include adrenoleukodystrophy, Refsum disease, spinocerebellar degeneration, and cerebral autosomal dominant arteriopathy with subcortical infarcts and leukoencephalopathy. Specific differentiation and diagnosis of MS versus these alternates requires specific evaluation and often relies on detailed laboratory testing.[124,125]

TREATMENT

Treatment can favorably affect MS by immune modulation, enhancement of myelination, improvement of conduction through demyelinated pathways, and providing symptomatic improvement without directly affecting the underlying disease (**Table 1**). Immune modulatory therapy diminishes the activation and proliferation of immune cells and their migration into the CNS by enhancing intrinsic suppressor activity or limiting the destruction caused by inflammatory processes. Such disease-modifying medications include injectable (interferon-beta and glatiramer acetate) and oral medications (fingolimod, teriflunomide, and dimethyl fumarate), monoclonal antibodies (natalizumab and alemtuzumab), and 1 chemotherapeutic

Table 1
Symptomatic MS treatment

Symptom	Treatments
Fatigue	Modafinil, amantadine, stimulants, SSRIs
Depression	SSRIs, SNRIs, bupropion, psychotherapy
Walking difficulty	Dalfampridine (Ampyra) is an oral agent that was approved on 1/22/2010 to help MS patients with walking. It helped about 40% of patients walk 25% faster than baseline, physical therapy, or mobility aids.
Nystagmus	Baclofen, clonazepam, gabapentin, memantine
Spasticity	Baclofen (either orally or via intrathecal pumps), Zanaflex, benzodiazepines, botulinum toxin.
Bladder dysfunction	Oxybutynin, terazosin, desmopressin, intravesicular botulinum toxin type A, self-catheterization
Pain or paresthesias	NSAIDs, anticonvulsants, antidepressants, surgery for trigeminal neuralgia
Tremor	Anticonvulsants, propranolol, clonazepam, deep brain stimulation
Pseudobulbar palsy	Dextromethorphan or quinidine (Nuedexta)
Sexual dysfunction	Phosphodiesterase 5 inhibitors (Sildenafil)

Abbreviations: NSAIDs, nonsteroidal antiinflammatory drugs, SSRIs, selective serotonin reuptake inhibitors; SNRIs, selective norepinephrine reuptake inhibitors.

agent (mitoxantrone). They are all indicated for patients with RRMS still in relapse, but, other than mitoxantrone, they do not have a role in the progressive phase of the illness. In patients with newly diagnosed MS and low disease activity, most authorities suggest starting treatment as soon as possible to influence the frequency of relapses, stabilize disease activity, and lessen long-term disability. The nonspecific immuno-suppressants azathioprine and cyclophosphamide have been used frequently without clearly established efficacy. Cladribine, mitoxantrone, antilymphocyte globulins, cyclosporine, and tacrolimus are chemotherapeutic agents with use as semispecific suppressors of MS disease activity. In extremely severe cases, total lymphoid irradi-ation may modulate the immune system, potentially benefiting MS, though controlled trials are lacking. Several peptides are being explored that interfere with binding within the trimolecular complex (T-cell receptor, antigen, and MHC class II molecule),[126] potentially leading to more specific agents decreasing the activity of the disease with minimal systemic immunosuppression.

Acute exacerbations are often initially treated with corticosteroids that enhance the resolution of symptoms and signs, though do not significantly affect the long-term outcome of an exacerbation. There are no certain dosing guidelines, although solume-drol 1g for 5 days is an appropriate course of treatment. Pulse therapy with corticoste-roids is associated with many temporary side effects such as insomnia, irritability, fluid retention, increased appetite, weight gain, hyperglycemia, hypertension, dyspepsia, depression, psychosis, bone fractures, and osteoporosis. In patients with poor venous access or otherwise intolerable reactions to corticosteroids, adrenocorticotropic hor-mone may be used instead. Plasmapheresis is sometimes used in severe relapses that are refractory to corticosteroids.

Therapies focused on improving conduction include 4-aminopyridine (4-AP) and 3, 4-diaminopyridine (3, 4-DAP), both potassium channel blockers that amplify and pro-long action potentials. Preliminary studies with 4-AP demonstrated improvement in may measures of neurologic function. However, when a large, multicenter, double-blind, placebo-controlled, study was performed, it failed to show an effect on the Expanded Disability Status Scale.[127] Unfortunately, higher levels of these medications can result in seizures and encephalopathy, potentially preventing sufficient dosage for demonstrable effect.[128]

Symptomatic therapy for MS is an important aspect of management.[129] Paresthesia may respond to antidepressants and anticonvulsants. Anticholinergic and β-blocker medications can improve bladder function, and fatigue can require amantadine and CNS stimulants. There are no medications currently available to treat muscle weakness, though physical therapy can optimize patient function. Spasticity, muscle cramps, and spasms respond to stretching and antispasticity medications, including baclofen, tizanidine, and benzodiazepines. If necessary, botulinum toxin can be introduced into specific muscles or, if generalized spasticity is refractory to other treatments, intrathecal baclofen administered by an implantable subcutaneous pump or dorsal root rhizotomy may be considered. Adaptive equipment includes ankle-foot orthoses for foot-drop dysfunction and canes, walkers, and wheelchairs for mobility. Tremor may respond to a variety of medications. Propranolol and primidone are often used initially, though isoniazid, buspirone, trazadone, baclofen, carbamazepine, gabapentin, benzodiazepines, and unilateral thalamotomy, can all be effective.[130]

REFERENCES

1. Poser CM, Brinar VV. The accuracy of prevalence rates of multiple sclerosis: a critical review. Neuroepidemiology 2007;29:150–5.
2. Poser C. Clinical diagnostic criteria in epidemiological studies of multiple sclerosis. Ann N Y Acad Sci 1965;122:506–19.
3. Evans C, Beland S-G, Kulaga S, et al. Incidence and prevalence of multiple sclerosis in the Americas: a systematic review. Neuroepidemiology 2013;40: 195–210.
4. Helmick C, Wrigley J, Zack M, et al. Multiple sclerosis in Key West, Florida. Am J Epidemiol 1989;130:935–49.
5. Wynn D, Rodriguez M, O'Fallon W, et al. A reappraisal of the epidemiology of multiple sclerosis in Olmstead County, Minnesota. Neurology 1990;40:780–6.
6. Hopkins R, Indian R, Pinnow E, et al. Multiple sclerosis in Galion, Ohio: prevalence and results of a case-control study. Neuroepidemiology 1991;10:192–9.
7. Mayr W, Pittock S, McClelland R, et al. Incidence and prevalence of multiple sclerosis in Olmstead County, Minnesota, 1985-2000. Neurology 2003;61: 1373–7.
8. Neuberger J, Lynch S, Sutton M, et al. Prevalence of multiple sclerosis in a residential area bordering an oil refinery. Neurology 2004;63:1796–802.
9. Cowen J, Sjostrom B, Doughty A, et al. Case-finding for MS prevalence studies in small communities requires a community-based approach. Neuroepidemiology 2007;28:246–52.
10. Williamson D, Henry J, Schiffer R, et al. Prevalence of multiple sclerosis in 19 Texas counties, 1998-2000. J Environ Health 2007;69:41–5.
11. Turabelidze G, Schootman M, Zhu B, et al. Multiple sclerosis prevalence and possible lead exposure. J Neurol Sci 2008;269:158–62.
12. Noonan C, Williamson D, Henry J, et al. The prevalence of multiple sclerosis in 3 US communities [abstract]. Prev Chronic Dis 2010;7:A1.
13. Pryse-Phillips W. The incidence and prevalence of multiple sclerosis in Newfoundland and Labrador, 1960-1986. Ann Neurol 1986;20:323–8.

14. Warren S, Warren K. Prevalence of multiple sclerosis in Barrhead County, Alberta, Canada. Can J Neurol Sci 1992;19:72–5.
15. Warren S, Warren K. Prevalence, incidence, and characteristics of multiple sclerosis in Westlock County, Alberta, Canada. Neurology 1993;43:1760–3.
16. Klein G, Rose M, Seland T. A prevalence study of multiple sclerosis in the Crownest Pass region of Southern Alberta. Can J Neurol Sci 1994;21:262–5.
17. Svenson L, Woodhead S, Platt G. Regional variations in the prevalence rates of multiple sclerosis in the province of Alberta, Canada. Neuroepidemiology 1994; 13:8–13.
18. Mirsattari S, Johnston J, McKenna R, et al. Aboriginal with multiple sclerosis HLA type and predominance of neuromyelitis optica. Neurology 2001;56: 317–23.
19. Beck C, Metz L, Svenson I, et al. Regional variation of multiple sclerosis prevalence in Canada. Mult Scler 2005;11:516–9.
20. Sloka J, Pryse-Phillips W, Stefanelle M. Incidence and prevalence of multiple sclerosis in Newfoundland and Labrador. Can J Neurol Sci 2005;32:37–42.
21. Svenson L, Warren S, Warren K, et al. Prevalence of multiple sclerosis in First Nations people of Alberta. Can J Neurol Sci 2007;34:175–80.
22. Hader W, Yee I. Incidence and prevalence of multiple sclerosis in Saskatoon, Saskatchewan. Neurology 2007;69:1224–9.
23. Warren S, Svenson L, Warren K. Contribution of incidence to increasing prevalence of multiple sclerosis in Alberta, Canada. Mult Scler 2008;14:872–9.
24. Marrie R, Yu N, Blanchard J, et al. The rising prevalence and changing age distribution of multiple sclerosis in Manitoba. Neurology 2010;74:465–71.
25. Warren S, Svenson L, Warren K, et al. Incidence of multiple sclerosis among First Nations people in Alberta, Canada. Neuroepidemiology 2007;28:21–7.
26. Callegaro D, Amaro De Lolio C, Radvany J, et al. Prevalence of multiple sclerosis in the city of Sao Paulo, Brazil, in 1990. Neuroepidemiology 1992;11:11–4.
27. Callegaro D, Goldbaum M, Morais L, et al. The prevalence of multiple sclerosis in the city of Sao Paulo, Brazil. Acta Neurol Scand 2001;104:208–13.
28. Toro J, Sarmiento O, Diaz del Castillo A, et al. Prevalence of multiple sclerosis in Bogota, Colombia. Neuroepidemiology 2007;28:33–8.
29. Melcon M, Gold L, Carra A, et al. Argentine Patagonia: prevalence and clinical features of multiple sclerosis. Mult Scler 2008;14:656–62.
30. Cristiano C, Patrucco L, Rojas J, et al. Prevalence of multiple sclerosis in Buenos Aires, Argentina using the capture-recapture method. Eur J Neurol 2009;16: 183–7.
31. Gracia F, Castillo L, Benzadon A, et al. Prevalence and incidence of multiple sclerosis in Panama (2000-2005). Neuroepidemiology 2009;32:287–93.
32. Simpson SJ, Blizzard L, Otahal P, et al. Latitude is significantly associated with the prevalence of multiple sclerosis: a meta-analysis. J Neurol Neurosurg Psychiatry 2011;82:1132–41.
33. Poppe A, Wolfson C, Zhu B. Prevalence of multiple sclerosis in Canada: a systematic review. Can J Neurol Sci 2008;35:593–601.
34. Risco J, Maldonado H, Luna L, et al. Latitudinal prevalence gradient of multiple sclerosis in Latin America. Mult Scler 2011;17:1055–9.
35. Orton S-M, Herrera B, Yee I, et al. Sex ratio of multiple sclerosis in Canada: a longitudinal study. Lancet Neurol 2006;5:932–6.
36. Kingwell E, Marriott JJ, Jette N, et al. Incidence and prevalence of multiple sclerosis in Europe: a systematic review. BMC Neurol 2013;13:128.

37. Sharpe G, Price SE, Last A, et al. Multiple sclerosis in island populations: prevalence in the Bailiwicks of Guernsey and Jersey. J Neurol Neurosurg Psychiatry 1995;58:22–6.
38. Rothwell PM, Charlton D. High incidence and prevalence of multiple sclerosis in south east Scotland: evidence of a genetic predisposition. J Neurol Neurosurg Psychiatry 1998;64:730–5.
39. Gray OM, McDonnell GV, Hawkins SA. Factors in the rising prevalence of multiple sclerosis in the north-east of Ireland. Mult Scler 2008;14:880–6.
40. Sotgiu S, Pugliatti M, Sanna A, et al. Multiple sclerosis complexity in selected populations: the challenge of Sardinia, insular Italy. Eur J Neurol 2002;9:329–41.
41. Casetta I, Granieri E, Marchi D, et al. An epidemiological study of multiple sclerosis in central Sardinia, Italy. Acta Neurol Scand 1998;98:391–4.
42. Granieri E, Casetta I, Govoni V, et al. The increasing incidence and prevalence of MS in a Sardinian province. Neurology 2000;55:842–7.
43. Montomolia C, Allemania C, Solinasa G, et al. An ecologic study of geographical variation in multiple sclerosis risk in central Sardinia, Italy. Neuroepidemiology 2002;21:187–93.
44. Pugliatti M, Sotgiu S, Solinas G, et al. Multiple sclerosis epidemiology in Sardinia: evidence for a true increasing risk. Acta Neurol Scand 2001;103:20–6.
45. Rosati G, Aiello I, Pirastru MI, et al. Epidemiology of multiple sclerosis in northwestern Sardinia: further evidence for higher frequency in Sardinians compared to other Italians. Neuroepidemiology 1996;15:10–9.
46. Rosati G, Aiello I, Mannu L, et al. Incidence of multiple sclerosis in the town of Sassari, Sardinia, 1965 to 1985: evidence for increasing occurrence of the disease. Neurology 1988;38:384–8.
47. Papathanasopoulos P, Gourzoulidou E, Messinis L, et al. Prevalence and incidence of multiple sclerosis in western Greece: a 23-year survey. Neuroepidemiology 2008;30:167–73.
48. Makhani N, Morrow SA, Fisk J, et al. MS incidence and prevalence in Africa, Asia, Australia and New Zealand: a systematic review. Mult Scler Relat Disord 2014;3:48–60.
49. Al-Din AS, Khogali M, Poser CM, et al. Epidemiology of multiple sclerosis in Arabs in Kuwait: a comparative study between Kuwaitis and Palestinians. J Neurol Sci 1990;100:137–41.
50. Alshubaili AF, Alramzy K, Ayyad YM, et al. Epidemiology of multiple sclerosis in Kuwait: new trends in incidence and prevalence. Eur Neurol 2005;53:125–31.
51. Alter M, Kahana E, Zilber N, et al. Multiple sclerosis frequency in Israel's diverse populations. Neurology 2006;66:1061–6.
52. Bharucha NE, Bharucha EP, Wadia NH, et al. Prevalence of multiple sclerosis in the Parsis of Bombay. Neurology 1988;38:727–9.
53. Cheng Q, Miao L, Zhang J, et al. A population-based survey of multiple sclerosis in Shanghai, China. Neurology 2007;68:1495–500.
54. El-Salem K, Al-Shimmery E, Horany K, et al. Multiple sclerosis in Jordan: a clinical and epidemiological study. J Neurol 2006;253:1210–6.
55. Etemadifar M, Janghorbani M, Shaygannejad V, et al. Prevalence of multiple sclerosis in Isfahan, Iran. Neuroepidemiology 2006;27:39–44.
56. Ghandehari K, Riasi HR, Nourian A, et al. Prevalence of multiple sclerosis in north east of Iran. Mult Scler 2010;16:1525–6.
57. Houzen H, Niino M, Hata D, et al. Increasing prevalence and incidence of multiple sclerosis in northern Japan. Mult Scler 2008;14:887–92.

58. Houzen H, Niino M, Kikuchi S, et al. The prevalence and clinical characteristics of MS in northern Japan. J Neurol Sci 2003;211:49–53.
59. Itoh T, Aizawa H, Hashimoto K, et al. Prevalence of multiple sclerosis in Asahikawa, a city in northern Japan. J Neurol Sci 2003;214:7–9.
60. Karni A, Kahana E, Zilber N, et al. The frequency of multiple sclerosis in Jewish and Arab populations in greater Jerusalem. Neuroepidemiology 2003;22:82–6.
61. Kim NH, Kim HJ, Cheong HK, et al. Prevalence of multiple sclerosis in Korea. Neurology 2010;75:1432–8.
62. Lai CH, Tseng HF. Population-based epidemiological study of neurological diseases in Taiwan: I. Creutzfeldt-Jakob disease and multiple sclerosis. Neuroepidemiology 2009;33:247–53.
63. Lau KK, Wong LK, Li LS, et al. Epidemiological study of multiple sclerosis in Hong Kong Chinese: questionnaire survey. Hong Kong Med J 2002;8:77–80.
64. Osoegawa M, Kira J, Fukazawa T, et al. Temporal changes and geographical differences in multiple sclerosis phenotypes in Japanese: nationwide survey results over 30 years. Mult Scler 2009;15:159–73.
65. Saadatnia M, Etemadifar M, Maghzi AH. Multiple sclerosis in Isfahan, Iran. Int Rev Neurobiol 2007;79:357–75.
66. Sahraian MA, Khorramnia S, Ebrahim MM, et al. Multiple sclerosis in Iran: a demographic study of 8,000 patients and changes over time. Eur Neurol 2010;64: 331–6.
67. Tsai CP, Yuan CL, Yu HY, et al. Multiple sclerosis in Taiwan. J Chin Med Assoc 2004;67:500–5.
68. Turk Boru U, Alp R, Sur H, et al. Prevalence of multiple sclerosis door-to-door survey in Maltepe, Istanbul, Turkey. Neuroepidemiology 2006;27:17–21.
69. Yu YL, Woo E, Hawkins BR, et al. Multiple sclerosis amongst Chinese in Hong Kong. Brain 1989;112:1445–67.
70. Svejgaard A. The immunogenetics of multiple sclerosis. Immunogenetics 2008; 60:275–86.
71. McFarland HF, Greenstein F, McFarlin DE, et al. Family and twin studies in multiple sclerosis. Ann N Y Acad Sci 1985;436:118–24.
72. Ebers GC, Bulman DE, Sadovnick AD, et al. A population based study of multiple sclerosis in twins. N Engl J Med 1986;315:1638–42.
73. Ebers GC. Genetics and multiple sclerosis: an overview. Ann Neurol 1994;36: S12–4.
74. Clinical demographics of multiplex families with multiple sclerosis. Multiple Sclerosis Genetics Group. Ann Neurol 1998;43:530–4.
75. Herrera BM, Ramagopalan SV, Lincoln MR, et al. Parent-of-origin effects in MS: observations from avuncular pairs. Neurology 2008;1:799–803.
76. Mumford CJ, Wood NW, Kellar-Wood H, et al. The British Isles survey of multiple sclerosis in twins. Neurology 1994;44:11–5.
77. Baranzini SE, Mudge J, van Velkinburgh JC, et al. Genome, epigenome and RNA sequences of monozygotic twins discordant for multiple sclerosis. Nature 2010;464:1351–6.
78. Bashinskaya VV, Kulakova OG, Boyko AN, et al. A review of genome-wide association studies for multiple sclerosis: classical and hypothesis-drive approaches. Hum Genet 2015;134:1143–62.
79. Burdett T, Hall PN, Hasting E, et al. The NHGRI-EBI Catalog of published genome-wide association studies. Available at: http://www.ebi.ac.uk/gwas. Accessed December 15, 2015.

80. DeJager PL, Jia X, Wang J, et al. Meta-analysis of genome scans and replication identify CD6, IRF8 and TNFRSF1A as new multiple sclerosis susceptibility loci. Nat Genet 2009;41:776–82.
81. De Jager PL, Baecher-Allan C, Maier LM, et al. The role of the CD58 locus in multiple sclerosis. Proc Natl Acad Sci U S A 2009;106:5264–9.
82. De Jager PL, Chibnik LB, Cui J, et al. Integration of genetic risk factors into a clinical algorithm for multiple sclerosis susceptibility: a weighted genetic risk score. Lancet Neurol 2009;8:1111–9.
83. Patsopoulos NA, Bayer Pharma MS Genetics Working Group, Steering Committees of Studies Evaluating IFNβ-1b and a CCR1-Antagonist, et al. Genome-wide meta-analysis identifies novel multiple sclerosis susceptibility loci. Ann Neurol 2011;70:897–912.
84. Online Mendelian Inheritance in Man, OMIM®. Johns Hopkins University, Baltimore, MD; OMIM Entry #126200-Multiple Sclerosis, susceptibility to; MS. World Wide Web URL. Available at: http://omim.org/DOI 5/30/16. Accessed December 15, 2015.
85. Calabresi PA, Fields NS, Farnon EC, et al. ELI-spot of Th-1 cytokine secreting PBMC's in multiple sclerosis: correlation with MRI lesions. J Neuroimmunol 1998;85:212–9.
86. Cox GM, Kithcart AP, Pitt D, et al. Macrophage migration inhibitory factor potentiates autoimmune-mediated neuroinflammation. J Immunol 2013;191:1043–54.
87. Langkamp M, Hörnig SC, Hörnig JB, et al. Detection of myelin autoantibodies: evaluation of an assay system for diagnosis of multiple sclerosis in differentiation from other central nervous system diseases. Clin Chem Lab Med 2009;47: 1395–400.
88. Tzartos JS, Khan G, Vossenkamper A, et al. Association of innate immune activation with latent Epstein-Barr virus in active MS lesions. Neurology 2012;78: 15–23.
89. Willis SN, Stadelmann C, Rodig SJ, et al. Epstein-Barr virus infection is not a characteristic feature of multiple sclerosis brain. Brain 2009;132:3318–28.
90. Sargsyan SA, Shearer AJ, Ritchie AM, et al. Absence of Epstein-Barr virus in the brain and CSF of patients with multiple sclerosis. Neurology 2010;74:1127–35.
91. Kurtzke JF, Beebe GW, Norman JE. Epidemiology of multiple sclerosis in U.S. veterans. 1. Race, sex, and geographic distribution. Neurology 1979;29: 1228–35.
92. Kurtzke JF, Beebe GW, Norman JE. Epidemiology of multiple sclerosis in U.S. veterans. 3. Migration and the risk of MS. Neurology 1985;35:672–8.
93. Smith CR, Scheinberg LC. Clinical features of multiple sclerosis. Semin Neurol 1985;5:85–93.
94. Chung SE, Cheong HK, Park JH, et al. Burden of disease of multiple sclerosis in Korea. Epidemiol Health 2012;34:e2012008.
95. Waxman SG. Membranes, myelin, and the pathophysiology of multiple sclerosis. N Engl J Med 1982;306:1529–33.
96. Popescu BF, Lucchinetti CF. Meningeal and cortical grey matter pathology in multiple sclerosis. BMC Neurol 2012;12:11.
97. Wolkorte R, Heersema DJ, Zijdewind I. Muscle fatigability during a sustained index finger abduction and depression scores are associated with perceived fatigue in patients with relapsing-remitting multiple sclerosis. Neurorehabil Neural Repair 2015;8:796–802.
98. Lublin FD, Reingold SC. Defining the clinical course of multiple sclerosis: results of an international survey. Neurology 1996;6:907–11.

99. McAlpine D. The benign form of multiple sclerosis: a study based on 241 cases seen with three years of onset and followed up until the tenth year or more of the disease. Brain 1961;84:185–203.

100. Detels R, Clark VA, Valdiviezo NL, et al. Factors associated with a rapid course of multiple sclerosis. Arch Neurol 1982;39:337–41.

101. Poser S, Kurtzke JF, Poser W, et al. Survival in multiple sclerosis. J Clin Epidemiol 1989;42:159–68.

102. Runmarker B, Andersen O. Prognostic factors in a multiple sclerosis incidence cohort with twenty-five years of follow-up. Brain 1993;116:117–34.

103. Poser CM, Paty DW, Scheinberg L, et al. New diagnostic criteria for multiple sclerosis: guidelines for research protocols. Ann Neurol 1983;13:227–31.

104. McDonald WI, Compston A, Edan G, et al. Recommended diagnostic criteria for multiple sclerosis: guidelines from the International Panel on the diagnosis of multiple sclerosis. Ann Neurol 2001;50:121–7.

105. Polman CH, Reingold Edan G, Edan G, et al. Diagnostic accuracy for multiple sclerosis: 2005 revisions to the "McDonald Criteria". Ann Neurol 2005;58:840–6.

106. Dalton CM, Brex PA, Miszkiel KA, et al. Application of the new McDonald criteria to patients with clinically isolated syndromes suggestive of multiple sclerosis. Ann Neurol 2002;52:47–53.

107. Montalban X, Tintore M, Swanton J, et al. MRI criteria for MS in patients with clinically isolated syndromes. Neurology 2010;74:427–34.

108. CHAMPS Study Group. MRI predictors of early conversion to clinically definite MS in the CHAMPS placebo group. Neurology 2002;59:998–1005.

109. Barkhof F, Rocca M, Francis G, et al. Validation of diagnostic magnetic resonance imaging criteria for multiple sclerosis and response to interferon beta-1a. Ann Neurol 2002;53:718–24.

110. Tintore M, Rovira A, Rio J, et al. New diagnostic criteria for multiple sclerosis: application in first demyelinating episode. Neurology 2003;60:27–30.

111. Polman CH, Reingold SC, Banwell B, et al. Diagnostic criteria for multiple sclerosis: 2010 revisions to the McDonald criteria. Ann Neurol 2011;69:292–302.

112. Swanton JK, Rovira A, Tintore M, et al. MRI criteria for multiple sclerosis in patients presenting with clinically isolated syndromes: a multicenter retrospective study. Lancet Neurol 2007;6:677–86.

113. Swanton JK, Fernando K, Dalton CM, et al. Modification of MRI criteria for multiple sclerosis in patients with clinically isolated syndromes. J Neurol Neurosurg Psychiatry 2006;77:830–3.

114. Inglese M, Grossman RI, Filippi M. Magnetic resonance imaging monitoring of multiple sclerosis lesion evolution. J Neuroimaging 2005;15(Suppl4):22S–9S.

115. Thompson AJ, Kaufman P, Shortman RC, et al. Oligoclonal immunoglobulins and plasma cells in spinal fluid of patients with multiple sclerosis. Br Med J 1979;1:16–7.

116. Kostulas VK, Link H, Lefvert AK. Oligoclonal IgG bands in cerebrospinal fluid. Principles for demonstration and interpretation based on findings in 1114 neurological patients. Arch Neurol 1987;44:1041–4.

117. Ingram DA, Thompson AJ, Swash M. Central motor conduction in multiple sclerosis: evaluation of abnormalities revealed by transcutaneous magnetic stimulation of the brain. J Neurol Neurosurg Psychiatry 1988;51:487–94.

118. Rubiera M, Rio J, Tintore M, et al. Neuromyelitis optica diagnosis in clinically isolated syndromes suggestive of multiple sclerosis. Neurology 2006;66:1568–70.

119. Lennon VA, Wingerchuk DM, Kryzer TJ, et al. A serum autoantibody marker of neuromyelitis optica: distinction from multiple sclerosis. Lancet 2004;364: 2106–12.
120. Weinshenker BG, Wingerchuk DM, Pittock SJ, et al. NMO-IgG: a specific biomarker for neuromyelitis optica. Dis Markers 2006;22:197–206.
121. Sellner J, Boggild M, Clanet M, et al. EFNS guidelines on diagnosis and management of neuromyelitis optica. Eur J Neurol 2010;17:1010–32.
122. Papadopoulos MC, Verkman A. Aquaporin 4 and neuromyelitis optica. Lancet Neurol 2012;11:535–44.
123. Jayakrishnan MP, Krishnakumar P. Clinical profile of acute disseminated encephalomyelitis in children. J Pediatr Neurosci 2010;5:111–4.
124. Younger DS, Younger APJ. Vasculitis and connective tissue disorders. In: Kalman B, Brannagan TH III, editors. Neuroimmunology in clinical practice. Hoboken (NJ): Wiley-Blackwell; 2008.
125. Younger DS, Younger APJ. CNS vasculitis. In: Coyle P, Rivzi S, editors. Clinical neuroimmunology: multiple sclerosis and related disorders. New York: Springer; 2011.
126. Vandenbark AA, Chou YK, Whitham R, et al. Treatment of multiple sclerosis with T-cell receptor peptides: results of a double-blind pilot trial. Nat Med 1996;2: 1109–15.
127. Van Diemen HAM, Polman CH, van Dongen TM, et al. The effect of 4-aminopyridine on clinical signs in multiple sclerosis: a randomized, placebo-controlled, double-blind, cross-over study. Ann Neurol 1992;32:123–30.
128. Bever CT, Young D, Anderson PA, et al. The effects of 4-aminopyridine in multiple sclerosis patients: results of a randomized, placebo-controlled, double-blind, concentration-controlled, crossover trial. Neurology 1994;44:1054–9.
129. Schapiro RT. Symptom management in multiple sclerosis. Ann Neurol 1994;36: S123–9.
130. Whittle IR, Haddow LJ. CT guided thalamotomy for movement disorders in multiple sclerosis: problems and paradoxes. Acta Neurochir 1995;64:S13–6.

Alzheimer Disease and Its Growing Epidemic

Risk Factors, Biomarkers, and the Urgent Need for Therapeutics

Richard A. Hickman, BMedSc (Hons), MBChB (Hons), MRCSEd[a,1],
Arline Faustin, MD[b,c,1], Thomas Wisniewski, MD[b,c,d,*]

KEYWORDS

- Alzheimer disease • Risk factors • Biomarkers • Epidemiology

KEY POINTS

- Alzheimer disease (AD) is increasing in prevalence worldwide.
- Many individuals have preclinical AD without symptoms.
- Biomarkers are currently in development for detecting preclinical AD that may be amenable to novel therapies.
- Addressing modifiable risk factors should also help to reduce the prevalence of AD in the future.

INTRODUCTION

Alzheimer disease (AD) represents one of the greatest medical challenges of this century; the condition is becoming increasingly prevalent worldwide and as yet, no effective treatments have been developed for this terminal disease. In the United States in 2016, more than 5 million people suffer with AD, costing an approximate $236 billion. Because the disease manifests at a late stage after a long period of clinically silent

None of the authors have anything to disclose.
Funding: NIH: AG08051; AG20245; NS073502.
[a] Department of Pathology, New York University School of Medicine, Alexandria ERSP, 450 East 29th Street, New York, NY 10016, USA; [b] Department of Pathology, The Center for Cognitive Neurology, New York University School of Medicine, Alexandria ERSP, 450 East 29th Street, New York, NY 10016, USA; [c] Department of Neurology, The Center for Cognitive Neurology, New York University School of Medicine, Alexandria ERSP, 450 East 29th Street, New York, NY 10016, USA; [d] Department of Psychiatry, The Center for Cognitive Neurology, New York University School of Medicine, Alexandria ERSP, 450 East 29th Street, New York, NY 10016, USA
[1] These authors contributed equally.
* Corresponding author. Department of Neurology, The Center for Cognitive Neurology, New York University School of Medicine, Alexandria ERSP, 450 East 29th Street, New York, NY 10016.
E-mail address: Thomas.wisniewski@nyumc.org

neurodegeneration, knowledge of the modifiable risk factors and the implementation of biomarkers is crucial in the primary prevention of the disease and presymptomatic detection of AD, respectively. This article discusses the growing epidemic of AD and antecedent risk factors in the disease process. Disease biomarkers are discussed and the implications that this may have for the treatment of this currently incurable disease.

EPIDEMIOLOGY

AD is the most common dementia in the elderly and is a growing epidemic across the globe. Although the risks associated with developing AD are multifactorial, the greatest risk factor by far is aging.[1] The age-specific risk of AD dramatically increases as individuals get older; findings from the Framingham study in the early 1990s showed that the incidence doubles every 5 years up to the age of 89 years.[2] Age-dependent increases have been seen in other studies.[3-5] Unsurprisingly, with global reductions in fertility and extended life expectancies, the number of patients with AD is expected to increase as populations age.[6] In the United States, it is estimated that approximately 5.3 million people had AD in 2015; a total of 5.1 million people being 65 years and older and approximately 200,000 people younger than age 65 years with early onset AD (EOAD).[7-9] It is estimated that the number of new cases of AD and other dementias will at least double by 2050 and substantially increase the socioeconomic burden worldwide.[7,10]

In 2010, it was estimated that dementia afflicted 35.6 million people worldwide, many of which will have AD, with the projection that this figure will double every 20 years.[11] The incidence of AD is generally lower in many less economically developed countries than in North America and Europe; however, sharp rises in prevalence have been predicted and seen in China, India, and Latin America.[12,13]

The effect of this increasing dementia has obvious socioeconomic consequences for each country affected, through costs of hospital care and also of caregivers. In the United States, the total payments were estimated at $226 billion of which Medicare and Medicaid provided 68%,[7,14] whereas out-of-pocket expenses for patients and their families were expected to be $44 billion.[7]

CLASSIFICATION AND STAGING

Revised criteria and guidelines by the National Institute on Aging and the Alzheimer Association published in 2011 have recognized three stages of AD: (1) preclinical AD, (2) mild cognitive impairment (MCI) caused by AD, and (3) dementia caused by AD.[8,15] These are described as follows[7]:

1. Preclinical AD: presymptomatic of AD with early AD-related brain changes as detected by neuroimaging or other biomarker studies
2. MCI caused by AD: mild cognitive decline but still able to perform activities of daily living
3. Dementia caused by AD: cognitive decline is more pronounced and interferes with activities of daily living

With this classification in mind, it follows that the actual number of individuals with active disease is a gross underestimate because it is based on approximations of diagnosed symptomatic patients and largely ignores the vast number of individuals who are preclinical, in whom the disease process is active but asymptomatic.[16] This long preclinical phase of AD is characterized by progressive neuronal loss, the formation of neurofibrillary tangles, and the deposition of amyloid plaques within the brain.[17-20] Although the exact pathogenesis of AD is debated, the prevailing hypothesis is that the neurodegeneration is the result of the amyloid cascade, in which aberrant digestion and processing of the amyloid precursor protein (APP) results in the accumulation of neurotoxic Aβ oligomeric proteins.[21–24] These proteins aggregate to form the insoluble amyloid plaques that are seen at microscopic examination of autopsy brains of patients with AD.

BIOMARKERS

It is widely believed that future therapeutics should be introduced during the preclinical and MCI stages of the disease course so as to preserve the existing functioning neural networks.[7,25] To provide effective recognition of preclinical AD, there will likely need to be widespread implementation of disease biomarkers, such as in national screening programs targeting specific age groups and other high-risk categories. Such screening may prove popular because many patients are keen to know their disease status at an earlier time point.[26–28]

Current disease biomarkers focus on indicators of cerebral amyloidosis or synaptic dysfunction. Markers of brain amyloidosis include reduced cerebrospinal fluid $A\beta_{42}$ concentrations and increased amyloid tracer uptake on PET.[29] These changes are followed after a period of time with markers of neuronal injury, notably increased cerebrospinal fluid tau levels and brain atrophy on MRI.[30,31] PET tau imaging has great promise as a biomarker and may be able to provide estimates of pathologic disease stage.[32] Validation is needed before introduction of these tests into the clinical setting, but would certainly be useful in providing a more complete overview of the current number of patients with AD and also in evaluating preclinical therapeutic response.

RISK FACTORS

The modifiable and nonmodifiable risk factors of AD are important because they provide insight into the predispositions of the disease process before onset and also provide stratification of individuals who may be at increased risk. Besides aging, which is the most significant risk factor, other determinants of AD include genetic risk factors and nongenetic modifiable risk factors.

NONMODIFIABLE GENETIC RISK FACTORS

Recent genome-wide association studies have revealed many new genes that increase the risk of developing AD.[33] This review, however, considers the most commonly discussed genetic influences on the disease, notably mutations in ApoE, APP, and presenilin mutations.

Apolipoprotein E

Of all of the mutations identified in AD, genome-wide association studies have demonstrated that it is the ε4 allele of the *APOE* gene that poses the greatest risk for AD.[34–38] ApoE is a 34-kDa astrocytic protein that is encoded on chromosome 19q13. The apoE gene has three alleles that result in the production of ε2, ε3, and ε4 isoforms. One of its principal functions within the central nervous system (CNS) is the delivery of cholesterol to neurons via the ApoE receptor.[39] ApoE3 is the most common variant, present in approximately 60% of the population, and is regarded as having no altered risk in AD.[7,35,36] However, the next most common allele is the ε4 followed by the ε2 allele. ApoE heterozygosity with ApoE4/E3 or ApoE4 homozygosity confers a significantly risk of developing AD, from 3-fold to 8- to 12-fold, respectively. In approximately 40% of cases of AD, ApoE4 is identified.[40] Furthermore, patients with ApoE4 have poorer cognitive performance in childhood and tend to develop the disease significantly earlier than those with ApoE3.[41] In a population-based study, patients who had suffered a head injury and carried the ApoE4 allele had a 10 times increased risk of developing AD, unlike those without the allele who were at two-fold increased risk.[42] The MIRAGE study demonstrated that patients who have suffered head injury are at markedly increased risk of developing AD.[43] Importantly, the ε2 isoform bestows a decreased risk of AD than the ε3 allele.[36] It comes as no surprise, therefore, that the ε2 allele is overrepresented in centenarians.[44]

Triggering Receptor on Myeloid Cells 2

Discovery of the triggering receptor on myeloid cells 2 (TREM2) allele as a rare genetic predisposition for AD has sparked interest because of its role in inflammation.[45] TREM2 is a receptor found on microglia that is important in phagocytosis and in dampening the CNS immune response.[46] Mutation in TREM2 is rare; however, the most common receptor mutation (R47H) increases the risk of late onset Alzheimer disease (LOAD) by approximately two-fold. Furthermore, mutations in TREM2 are associated with more severe degrees of atrophy in AD than those without.[47] Mutations in TREM2 that increase the risk and severity of AD may result from derangements in neuroinflammation and amyloid clearance.

Amyloid Precursor Protein and Presenilin Mutations

EOAD, which usually begins in patients younger than 65 years of age, represents less than 1% of cases of AD.[48] EOAD is often caused by autosomal-dominant mutations, such as mutations in APP, presenilin-1, and presenilin-2 genes.[48]

Mutations in proteins that are involved in the synthesis of Aβ result in downstream overproduction of the pathologic Aβ. APP is encoded on chromosome 21q21.3 and comprises three transcript variants, the most common of which protein within the CNS is 695 amino acids long.[49] More than 30 coding APP mutations have been identified that usually result in an autosomal-dominant EOAD because of increased Aβ production, shifts in synthesis of pathologic $A\beta_{1-42}$, or production of Aβ that may have increased susceptibility to aggregation.[50] Of interest, not all APP mutations result in AD preponderance; actually, one mutation was found to be protective.[50]

Presenilin is one of the proteins that constitute the active site of γ-secretase and therefore mutations alter the efficacy of this enzyme increasing the amount of $A\beta_{1-42}$ production. Presenilin mutations account for most cases of familial AD.[48]

Down Syndrome

Down syndrome is the most common chromosomal abnormality with an incidence of 1 per 733 live births and is characterized by trisomy 21.[49] Because APP is encoded on chromosome 21q21.3, this results in three copies of the APP protein. This increased abundance of APP expression, production of Aβ is considered to be one of the mechanisms as to why many of these patients develop EOAD. Given that the lifespan of patients with Down syndrome is now 55 to 60 years of age, approximately 70% of patients will suffer from AD.[51]

Cardiovascular Health

A large body of evidence suggests that cardiovascular disease increases the risk of dementia. Studies that have investigated patients with clinical and subclinical cardiovascular disease have poorer cognitive function than those without.[52,53] Cortical ischemic changes can increase the risk of dementia.[54] However, studying the role of cardiovascular disease and AD is complicated by several issues, notably that extensive cardiovascular disease and dementia may preclude from a clinical diagnosis of AD and may instead favor a diagnosis of multi-infarct dementia.[55]

Studies have shown mixed results with regard to the influence of hypertension and this is in part caused by differences in study design.[54,56–58] Observational studies, however, have generally shown that increased hypertension is associated with cognitive decline and an increased likelihood of developing AD, possibly through blood vessel injury, protein extravasation, neuronal injury, and subsequent Aβ accumulation.[59]

Diabetes Mellitus

Diabetes mellitus (DM) is associated with an increased risk of cognitive decline and AD later in life. Observational studies of type 2 DM (T2DM) have found that T2DM nearly doubles the risk of AD.[60–62] In the Religious Orders Study, 824 individuals who were older than 55 years of age were evaluated for cognitive decline and AD, and it was found that those with DM had a 65% increased risk of developing AD after a mean 5.5-year period.[63] The cognitive decline was found to be mainly in perceptual speed. Several meta-analyses have further confirmed an increased risk of AD in DM. The biologic mechanism for this association may relate to competition of Aβ and insulin for insulin-degrading enzyme, thereby reducing Aβ clearance. Alternatively, increased Aβ aggregation has been demonstrated through increased age-related glycation end-products that can occur in DM.

Antidiabetic therapies in patients with DM and cognitive impairment and also in patients with AD have shown improvement in cognition, which may be related to the anti-inflammatory properties of these drugs.

Traumatic Brain Injury

Traumatic brain injury (TBI) is a growing public health concern worldwide because the incidence is rising and it carries a significant health care and socioeconomic burden for society.[64–68] For patients who survive TBI, the average life expectancy is considerably shortened and many cases of TBI suffer chronic neurologic and psychological morbidity that reduces quality of life.[69–72] More data are now showing that there are ongoing chronic changes within the brain following TBI and that these ensuing processes may result in further damage with possible neurodegenerative sequelae.[73]

The first documentation of a syndrome that directed attention toward a neurodegenerative phenomenon after head injury was "punch drunk syndrome." This syndrome described degenerative changes after repeated episodes of sublethal head injuries in professional boxers.[74] This condition is now termed chronic traumatic encephalopathy and afflicts a diverse range of people including professional and amateur players of contact sports and military veterans.[75–78] Chronic traumatic encephalopathy has pathologic features that overlap with AD and TBI is recognized to shorten the time to onset of AD.[79] Furthermore, it is now considered that TBI is the most significant environmental risk factor for AD.[76,80]

Recent data have demonstrated that in long-standing TBI and AD there is chronic inflammation within the brain parenchyma and this persistent inflammatory milieu within the brain parenchyma could be where the pathophysiology of TBI and AD converge.[81,82]

Following TBI the amyloid levels increase because of several factors. First, APP expression is noticeably increased post-TBI.[83,84] APP is particularly prominent at the axon terminals where there has been axonal transection and axonal transection is known to occur even in mild cases of TBI.[85,86] Second, β-secretase and γ-secretase, enzymes that contribute to the digestion of APP and formation of Aβ, are also upregulated.[87–89] These increases in substrate and enzymes result in increased deposition of amyloid at the axon bulbs and offers one explanation as to how the risk of AD is increased after TBI.[90]

The Influence of Neprilysin and Traumatic Brain Injury

Removal of cerebral amyloid is likely to be multifactorial, involving partly passive diffusion of soluble amyloid, active transport mechanisms, and cellular digestion.[91,92] The degree of amyloid pathology post-TBI and in AD is particularly influenced by neprilysin. Neprilysin is a membrane zinc metalloprotease that is capable of digesting Aβ peptide and thus has the capability of reducing the amyloid load within the brain.[93] Neprilysin knockout mice demonstrate increased amyloid burden in a gene–dose dependent correlation.[94] Johnson and colleagues[95] demonstrated that in postmortem subjects, the degree of amyloid burden was most in patients who had more than 41 GT repeats in the promoter region of the neprilysin gene, which was considered to be related to defective amyloid clearance. Curiously, neprilysin expression increases post-TBI and this may be a mechanism by which Aβ and amyloid plaques are cleared months after injury, despite increased intra-axonal APP and presenilin-1 expression.[96] With age-related reduction in neprilysin, the balance between formation of amyloid and its breakdown may shift toward accumulation of amyloid and this may be responsible for the preponderance to AD post-TBI.[97]

There is also likely to be a contribution to amyloid breakdown from microglial activation. Neprilysin, metalloproteinase-9, and several other factors that are released by healthy microglia digest Aβ.[98] There is a heightened neuroinflammatory response following TBI that persists, and the activation of microglia most likely releases factors that assist in the digestion of Aβ. However, with aging, the efficacy of microglial breakdown is likely to be lost, and may even accentuate the accumulation, thereby causing a gradual shift toward accumulation of amyloid in the dynamic Aβ turnover.[99]

Previous Amyloid Exposure

One of the most concerning developments over the past few years has been the accumulation of evidence that suggests infectivity of amyloid in a prion-like fashion. In a recent case series of iatrogenic Creutzfeldt-Jakob disease, a proportion of patients who received homogenized human pituitaries for growth hormone replacement were found to have significant cerebral amyloid angiopathy at autopsy, to an extent that was inconsistent with age.[100] Given that pituitaries may have amyloid deposits, there is the possibility that amyloid could seed through peripheral injection with proteopathic spread over subsequent decades.[100,101] The proteopathic spread of amyloid in the brain has been demonstrated in numerous animal models and in human AD pathologic staging.[102]

The main fear that stems from these findings is that iatrogenic infection may occur from reused surgical instruments, because amyloid is difficult to remove from metal devices.[103] Further research is needed in this area to gauge the significance of these findings on amyloid infectivity.

Protective Factors

In general, environmental influences that are anti-inflammatory seem to be beneficial at reducing the likelihood of developing AD. Low-calorie diets that are sustained for a protracted period of time are associated with reduced free radical production and increased brain neurogenesis and brain-derived neurotrophic factor (BDNF) concentrations, all of which are recognized to promote healthier brain aging.[44,104] Data regarding diets that are rich in antioxidants and polyunsaturated fatty acids have proved inconclusive with some studies demonstrating a reduction in the risk of AD, whereas others show no such association.[105–107]

Other protective influences include cognitive stimulation and a high educational achievement, which improves cognitive reserve.[108,109] Physical exercise does seem to reduce the risk of developing dementia and can show improvements in cognition in patients with dementia.[110–114]

PERSPECTIVES

Although the incidence of AD seems to be increasing worldwide, the age-specific risk of developing AD in high-income countries may be decreasing. Changes in diet, exercise, education, and management of chronic conditions, such as DM, seem to be improving the individual age-specific risk of AD within the United States.[115] However, in view of longer life expectancies and worldwide increases in the prevalence of other risk factors, such as obesity and DM, the incidence of AD is most likely set to increase considerably with significant socioeconomic impact.

Future work on the development and validation of biomarkers and on the introduction of therapeutics into the preclinical phase of AD has the greatest promise in the effective treatment of this otherwise incurable disease.

REFERENCES

1. Esiri MM, Chance SA. Cognitive reserve, cortical plasticity and resistance to Alzheimer's disease. Alzheimers Res Ther 2012;4(2):7.
2. Bachman DL, Wolf PA, Linn RT, et al. Incidence of dementia and probable Alzheimer's disease in a general population: the Framingham Study. Neurology 1993;43(3 Pt 1):515–9.
3. Vardarajan BN, Faber KM, Bird TD, et al. Age-specific incidence rates for dementia and Alzheimer disease in NIA-LOAD/NCRAD and EFIGA families: National Institute on Aging Genetics Initiative for Late-Onset Alzheimer Disease/National Cell Repository for Alzheimer Disease (NIA-LOAD/NCRAD) and Estudio Familiar de Influencia Genetica en Alzheimer (EFIGA). JAMA Neurol 2014; 71(3):315–23.
4. Edland SD, Rocca WA, Petersen RC, et al. Dementia and Alzheimer disease incidence rates do not vary by sex in Rochester, Minn. Arch Neurol 2002; 59(10):1589–93.
5. Ott A, Breteler MM, van Harskamp F, et al. Prevalence of Alzheimer's disease and vascular dementia: association with education. The Rotterdam study. BMJ 1995;310(6985):970–3.
6. Prince M, Wimo A, Guerchet M, et al. World Alzheimer Report 2015: the Global Impact of Dementia; 2015. Available at: https://www.alz.co.uk/research/WorldAlzheimerReport2015.pdf.
7. Alzheimer's Association. 2015 Alzheimer's disease facts and figures. Alzheimers Dement 2015;11(3):332–84.
8. Hebert LE, Weuve J, Scherr PA, et al. Alzheimer disease in the United States (2010-2050) estimated using the 2010 census. Neurology 2013;80(19):1778–83.
9. Alzheimer's Association. Early-onset dementia: a national challenge, a future crisis. Washington, DC: Alzheimer's Association; 2006.
10. Brookmeyer R, Johnson E, Ziegler-Graham K, et al. Forecasting the global burden of Alzheimer's disease. Alzheimers Dement 2007;3(3):186–91.
11. Prince M, Bryce R, Albanese E, et al. The global prevalence of dementia: a systematic review and metaanalysis. Alzheimers Dement 2013;9(1):63–75.e2.

12. Kalaria RN, Maestre GE, Arizaga R, et al. Alzheimer's disease and vascular dementia in developing countries: prevalence, management, and risk factors. Lancet Neurol 2008;7(9):812–26.

13. Ferri CP, Prince M, Brayne C, et al. Global prevalence of dementia: a Delphi consensus study. Lancet (London, England) 2005;366(9503):2112–7.

14. Hurd MD, Martorell P, Langa KM. Monetary costs of dementia in the United States. N Engl J Med 2013;369(5):489–90.

15. Jack CR Jr, Albert MS, Knopman DS, et al. Introduction to the recommendations from the National Institute on Aging-Alzheimer's Association workgroups on diagnostic guidelines for Alzheimer's disease. Alzheimers Dement 2011;7(3):257–62.

16. McKhann G, Drachman D, Folstein M, et al. Clinical diagnosis of Alzheimer's disease: report of the NINCDS-ADRDA Work Group under the auspices of Department of Health and Human Services Task Force on Alzheimer's Disease. Neurology 1984;34(7):939–44.

17. Nelson PT, Alafuzoff I, Bigio EH, et al. Correlation of Alzheimer disease neuropathologic changes with cognitive status: a review of the literature. J Neuropathol Exp Neurol 2012;71(5):362–81.

18. Consensus recommendations for the postmortem diagnosis of Alzheimer's disease. The National Institute on Aging, and Reagan Institute Working Group on Diagnostic Criteria for the Neuropathological Assessment of Alzheimer's Disease. Neurobiol Aging 1997;18(4 Suppl):S1–2.

19. Brier MR, McCarthy JE, Benzinger TL, et al. Local and distributed PiB accumulation associated with development of preclinical Alzheimer's disease. Neurobiol Aging 2016;38:104–11.

20. Saito S, Yamamoto Y, Ihara M. Mild cognitive impairment: at the crossroad of neurodegeneration and vascular dysfunction. Curr Alzheimer Res 2015;12(6):507–12.

21. Hardy J, Allsop D. Amyloid deposition as the central event in the aetiology of Alzheimer's disease. Trends Pharmacol Sci 1991;12(10):383–8.

22. Tanzi RE, Bertram L. Twenty years of the Alzheimer's disease amyloid hypothesis: a genetic perspective. Cell 2005;120(4):545–55.

23. Wisniewski T, Goni F. Immunotherapeutic approaches for Alzheimer's disease. Neuron 2015;85(6):1162–76.

24. Di Paolo G, Kim TW. Linking lipids to Alzheimer's disease: cholesterol and beyond. Nat Rev Neurosci 2011;12(5):284–96.

25. Bloudek LM, Spackman DE, Blankenburg M, et al. Review and meta-analysis of biomarkers and diagnostic imaging in Alzheimer's disease. J Alzheimers Dis 2011;26(4):627–45.

26. Wikler EM, Blendon RJ, Benson JM. Would you want to know? Public attitudes on early diagnostic testing for Alzheimer's disease. Alzheimers Res Ther 2013;5(5):43.

27. Neumann PJ, Cohen JT, Hammitt JK, et al. Willingness-to-pay for predictive tests with no immediate treatment implications: a survey of US residents. Health Econ 2012;21(3):238–51.

28. Kopits IM, Chen C, Roberts JS, et al. Willingness to pay for genetic testing for Alzheimer's disease: a measure of personal utility. Genet Test Mol Biomarkers 2011;15(12):871–5.

29. Jack CR Jr, Knopman DS, Jagust WJ, et al. Hypothetical model of dynamic biomarkers of the Alzheimer's pathological cascade. Lancet Neurol 2010;9(1):119–28.

30. Toledo JB, Xie SX, Trojanowski JQ, et al. Longitudinal change in CSF Tau and Abeta biomarkers for up to 48 months in ADNI. Acta Neuropathol 2013; 126(5):659–70.
31. Vemuri P, Wiste HJ, Weigand SD, et al. Serial MRI and CSF biomarkers in normal aging, MCI, and AD. Neurology 2010;75(2):143–51.
32. James OG, Doraiswamy PM, Borges-Neto S. PET imaging of tau pathology in Alzheimer's disease and tauopathies. Front Neurol 2015;6:38.
33. Karch CM, Goate AM. Alzheimer's disease risk genes and mechanisms of disease pathogenesis. Biol Psychiatry 2015;77(1):43–51.
34. Corder EH, Saunders AM, Strittmatter WJ, et al. Gene dose of apolipoprotein E type 4 allele and the risk of Alzheimer's disease in late onset families. Science 1993;261(5123):921–3.
35. Potter H, Wisniewski T. Apolipoprotein E: essential catalyst of the Alzheimer amyloid cascade. Int J Alzheimers Dis 2012;2012:489428.
36. Raber J, Huang Y, Ashford JW. ApoE genotype accounts for the vast majority of AD risk and AD pathology. Neurobiol Aging 2004;25(5):641–50.
37. Holtzman DM, Herz J, Bu G. Apolipoprotein E and apolipoprotein E receptors: normal biology and roles in Alzheimer disease. Cold Spring Harb Perspect Med 2012;2(3):a006312.
38. Spinney L. Alzheimer's disease: the forgetting gene. Nature 2014;510(7503): 26–8.
39. Bu G. Apolipoprotein E and its receptors in Alzheimer's disease: pathways, pathogenesis and therapy. Nat Rev Neurosci 2009;10(5):333–44.
40. Farrer LA, Cupples LA, Haines JL, et al. Effects of age, sex, and ethnicity on the association between apolipoprotein E genotype and Alzheimer disease. A meta-analysis. APOE and Alzheimer Disease Meta Analysis Consortium. JAMA 1997; 278(16):1349–56.
41. Deary IJ, Whiteman MC, Pattie A, et al. Apolipoprotein e gene variability and cognitive functions at age 79: a follow-up of the Scottish mental survey of 1932. Psychol Aging 2004;19(2):367–71.
42. Mayeux R, Ottman R, Maestre G, et al. Synergistic effects of traumatic head injury and apolipoprotein-epsilon 4 in patients with Alzheimer's disease. Neurology 1995;45(3 Pt 1):555–7.
43. Guo Z, Cupples LA, Kurz A, et al. Head injury and the risk of AD in the MIRAGE study. Neurology 2000;54(6):1316–23.
44. Esiri MM. Ageing and the brain. J Pathol 2007;211(2):181–7.
45. Guerreiro R, Wojtas A, Bras J, et al. TREM2 variants in Alzheimer's disease. N Engl J Med 2013;368(2):117–27.
46. Rohn TT. The triggering receptor expressed on myeloid cells 2: "TREM-ming" the inflammatory component associated with Alzheimer's disease. Oxid Med Cell Longev 2013;2013:860959.
47. Rajagopalan P, Hibar DP, Thompson PM. TREM2 and neurodegenerative disease. N Engl J Med 2013;369(16):1565–7.
48. Blennow K, de Leon MJ, Zetterberg H. Alzheimer's disease. Lancet (London, England) 2006;368(9533):387–403.
49. Bayer TA, Cappai R, Masters CL, et al. It all sticks together: the APP-related family of proteins and Alzheimer's disease. Mol Psychiatry 1999;4(6):524–8.
50. Jonsson T, Atwal JK, Steinberg S, et al. A mutation in APP protects against Alzheimer's disease and age-related cognitive decline. Nature 2012;488(7409): 96–9.

51. Hartley D, Blumenthal T, Carrillo M, et al. Down syndrome and Alzheimer's disease: common pathways, common goals. Alzheimers Dement 2015;11(6): 700–9.

52. Breteler MM, Claus JJ, Grobbee DE, et al. Cardiovascular disease and distribution of cognitive function in elderly people: the Rotterdam Study. BMJ 1994; 308(6944):1604–8.

53. Kuller LH, Shemanski L, Manolio T, et al. Relationship between ApoE, MRI findings, and cognitive function in the Cardiovascular Health Study. Stroke 1998; 29(2):388–98.

54. Reitz C, Brayne C, Mayeux R. Epidemiology of Alzheimer disease. Nat Rev Neurol 2011;7(3):137–52.

55. Stampfer MJ. Cardiovascular disease and Alzheimer's disease: common links. J Intern Med 2006;260(3):211–23.

56. Kivipelto M, Helkala EL, Hanninen T, et al. Midlife vascular risk factors and late-life mild cognitive impairment: a population-based study. Neurology 2001; 56(12):1683–9.

57. Launer LJ, Masaki K, Petrovitch H, et al. The association between midlife blood pressure levels and late-life cognitive function. The Honolulu-Asia Aging Study. JAMA 1995;274(23):1846–51.

58. Swan GE, Carmelli D, Larue A. Systolic blood pressure tracking over 25 to 30 years and cognitive performance in older adults. Stroke 1998;29(11):2334–40.

59. Kalaria RN. Vascular basis for brain degeneration: faltering controls and risk factors for dementia. Nutr Rev 2010;68(Suppl 2):S74–87.

60. Leibson CL, Rocca WA, Hanson VA, et al. The risk of dementia among persons with diabetes mellitus: a population-based cohort study. Ann N Y Acad Sci 1997; 826:422–7.

61. Luchsinger JA, Tang MX, Stern Y, et al. Diabetes mellitus and risk of Alzheimer's disease and dementia with stroke in a multiethnic cohort. Am J Epidemiol 2001; 154(7):635–41.

62. Ott A, Stolk RP, van Harskamp F, et al. Diabetes mellitus and the risk of dementia: the Rotterdam Study. Neurology 1999;53(9):1937–42.

63. Arvanitakis Z, Wilson RS, Bienias JL, et al. Diabetes mellitus and risk of Alzheimer disease and decline in cognitive function. Arch Neurol 2004;61(5):661–6.

64. Roozenbeek B, Maas AI, Menon DK. Changing patterns in the epidemiology of traumatic brain injury. Nat Rev Neurol 2013;9(4):231–6.

65. Maas AI, Stocchetti N, Bullock R. Moderate and severe traumatic brain injury in adults. Lancet Neurol 2008;7(8):728–41.

66. Langlois JA, Rutland-Brown W, Wald MM. The epidemiology and impact of traumatic brain injury: a brief overview. J Head Trauma Rehabil 2006;21(5):375–8.

67. Coronado VG, McGuire LC, Sarmiento K, et al. Trends in traumatic brain injury in the U.S. and the public health response: 1995-2009. J Safety Res 2012;43(4): 299–307.

68. Bruns J Jr, Hauser WA. The epidemiology of traumatic brain injury: a review. Epilepsia 2003;44(Suppl 10):2–10.

69. Dutton RP, Stansbury LG, Leone S, et al. Trauma mortality in mature trauma systems: are we doing better? An analysis of trauma mortality patterns, 1997-2008. J Trauma 2010;69(3):620–6.

70. Selassie AW, McCarthy ML, Ferguson PL, et al. Risk of posthospitalization mortality among persons with traumatic brain injury, South Carolina 1999-2001. J Head Trauma Rehabil 2005;20(3):257–69.

71. Ferguson PL, Smith GM, Wannamaker BB, et al. A population-based study of risk of epilepsy after hospitalization for traumatic brain injury. Epilepsia 2010; 51(5):891–8.

72. Fazel S, Wolf A, Pillas D, et al. Suicide, fatal injuries, and other causes of premature mortality in patients with traumatic brain injury: a 41-year Swedish Population Study. JAMA Psychiatry 2014;71(3):326–33.

73. Masel BE, DeWitt DS. Traumatic brain injury: a disease process, not an event. J Neurotrauma 2010;27(8):1529–40.

74. Martland HS. Punch drunk. JAMA 1928;91(15):1103–7.

75. McKee AC, Stern RA, Nowinski CJ, et al. The spectrum of disease in chronic traumatic encephalopathy. Brain 2013;136(Pt 1):43–64.

76. Shively S, Scher AI, Perl DP, et al. Dementia resulting from traumatic brain injury: what is the pathology? Arch Neurol 2012;69(10):1245–51.

77. Goldstein LE, Fisher AM, Tagge CA, et al. Chronic traumatic encephalopathy in blast-exposed military veterans and a blast neurotrauma mouse model. Sci Transl Med 2012;4(134):134ra160.

78. McKee AC, Cantu RC, Nowinski CJ, et al. Chronic traumatic encephalopathy in athletes: progressive tauopathy after repetitive head injury. J Neuropathol Exp Neurol 2009;68(7):709–35.

79. Plassman BL, Havlik RJ, Steffens DC, et al. Documented head injury in early adulthood and risk of Alzheimer's disease and other dementias. Neurology 2000;55(8):1158–66.

80. Fleminger S, Oliver DL, Lovestone S, et al. Head injury as a risk factor for Alzheimer's disease: the evidence 10 years on; a partial replication. J Neurol Neurosurg Psychiatry 2003;74(7):857–62.

81. Johnson VE, Stewart JE, Begbie FD, et al. Inflammation and white matter degeneration persist for years after a single traumatic brain injury. Brain 2013;136(Pt 1):28–42.

82. Smith C, Gentleman SM, Leclercq PD, et al. The neuroinflammatory response in humans after traumatic brain injury. Neuropathol Appl Neurobiol 2013;39(6): 654–66.

83. Pierce JE, Trojanowski JQ, Graham DI, et al. Immunohistochemical characterization of alterations in the distribution of amyloid precursor proteins and beta-amyloid peptide after experimental brain injury in the rat. J Neurosci 1996; 16(3):1083–90.

84. Van den Heuvel C, Blumbergs PC, Finnie JW, et al. Upregulation of amyloid precursor protein messenger RNA in response to traumatic brain injury: an ovine head impact model. Exp Neurol 1999;159(2):441–50.

85. Gentleman SM, Nash MJ, Sweeting CJ, et al. Beta-amyloid precursor protein (beta APP) as a marker for axonal injury after head injury. Neurosci Lett 1993; 160(2):139–44.

86. Oppenheimer DR. Microscopic lesions in the brain following head injury. J Neurol Neurosurg Psychiatry 1968;31(4):299–306.

87. Cribbs DH, Chen LS, Cotman CW, et al. Injury induces presenilin-1 gene expression in mouse brain. Neuroreport 1996;7(11):1773–6.

88. Nadler Y, Alexandrovich A, Grigoriadis N, et al. Increased expression of the gamma-secretase components presenilin-1 and nicastrin in activated astrocytes and microglia following traumatic brain injury. Glia 2008;56(5):552–67.

89. Blasko I, Beer R, Bigl M, et al. Experimental traumatic brain injury in rats stimulates the expression, production and activity of Alzheimer's disease beta-secretase (BACE-1). J Neural Transm 2004;111(4):523–36.

90. Clinton J, Roberts GW, Gentleman SM, et al. Differential pattern of beta-amyloid protein deposition within cortical sulci and gyri in Alzheimer's disease. Neuropathol Appl Neurobiol 1993;19(3):277–81.

91. Deane R, Sagare A, Zlokovic BV. The role of the cell surface LRP and soluble LRP in blood-brain barrier Abeta clearance in Alzheimer's disease. Curr Pharm Des 2008;14(16):1601–5.

92. Turner AJ, Fisk L, Nalivaeva NN. Targeting amyloid-degrading enzymes as therapeutic strategies in neurodegeneration. Ann N Y Acad Sci 2004;1035:1–20.

93. Iwata N, Tsubuki S, Takaki Y, et al. Identification of the major Abeta1-42-degrading catabolic pathway in brain parenchyma: suppression leads to biochemical and pathological deposition. Nat Med 2000;6(2):143–50.

94. Iwata N, Tsubuki S, Takaki Y, et al. Metabolic regulation of brain Abeta by neprilysin. Science 2001;292(5521):1550–2.

95. Johnson VE, Stewart W, Graham DI, et al. A neprilysin polymorphism and amyloid-beta plaques after traumatic brain injury. J Neurotrauma 2009;26(8):1197–202.

96. Chen XH, Johnson VE, Uryu K, et al. A lack of amyloid beta plaques despite persistent accumulation of amyloid beta in axons of long-term survivors of traumatic brain injury. Brain Pathol 2009;19(2):214–23.

97. Hellstrom-Lindahl E, Ravid R, Nordberg A. Age-dependent decline of neprilysin in Alzheimer's disease and normal brain: inverse correlation with A beta levels. Neurobiol Aging 2008;29(2):210–21.

98. Yan P, Hu X, Song H, et al. Matrix metalloproteinase-9 degrades amyloid-beta fibrils in vitro and compact plaques in situ. J Biol Chem 2006;281(34):24566–74.

99. Hickman SE, Allison EK, El Khoury J. Microglial dysfunction and defective beta-amyloid clearance pathways in aging Alzheimer's disease mice. J Neurosci 2008;28(33):8354–60.

100. Jaunmuktane Z, Mead S, Ellis M, et al. Evidence for human transmission of amyloid-beta pathology and cerebral amyloid angiopathy. Nature 2015;525(7568):247–50.

101. Irwin DJ, Abrams JY, Schonberger LB, et al. Evaluation of potential infectivity of Alzheimer and Parkinson disease proteins in recipients of cadaver-derived human growth hormone. JAMA Neurol 2013;70(4):462–8.

102. Eisele YS, Obermuller U, Heilbronner G, et al. Peripherally applied Abeta-containing inoculates induce cerebral beta-amyloidosis. Science 2010;330(6006):980–2.

103. Prusiner SB. Biology and genetics of prions causing neurodegeneration. Annu Rev Genet 2013;47:601–23.

104. Mattson MP, Maudsley S, Martin B. BDNF and 5-HT: a dynamic duo in age-related neuronal plasticity and neurodegenerative disorders. Trends Neurosci 2004;27(10):589–94.

105. Kalmijn S, Launer LJ, Ott A, et al. Dietary fat intake and the risk of incident dementia in the Rotterdam Study. Ann Neurol 1997;42(5):776–82.

106. Roberts RO, Cerhan JR, Geda YE, et al. Polyunsaturated fatty acids and reduced odds of MCI: the Mayo Clinic Study of Aging. J Alzheimers Dis 2010;21(3):853–65.

107. Engelhart MJ, Geerlings MI, Ruitenberg A, et al. Diet and risk of dementia: does fat matter?: The Rotterdam Study. Neurology 2002;59(12):1915–21.

108. Carlson MC, Helms MJ, Steffens DC, et al. Midlife activity predicts risk of dementia in older male twin pairs. Alzheimers Dement 2008;4(5):324–31.

109. Fratiglioni L, Wang HX. Brain reserve hypothesis in dementia. J Alzheimers Dis 2007;12(1):11–22.
110. Groot C, Hooghiemstra AM, Raijmakers PG, et al. The effect of physical activity on cognitive function in patients with dementia: a meta-analysis of randomized control trials. Ageing Res Rev 2016;25:13–23.
111. Abbott RD, White LR, Ross GW, et al. Walking and dementia in physically capable elderly men. JAMA 2004;292(12):1447–53.
112. Fratiglioni L, Paillard-Borg S, Winblad B. An active and socially integrated lifestyle in late life might protect against dementia. Lancet Neurol 2004;3(6): 343–53.
113. Rovio S, Kareholt I, Helkala EL, et al. Leisure-time physical activity at midlife and the risk of dementia and Alzheimer's disease. Lancet Neurol 2005;4(11):705–11.
114. Akbaraly TN, Portet F, Fustinoni S, et al. Leisure activities and the risk of dementia in the elderly: results from the Three-City Study. Neurology 2009;73(11): 854–61.
115. Langa KM. Is the risk of Alzheimer's disease and dementia declining? Alzheimers Res Ther 2015;7(1):34.

Epidemiology of Parkinson Disease

Andrea Lee, MD[a], Rebecca M. Gilbert, MD, PhD[a,b],*

KEYWORDS

- Parkinson disease • Epidemiology • Neuroepidemiology
- Neurodegenerative disorder

KEY POINTS

- Parkinson disease (PD) is the second most common neurodegenerative disorder, presenting with bradykinesia, rigidity, tremor, and postural instability.
- Incidence rates of PD are 8 to 18 per 100,000 person-years based on prospective population-based studies with either record-based or in-person case finding.
- Nonmotor symptoms include autonomic dysfunction, sleep disorders, mood disorders, cognitive abnormalities, and pain and sensory disorders. Hallucinations and dementia predict later nursing home placement.
- There are 18 PD-related gene loci that have been identified to date, with at least 7 disease-causing genes.
- PD is a very complicated condition for physicians to optimally manage, with specific rehabilitation needs and complicated psychosocial dynamics, all that evolve with time.

INTRODUCTION
Epidemiology

Parkinson disease (PD) is the second most common neurodegenerative disorder after Alzheimer disease and refers to the clinical presentation of bradykinesia, rigidity, tremor, and postural instability. The main known risk factor is increased age. The estimated prevalence of PD in industrialized countries is 0.3% in the general population, 1.0% in people older than 60 years, and 3.0% in those aged 80 years and older, with incidence rates of PD of 8 to 18 per 100,000 person-years based on prospective population-based studies with either record-based or in-person case finding.[1–3] The median age of onset is 60 years; the mean duration of the disease from diagnosis

The authors have nothing to declare.

[a] Department of Neurology, New York University School of Medicine, 240 East 38th Street, 20th Floor, New York, NY 10016, USA; [b] The Marlene and Paolo Fresco Institute for Parkinson's and Movement Disorders, New York University Langone Medical Center, 240 East 38th Street, 20th Floor, New York, NY 10016, USA

* Corresponding author. The Marlene and Paolo Fresco Institute for Parkinson's and Movement Disorders, New York University Langone Medical Center, 240 East 38th Street, 20th Floor, New York, NY 10016.

E-mail address: Rebecca.Gilbert2@nyumc.org

to death is 15 years, although patients can live for decades with PD.[4,5] Sex differences exist in PD.[6] In addition to older age, male sex is recognized as a prominent risk factor in developing PD. Both incidence and prevalence of PD are 1.5 to 2.0 times higher in men than in women.[7] Age at onset is 2.1 years later in women (53.4 years) than in men (51.3 years). Women present with a milder PD phenotype, as evidenced by higher presentation of tremor (67%) than men (48%) and a slower rate of motor impairment. Animal studies suggest that estrogen may play a neuroprotective role against cell death of striatal dopaminergic neurons. Nonmotor symptoms that are more prevalent in women are anxiety, depression, and constipation, whereas men suffered more from daytime sleepiness, drooling, and sexual symptoms.[8]

Natural History

The natural history of disability and progression of motor symptoms in PD has been well studied since the seminal article by Hoehn and Yahr in 1967.[9] The Hoehn and Yahr (H&Y) scale is the most commonly used system for describing the progression of PD. The transition from H&Y scale stage II to stage III is considered a pivotal milestone in PD when gait and balance impairment result in disability in many gait-dependent activities, such as walking, dressing, bathing, and housework. In one longitudinal study, the time to reach H&Y scale III was 7.73 years.[10] Male sex, gait disorder, lack of tremor, and lack of asymmetry as presenting clinical features are associated with poorer long-term survival.[11]

Clinical Subtypes

Subtypes of PD have emerged, with patients classified according to distinct clinical features, such as motor phenotype, or age of onset.[12] Patients presenting with tremor at onset have a slower progression of disease than those with a postural-instability-gait difficulty (PIGD) phenotype.[13] The PIGD form of PD is associated with a faster rate of cognitive decline and a higher incidence of dementia, whereas those with tremor-predominant PD start to show signs of dementia only after PIGD symptoms develop.[14] Patients with late-onset PD (aged >60 years) are often characterized by the PIGD subtype,[15] whereas young-onset PD (aged 20–40 years) presents more often with tremor, rigidity, dystonia and a higher rate of levodopa-related motor complications, such as dyskinesias.[12]

Nonmotor Symptoms

In addition to motor dysfunction, nonmotor symptoms (NMSs) of PD are recognized to play an extremely important role in adversely affecting the quality of life of patients with PD and may precede the formal diagnosis by decades.[17] The Braak hypothesis[16] suggests that Lewy bodies, the cellular abnormalities seen in neurons of Parkinson diseased brains, are found in multiple brain stem nuclei, causing non motor symptoms prior to their appearance in the areas of the brain that cause motor symptoms. In recent studies, at least one NMS was reported by almost 100% of patients with PD.[18–20] Some suggest that the NMSs of dementia and hallucinations are the strongest predictors of nursing home placement for patients with PD.[18] NMSs are broadly classified as autonomic dysfunction, sleep disorders, mood disorders, cognitive abnormalities, and pain and sensory disorders. Of these, dysautonomia, rapid eye movement (REM) sleep behavior disorder (RBD), depression, and olfactory disturbance have been shown to often predate the onset of motor symptoms of PD.

Dysautonomia

Dysautonomia associated with PD mainly consists of gastrointestinal dysfunction, genitourinary abnormalities, and cardiovascular dysfunction with orthostatic hypotension. Constipation is one of the most common NMSs with a prevalence ranging from 50% to 70%.[21,22] It was even described in James Parkinson's[23] original essay on PD and often precedes the development of motor symptoms.[22] Genitourinary dysfunction due to detrusor overactivity is the most frequent urodynamic abnormality,[24] which leads to urinary urgency, frequency, incontinence, and nocturia; it is estimated to have a prevalence of 25% to 50%.[25] Sexual dysfunction in men with PD presents mainly as erectile dysfunction, although decreased sexual drive and difficulty with arousal and orgasm have been reported in both sexes. Cardiovascular dysfunction is present in almost 60% of patients with PD.[18] Orthostatic hypotension can be one of the most debilitating cardiovascular NMSs and may manifest in an array of symptoms, including lightheadedness, fatigue, dyspnea on exertion, foggy thinking, or blurred vision.

Sleep disturbances
Sleep disturbances are exceedingly common in PD, and its prevalence may approach 90%.[26] These disturbances include RBD, restless legs syndrome, periodic limb movements of sleep, insomnia, and excessive daytime somnolence.[27] The most common form of sleep disturbance is sleep fragmentation with frequent awakenings, leading to excessive daytime somnolence. The problem is multifactorial and compounded by impaired ability to turn in bed due to rigidity and bradykinesia, nocturia, medication effects, and periodic limb movements.[18] Similar to constipation, RBD often precedes the motor onset of PD and has gained attention as a possible predictor for the development of the disease. RBD is characterized by acting out a dream during characteristic REM sleep, when there should be atonia on polysomnography.[28] The prevalence of RBD in PD may be in the range of 25% to 50%, and some studies suggest that patients with RBD have an 80% to 90% risk of eventually developing PD.[18] It is important to identify RBD in patients with PD because it can potentially be dangerous to the bed partner and can be effectively treated with medication.

Mood disorders
Mood disorders, such as depression, anxiety, and apathy, are common in PD. Like constipation and RBD, depression may precede motor manifestations and be an early prodromal sign of PD. One meta-analysis reported a prevalence of major depressive disorder in 17%, minor depression in 22%, and dysthymia in 13% of patients with PD.[29] Anxiety disorders, including generalized anxiety disorder, agoraphobia, panic disorder, and social phobia, are present in individuals with PD at a prevalence of 20% to 40%.[21] One meta-analysis suggests that apathy may be present in 40% of individuals with PD.[30] The lack of motivation marked by reduced goal-oriented behavior and decreased emotional expressivity has been shown to contribute significantly to caregiver burden and has negative implications for treatment and long-term care.

Cognitive disturbances
One of the most feared complications of PD for patients and their caregivers is the development of dementia. Cognitive dysfunction in PD may present in varying degrees.[31] The prevalence of dementia is greater than 75% in individuals who survive 10 years with the PD diagnosis.[32] Mild cognitive impairment affects 18.9% to 38.2% of patients in the early stages of the disorder.[33]

Pain and sensory disturbances
Several sensory abnormalities have been described in individuals in PD. Olfactory impairment is among the earliest NMSs of PD and is present in approximately 90% of early stage PD cases.[34] Vision problems occur in the PD population in the form

of reduced contrast sensitivity, color discrimination, and dry eye syndrome. Issues affecting structures around the eye occur in those with PD, such as seborrheic blepharitis and meibomian gland disease.[35] Pain is a frequent problem in PD that worsens over the course of the disease, and patients who have pain are more depressed and have a poorer quality of life than those who do not. Pain was present in 76% of patients with PD in one cross-sectional study[36] and can be categorized as musculoskeletal, dystonic, central neuropathic, radicular, and other (nonradicular low back pain, arthritic, visceral).

Neurogenetics

Over the past 2 decades there has been an explosion of research on the genetics of PD; 18 PD-related gene loci have been identified to date, with at least 7 disease-causing genes, including alpha-synuclein-synuclein, leucine-rich repeat kinase 2 (LRRK2), Parkin, PTEN-induced putative kinase-1 (PINK1), DJ-1, ATPase type 13A2 (ATP3A2), and glucocerebrosidase. Mutations of these genes have been identified as the cause of rare familial forms of PD. It is estimated that monogenic PD accounts for about 5% of all PD cases in either an autosomal dominant or autosomal recessive inheritance pattern. LRRK2 mutations are the most common and have been associated with 1% of sporadic PD cases and account for 4% of hereditary parkinsonism cases. LRRK2 mutations generally give rise to a benign tremor-predominant disease phenotype that resembles sporadic PD,[37] particularly asymmetric parkinsonism with tremor but with a decreased risk of cognitive and olfactory impairment.[12] Mutations in 4 genes (Parkin, DJ-1, PINK1, and ATP13A2) cause recessive early onset parkinsonism (age of onset <40 years). Parkin mutations are the second most common genetic cause of L-dopa responsive parkinsonism and account for one-third to one-half of all young-onset PD, whereas mutations in the other 3 genes are more rare.[4] The Parkin mutation phenotype has a slow and benign course compared with sporadic PD, with good response to dopaminergic drugs and sleep benefit (patients do better in the morning).

Management in Different Settings to Modify Outcome

PD is a very complicated condition for physicians to optimally manage, with multiple motor and nonmotor manifestations, specific rehabilitation needs, and complicated psychosocial dynamics that evolve with time. Despite this, recent data demonstrated that only 58% of patients with PD saw a neurologist (as opposed to an internist, family medicine physician, or geriatrician) in the 3 years under study. Those who were cared for by a neurologist, however, had lower rates of admission to nursing home, lower rates of hip fracture, and improved survival.[38] Women and minorities were less likely to be seen by a neurologist than white men.

Although evidence strongly suggests that outcomes improve with treatment by a neurologist, it is less clear whether specialty within neurology offers benefits over general neurology. For example, there are movement disorder fellowships that train board certified neurologists in PD care, PD centers that offer comprehensive multidisciplinary care for patients, and PD-specific hospital units. These programs are being closely studied to determine whether these types of specific care lead to better outcomes for patients, lower health care costs, or both. If they do, methods to deliver this specialized care to larger numbers of people will be necessary. To that end, PD-specific telemedicine is currently being studied.

Clinic based

A recent randomized controlled study compared patients who received care from a general neurologist with those who received care from a movement disorders physician who was part of a multidisciplinary outpatient setting with dedicated PD nurses and social workers. Patients followed by the multidisciplinary team had improved scores on measures of quality of life as well as motor performance.[39] The study investigators discussed that the study design did not allow separation of the benefits conferred by seeing a movement disorders physician from the benefits conferred by the multidisciplinary nature of the program. Nevertheless, if this finding holds in future studies, it will become necessary to scale up this type of care to reach larger numbers of patients.

Hospital based

Hospitalization offers unique challenges to patients with PD. It is very difficult for a traditional hospital floor to dispense medications as frequently and as on time as patients with PD often need. If doses are late or missed, motor function, including ability to swallow, can be severely affected, which, in turn, can increase deconditioning, increase fall risk, impede inpatient physical therapy efforts, and potentially keep patients from swallowing their next doses of medication, which can all lead to a downward spiral. Patients with PD are at an increased risk for dysautonomia and hallucinations when medically ill, which can be difficult to manage. Finally, patients with PD may be given medications while hospitalized, for nausea or psychosis, that can worsen their parkinsonism. For these reasons, a pilot PD-specific hospital unit, in which physicians and staff had PD-specific training and on which PD medications were readily available, was created and its outcomes were studied.[40] The PD unit had more accurate and on-time medication delivery to patients, shorter lengths of stay, and better patient satisfaction scores.

Telemedical

The way to increase the number of patients able to be seen by PD specialists is through telemedicine. This method of providing care is developing rapidly and is improving in its scope and possibilities alongside the technologies available to support it. The studies that have been performed so far to evaluate telemedicine have been small and most were not performed in randomized, controlled trials (RCTs). Nevertheless, the studies have been promising, demonstrating patient satisfaction with the method, vast savings in travel and time, and improvements in motor performance and quality of life, likely to the same degree as face-to-face encounters.[41] So far, telemedicine for PD has been used exclusively in wealthy countries, although the potential for meeting needs in the developing world is exciting.

PUBLIC HEALTH ASPECTS
Risk Factors

Factors that may increase risk of Parkinson disease

The cause or causes of PD have not been firmly established and, like most chronic diseases, are expected to be a combination of modifiable (eg, environmental exposures that increase or mitigate risk) and nonmodifiable factors (eg, genetic factors). Understanding the modifiable causes is vital to a public health policy of PD management. However, conflicting data exist for most of these factors making it difficult to formulate a public health response without further study.

Pesticides The observation that 1-methyl-4-phenyl-1,2,3,6-tetrahydropyridine (MPTP), an accidental byproduct of the manufacturing of the synthetic opioid 1-methyl-4-phenyl-4-propionoxypiperidine (MPPP), could cause a PD phenotype sparked interest in the possibility that other environmental toxins could be damaging to dopaminergic cells as well.[42] Toxins that resemble MPTP were suspected, including 2 pesticides, paraquat and rotenone. Most human data concerning the relationship between these and other pesticides comes from case-control studies in which patients and controls were asked via a questionnaire about their exposures. Recall bias is a particular concern in this type of study, as patients who have PD are invested in finding a cause of their condition and may over-report exposure. The data collection varies widely among studies in the level of detail concerning amount and type of exposure as well as analysis of confounding factors, such as smoking, which has shown to have a protective effect.[43]

Occupation related Additional studies have shown that farming as an occupation may also confer an increased risk of PD, although this is difficult to separate from exposure to pesticides. Welding, with its exposure to manganese, has also been studied as a risk factor for PD. An interesting recent study that collected occupational history of cases and controls found that artistic occupations tend to be protective from PD. The hypothesis given for this finding is that patients with premotor PD and lower dopamine levels may have subtle cognitive and behavioral changes that limit novelty seeking and, therefore, may gravitate to more structured occupations.[44]

Traumatic brain injury Traumatic brain injury (TBI) may predispose a person to develop PD later in life. The data exploring this correlation have been contradictory, and recall bias (those with PD are more likely to remember a past head trauma) as well as reverse causation (those with imbalance from PD are more likely to suffer from a head trauma) have been cited as reasons that studies have been faulty. Two recent studies explored this issue. One followed the medical records of patients who presented to an emergency department with head trauma versus trauma that did not involve the head. Patients with TBI had a higher likelihood of developing PD later in life.[45] The second study administered questionnaires to patients with PD and controls and determined, unlike other case-control studies of similar design, that there was no increased history of TBI in the PD population.[46]

Factors that may mitigate risk of Parkinson disease

Caffeine The first suggestion that caffeine could be protective in PD came in 1996 with a questionnaire-based study examining ingestion of specific foods in a case-controlled manner. Patients with PD reported drinking less coffee than controls.[47] This study was followed up by prospective data collection. In 2 large cohorts followed over time, an inverse association was found between PD and caffeine consumption in the forms of coffee, tea, and other caffeine sources.[48] Recommending caffeine for patients who already have PD can be difficult because caffeine can worsen tremor. Molecularly, caffeine inhibits the adenosine receptor, and adenosine inhibitors have since been developed for the treatment of PD. Istradefylline is one such compound, already approved for use in Japan and being studied in a clinical trial in the United States. Other adenosine inhibitors are also in clinic trials in the United States.

Cigarette smoking Numerous studies have identified an inverse association between smoking and PD. Because smoking itself cannot be recommended to patients with PD, as it presents numerous health risks, researchers have tried to harness the seeming protective effect of smoking in other ways. A clinical trial of the nicotine patch as a neuroprotective agent in PD is set to start. However, the assertion that smoking is protective in PD came under question in a recent study that suggested that patients with PD had lower smoking rates because low dopamine levels make it easier to quit and harder to become addicted.[49] This theory suggests that prodromal PD is protective of smoking addiction and not the other way around.

Alcohol consumption Because epidemiologic data suggested that smoking and coffee intake may reduce the risk of developing PD, alcohol consumption was studied as well. A recent review of all the studies performed from 2000 to 2014 looked at this relationship and found conflicting results. In general, prospective studies showed an increased risk of PD in the setting of moderate alcohol use, whereas case control studies showed a decreased risk. The question of alcohol's relationship to PD is, therefore, still not fully understood.[50]

Nonsteroidal antiinflammatory drugs Laboratory data suggest that neuroinflammation can play a role in the eventual death of neurons in PD, and that decreasing this inflammation could be neuroprotective. Several studies have tried to determine whether ingestion of nonsteroidal antiinflammatory drugs (NSAIDs) could reduce the risk of developing PD. A recent Cochrane review of these data concluded that nonaspirin NSAIDs, with the most data on ibuprofen, may reduce the risk of developing PD.[51]

Statins Statins have been shown to have antiinflammatory properties and the hypothesis was developed that they may be potential neuroprotective agents. Statins are already one of the most commonly prescribed drugs, which increase the interest in these medications. A recent analysis of statin use and its correlation to PD rates was prospectively studied in 2 ongoing large cohorts. Regular use of statins was associated with a modest reduction of PD risk.[52]

Calcium channel blockers Calcium channel blockade can protect neurons from excitotoxicity in cell culture and animal models of PD. These data led to a phase II trial testing the neuroprotective effects of the calcium channel blocker isradipine in patients with early PD.[53] Despite the propensity of patients with PD to have low blood pressures, the drug was tolerated and the results led to the development of a larger phase III clinical trial, which is ongoing.[54]

Hyperuricemics Preclinical data suggested that elevated plasma levels of uric acid was protective against PD. In large cohorts of patients with PD followed over time, higher urate levels predicted a more benign disease course. In addition, prospectively collected data of healthy individuals correlated higher urate levels to lower rates of PD. Because of these findings, a phase II trial of inosine, a precursor of urate, was conducted in patients with early PD.[55] Results showed that elevating uric acid was possible and safe in patients with early PD. Although not powered to determine whether there was a clinical improvement in patients with elevated urate levels, preliminary data was promising and will likely lead to a phase III trial.

Exercise Recent studies have demonstrated that exercise can improve motor function in PD as well as some of the nonmotor symptoms of PD, such as fatigue, cognition, and depression. A recent meta-analysis reviewed the evidence of RCTs controlled studies of exercise of all types conducted between the years of 2013 and 2015.[56] Thirty-three studies of exercise and physical therapy techniques of various modalities, including aerobic exercise, strength training, and balance training, were conducted. Benefits were found in different exercise paradigms. One particular study highlighted the phenomenon that exercises of diverse types had benefits on functioning in PD. Shulman and colleagues[57] conducted a trial with 3 arms: high-intensity treadmill training, low-intensity treadmill training, and stretching and resistance exercises. All groups increased gait speed; but interestingly, the stretching and resistance group increased by the biggest margin.

Infectious Disease Causation: Implications for Public Health

In recent years, a series of new theories have been proposed to explain the root cause of PD. They introduce the possibility of additional modifiable risk factors for PD and present new challenges from a public health perspective. Public health implications of this theory would be profound as it suggests that PD could be transmitted person to person.

Enteric-pathogen

In addition to the understanding that Lewy bodies affects multiple brain areas, it has also been long established that Lewy bodies can be found in neurons far from the brain, most notably the enteric nervous system and autonomic ganglion.[48] One recent theory posits that PD is caused by an enteric pathogen, which then traverses up the vagus nerve to gain entry into the brain. A recent epidemiologic study analyzed PD rates in patients who had previously received a complete vagotomy or a selected vagotomy to treat peptic ulcer disease from 1977 to 1995 in Demark. Results showed a lower incidence of PD in those who had received a complete vagotomy as compared both with controls and with those who received a selected vagotomy.[58] The data were interpreted to mean that lacking the vagus nerve was protective of PD as it prevented transmission of microorganisms from the gut to the brain. A related theory argues that intestinal flora plays an important role in PD and that the microbiome of patients with PD differs from that of controls.[59] These theories substantiate the need to search for a potential infectious agent, introduced through the gut, which could contribute to the development of PD.

Prions

The Braak hypothesis suggests that the pathologic hallmark of PD, the abnormal accumulation of alpha-synuclein into Lewy bodies, occurs in a stepwise fashion from the lower brainstem to the midbrain to the cortex. The lower brain stem contains centers of parasympathetic function, sleep regulation, and mood, which are affected by the disease before the midbrain, where the substantia nigra and the dopaminergic neurons responsible for the motor symptoms of PD are located.[16] Therefore, although it seems that Parkinson pathology travels from one neuronal region to another, it is not yet clear how that movement occurs. A new theory that is gaining traction is that the responsible agent is abnormally aggregated alpha-synuclein itself, which would make PD transmission akin to that of a prion disease. It was recently shown that alpha-synuclein can take on different conformations with different potentials to propagate their conformations,[60] the hallmark of a prion. In addition, autopsies of patients who received fetal cell transplants under experimental protocols in the early 1990s revealed that Lewy bodies were present in the fetal transplant as well.[61] One way to explain how the relatively young cells had the identical Lewy body pathology as their elderly neighbors was to hypothesize that the Lewy body migrated from 1 cell to the other.

CONCLUSION

Although much is understood about PD, much is yet a mystery. As more research uncovers the basic biology of how PD develops, this will translate into public health opportunities to prevent or improve this difficult and multi-faceted disease.

REFERENCES

1. De Lau LML, Breteler MMB. Epidemiology of Parkinson's disease. Lancet Neurol 2006;5:525–38.

2. Nussbaum RL, Ellis CE. Alzheimer's disease and Parkinson's disease. N Engl J Med 2003;348:1356–64.
3. Tanner CM, Goldman SM. Epidemiology of Parkinson's disease. Neurol Clin 1996; 14:317–35.
4. Lees AJ, Hardy J, Revesz T. Parkinson's disease. Lancet 2009;373:2055–66.
5. Katzenschlager R, Head J, Schraq A, et al. Fourteen-year final report of the randomized PDRG-UK trial comparing three initial treatments in PD. Neurology 2008; 71:474–80.
6. Gillies GE, Pienaar IS, Vohra S, et al. Sex differences in Parkinson's disease 2014. Front Neuroendocrinol 2014;35:370–84.
7. Haaxma CA, Bloem BR, Borm GF, et al. Gender differences in Parkinson's disease. J Neurol Neurosurg Psychiatry 2007;78:819–24.
8. Martinez-Martin P, Falup Pecurariu C, Odin P, et al. Gender-related differences in the burden of non-motor symptoms in Parkinson's disease. J Neurol 2013;259: 1639–47.
9. Hoehn MM, Yahr MD. Parkinsonism: onset, progression and mortality. Neurology 1967;17(5):427–42.
10. Duarte J, Olmos LMG, Mendoza A, et al. Natural history of Parkinson's disease in the province of Segovia: disability in a 20 years longitudinal study. Neurodegener Dis 2015;15:87–92.
11. Diem Zangerl A, Seppi K, Wenning G, et al. Mortality in Parkinson's disease: a 20 year follow-up study. Mov Disord 2009;24:819–25.
12. Thengannat MA, Jankovic J. Parkinson disease subtypes. JAMA Neurol 2014;71: 499–504.
13. Jankovic J, Kapadia AS. Functional decline in Parkinson disease. Arch Neurol 2001;58:1611–5.
14. Alves G, Larsen JP, Emre M, et al. Changes in motor subtype and risk for incident dementia in Parkinson's disease. Mov Disord 2006;21:1123–30.
15. Wickremaratchi MM, Knipe MD, Sastry BS, et al. The motor phenotype of Parkinson's disease in relation to age at onset. Mov Disord 2011;26:457–63.
16. Braak H, Del Tredici K, Rüb U, et al. Staging of brain pathology related to sporadic Parkinson's disease. Neurobiol Aging 2003;24:197–211.
17. Berg D, Postume RB, Adler CH, et al. MDS research criteria for prodromal Parkinson's disease. Mov Disord 2015;3:1600–9.
18. Pfeiffer RF. Non-motor symptoms in Parkinson's disease. Parkinsonism Relat Disord 2016;22(Suppl 1):S119–22.
19. Kim HS, Cheon SM, Seo JW, et al. Nonmotor symptoms more closely relate to Parkinson's disease: comparison with normal elderly. J Neurol Sci 2013;324:70–3.
20. Krishnan. Do nonmotor symptoms in Parkinson's disease differ from normal aging? Mov Disord 2011;26:2110–3.
21. Sung VW, Nicholas AP. Nonmotor symptoms of Parkinson's disease. Neurol Clin 2013;31:1–16.
22. Martinez-Martin P, Schapira AH, Stocchi F, et al. Prevalence of nonmotor symptoms in Parkinson's disease in an international setting; study using nonmotor symptoms questionnaire in 545 patients. Mov Disord 2007;22:1623–9.
23. Parkinson J. An essay on the shaking palsy. 1817.
24. Sakakibara R, Panicker J, Finazzi-Agro E, et al. A guideline for the management of bladder dysfunction in Parkinson's disease and other gait disorders. Neurourol Urodyn 2015. http://dx.doi.org/10.1002/nau.22764.
25. Winge K. Lower urinary tract dysfunction in patients with parkinsonism and other neurodegenerative disorders. Handb Clin Neurol 2015;130:335–56.

26. Kurtis MM, Rodriguez-Blazquez C, Martinez-Martin P, ELEP group. Relationship between sleep disorders and other nonmotor symptoms in Parkinson's disease. Parkinsonism Relat Disord 2013;19:1152–5.

27. Stocchi F, Barbato L, Nordera G, et al. Sleep disorders in Parkinson's disease. J Neurol 1998;245(Supp 1):S15–8.

28. McCarter SJ, St. Louis EK, Boeve BF. REM sleep behavior disorder and REM sleep without atonia as an early manifestation of degenerative neurological disease. Curr Neurol Neurosci Rep 2012;12:226.

29. Riejinders JS, Ehrt U, Weber WE, et al. A systematic review of prevalence studies of depression in Parkinson's disease. Mov Disord 2008;23:183–9.

30. Den Brock MG, Van Dalen JW, van Gool WA, et al. Apathy in Parkinson's disease: a systematic review and meta-analysis. Mov Disord 2015;30:759–69.

31. Aarsland D, Andersen K, Larsen JP, et al. Prevalence and characteristics of dementia in Parkinson disease: an 8-year prospective study. Arch Neurol 2003;60: 387–92.

32. Hely MA, Reid WG, Adena MA, et al. The Sydney multicenter study of Parkinson's disease: the inevitability of dementia at 20 years. Mov Disord 2008;23:837–44.

33. Litvan I, Aarsland D, Adler C, et al. MDS task force on mild cognitive impairment in Parkinson's disease: critical review of PD-MCI. Mov Disord 2011;26:1814–24.

34. Doty RL. Olfactory dysfunction in Parkinson disease. NatRev Neurol 2012;8: 329–39.

35. Nowacka B, Lubiński W, Honczarenko K, et al. Ophthalmological features of Parkinson disease. Med Sci Monit 2014;20:2243–9.

36. Valkovic P, Minar M, Singliarova H, et al. Pain in Parkinson's disease: a cross-sectional study of its prevalence, types, and relationship to depression and quality of life. PLoS One 2015;10(8):e0136541.

37. Gasser T. Milestones in PD genetics. Mov Disord 2011;26(6):1042–8.

38. Willis AW, Schootman M, Evanoff BA, et al. Neurologist care in Parkinson disease: a utilization, outcomes and survival study. Neurology 2011;77:851–7.

39. Van der Marck MA, Bloem BR, Borm GF, et al. Effectiveness of multi-disciplinary care for Parkinson's disease: a randomized controlled trial. Mov Disord 2013;28: 605–11.

40. Skelly R. Does a specialist unit improve outcomes for hospitalized patients with Parkinson's disease. Parkinsonism Relat Disord 2014;20:1242–7.

41. Achey M, Aldred JL, Aljehani N, et al. The past, present and future of telemedicine for Parkinson's disease. Mov Disord 2014;29:871–83.

42. Brown TP, Rumsby PC, Capleton AC, et al. Pesticides and Parkinson's disease—is there a link? Environ Health Perspect 2006;114:156–64.

43. Moretto A, Colosio C. The role of pesticide exposure in the genesis of Parkinson's disease: epidemiological studies and experimental data. Toxicology 2013;307: 24–34.

44. Haaxma CA, Borm GF, van der Linden D, et al. Artistic occupations are associated with a reduced risk of Parkinson's disease. J Neurol 2015;262:2171–6.

45. Gardner RC, Burke JF, Nettiksimmons J, et al. Traumatic brain injury in later life increases risk for Parkinson's disease. Ann Neurol 2015;77:987–95.

46. Kenborg L, Rugbjerg K, Lee PC, et al. Head injury and risk for Parkinson disease: results from a Danish case-control study. Neurology 2015;84:1098–103.

47. Hellenbrand W, Seidler A, Boeing H, et al. Diet and Parkinson's disease. I: A possible role for the past intake of specific foods and food groups. Results from a self-administered food-frequency questionnaire in a case-control study. Neurology 1996;47:636–43.

48. Braak H, de Vos RA, Bohl J, et al. Gastric alpha-synuclein immunoreactive inclusions in Meissner's and Auerbach's plexuses in cases staged for Parkinson's disease-related brain pathology. Neurosci Lett 2006;396:67–72.

49. Ritz B, Lee PC, Lassen CF, et al. Parkinson disease and smoking revisited: ease of quitting is an early sign of the disease. Neurology 2014;83:1396–402.

50. Bettiol SS, Rose TC, Hughes CJ, et al. Alcohol consumption and Parkinson's disease risk: a review of recent findings. J Parkinsons Dis 2015;5:425–42.

51. Rees K, Stowe R, Patel S, et al. Non-steroidal anti-inflammatory drugs as disease-modifying agents for Parkinson's disease: evidence from observational studies. Cochrane Database Syst Rev 2011;(11):CD008454.

52. Gao X, Simon KC, Schwarzschild MA, et al. Prospective study of statin use of risk of Parkinson disease. Arch Neurol 2012;69:380–4.

53. Parkinson Study Group. Phase II safety, tolerability and dose selection study of isradipine as a potential disease-modifying intervention in early Parkinson's disease (STEADY-PD). Mov Disord 2013;28:1823–31.

54. ClinicalTrials.gov. Identifier: NCT02168842.

55. The Parkinson Study Group SURE-PD Investigators, Schwarzschild MA, Ascherio A, et al. Inosine to increase serum and CSF urate in Parkinson disease: a randomized, placebo controlled trial. JAMA Neurol 2013;71:141–59.

56. Bloem BR, de Vries NM, Ebersbach G, et al. Nonpharmacological treatments for patients with Parkinson's disease. Mov Disord 2015;30:1504–20.

57. Shulman LM, Katzel LI, Ivey FM, et al. Randomized clinical trial of 3 types of physical exercise for patients with Parkinson disease. JAMA Neurol 2013;70:183–90.

58. Svensson E, Horváth-Puhó E, Thomsen RW, et al. Vagotomy and subsequent risk of Parkinson's disease. Ann Neurol 2015;78:522–9.

59. Scheperjans F, Aho V, Pereira PA, et al. Gut microbiota are related to Parkinson's disease and clinical phenotype. Mov Disord 2015;30:350–8.

60. Peelaerts W, Bousset L, Van der Perren A, et al. Alpha-synuclein strains cause distinct synucleinopathies after local and systemic administration. Nature 2015; 522:340–4.

61. Kordower JH, Chu Y, Hauser RA, et al. Lewy body-like pathology in long term embryonic nigral transplants in Parkinson's disease. Nat Med 2008;14:504–6.

Epidemiology of Ischemic Stroke

Albert S. Favate, MD[a], David S. Younger, MD, MPH, MS[a,b,]*

KEYWORDS

- Stroke • Public health • Epidemiology

KEY POINTS

- The burden of ischemic stroke is considerably impacting populations of every age group, ethnicity, race, and country.
- Genetic factors are important in the development of ischemic stroke that may be unique or differentially impact on individuals or populations.
- Large, well-powered genome-wide association study analyses have uncovered significant associations in ischemic stroke.
- The domestic and global burden of ischemic stroke makes it an important public health concern.

INTRODUCTION

Ischemic stroke (IS) is a heterogeneous multifactorial disorder recognized by the sudden onset of neurologic signs related directly to the sites of injury in the brain where the morbid process occurs. The evaluation of complex neurologic disorders, such as stroke, in which multiple genetic and epigenetic factors interact with environmental risk factors to increase the risk has been revolutionized by the genome-wide association studies (GWAS) approach. This approach has the potential to provide insight into appropriate individual and population risk reduction and public health policy approaches to avert irreversible sequela and burden of stroke.

The importance of addressing stroke through well-devised epidemiologic studies was underscored by the Global Burden of Disease 2013 Study (GBD 2013). The GBD 2013 used world mapping to visualize stroke burden and its trends in various regions and countries using epidemiologic measures of age-standardized incidence, mortality, prevalence, disability-adjusted life years, and years lived with disability associated with stroke from 1990 to 2013.[1] Their findings showed that the absolute

The authors have nothing to disclose.
[a] Division of Neuroepidemiology, Department of Neurology, New York University School of Medicine, New York, NY, USA; [b] College of Global Public Health, New York University, New York, NY, USA
* Corresponding author. 333 East 34th Street, 1J, New York, NY 10016.
E-mail address: david.younger@nyumc.org

Neurol Clin 34 (2016) 967–980
http://dx.doi.org/10.1016/j.ncl.2016.06.013
0733-8619/16/$ – see front matter © 2016 Elsevier Inc. All rights reserved.

neurologic.theclinics.com

number of people affected by stroke substantially increased across all countries in spite of dramatic declines in age-standardized incidence, prevalence, mortality rates, and disability. Population growth and aging have played an important role in the observed increase in stroke. With significant geographic country and regional differences and developing countries sharing in the impact of stroke, the domestic and global burden of this disease may actually be borne by low- and middle-income populations making it a public health concern. This article addresses the epidemiologic approaches to stroke and its present domestic and global burden.

EPIDEMIOLOGY OF STROKE

Stroke is the leading cause of morbidity and mortality in industrialized countries. Residents of northern Manhattan have been the source of epidemiologic interest since 1998 when the Northern Manhattan Stroke Study (NOMASS)[2] conducted a population-based study designed to determine stroke incidence, risk factors, and prognosis in the multiethnic urban population of northern Manhattan. Based on the 1990 census,[3] the initial population of about 260,000 people were 40% older than 39 years, 20% black, 63% Hispanic, and 15% white. This community has been exhaustively studied for nearly 2 decades by investigators at the New York Presbyterian/Columbia Presbyterian Medical Center, the only hospital in the region. The later 2000 US census served as a model for race-ethnicity questionnaires in establishing baseline demographics of the northern Manhattan study cohort. The 2006 Take Care New York (TCNY) community health appraisal of northern Manhattan published by the New York City Department of Health and Mental Hygiene[4] added useful sociodemographic information for this ethnically and racially diverse community that now comprises 71% Hispanics, 14% blacks, 11% whites, and 2% Asians or others. With nearly 1 in 10 Inwood and Washington Heights residents of northern Manhattan using the emergency department when sick or in need of health advice, and about a third lacking a regular health care provider, the health needs of the community have been adequately addressed by the consortium of New York Presbyterian/Columbia Presbyterian Medical Center satellite hospitals and clinics. According to TCNY[4] there was a decrease in the annual mortality rate of 20% in the past decade mirroring that of New York City (NYC) overall. Between 2003 and 2004, the average annual mortality rate in Inwood and Washington Heights was 8% lower than in Manhattan and greater than 10% lower than NYC with respective annual mortality rates of 640, 697, and 718 per 100,000.

For almost 2 decades, NOMASS collaborators from the Departments of Neurology and public health at Columbia University, Miller School of Medicine, and the College of Global Public Health of New York University have evaluated risk factors related to IS. The initial study by Sacco and colleagues[2] enrolled 924 northern Manhattan residents aged 20 years or more, of white, black, or Hispanic race and ethnicity with neurologic symptoms deemed due to stroke over a 4-year period from 1993 to 1997 and provided insight into racial and ethnic differences associated with stroke. A comparison of the incidences of subtype- and age-specific stroke rates stratified by sex, race, and ethnicity detected 2- to 3-fold differences in stroke incidence rates with blacks and Hispanics at greater stroke risk than white residing in the same urban community. Although overall stroke cases comprised mainly cerebral infarction (CI) in 77%, hemorrhagic stroke cases, including intracerebral hemorrhage (ICH) and subarachnoid hemorrhage (SAH), were encountered among blacks with a 1.4- and 2.1-fold greater risk, respectively. A weakness of the study was the exclusion of patients with milder stroke who were not hospitalized. Later studies by the same investigators[5] noted that in adults aged 20 to 44 years, only 45% of strokes were caused by CI, with 31% ICH and 24% SAH, compared with 80%, 14%, and 5%, respectively, in older individuals. A cryptogenic etiopathogenesis of stroke occurred more frequently in younger than older adults, 55% versus 42%; cardio-embolic stroke occurred less frequency: 6% versus 22% in young versus older. However, extracranial and intracranial atherosclerosis and lacunar infarction occurred with about equal frequency. Men had a case fatality rate of 21% compared with 11% for women. The relative risk of any stroke was greater in younger blacks and Hispanics than in whites, with an overall case fatality rate that was highest in ICH followed by SAH and infarct. NOMASS has investigated other risk factors associated with stroke in northern Manhattan using increasingly more sophisticated epidemiologic study designs and complex questions commensurate with the increasing body of knowledge associated with stroke morbidity and mortality.

Sacco and colleagues[6] carried out a population-based case-control study between 1993 and 1997 examining alcohol consumption. They detected the beneficial protective effects of moderate alcohol consumption of up to 2 drinks per day for IS after adjustment for risk factors of cardiac disease, hypertension, diabetes mellitus (DM), current smoking, body mass index, and education in younger and older men and women and in whites, blacks, and Hispanics. A weakness of the study was the lack of distinction between consumption of red wine and white wine and a variety of biases with a possible trend toward alcohol use in the community. Elkind and colleagues[7] provided additional insight into the role of moderate alcohol consumption noting that after adjusting for risk factors compared with those who did not drink in the past year, moderate drinkers had a reduced risk of IS (0.67; 95% confidence interval, 0.46–0.99). Their results were similar when never-drinkers were used as referent group. The salutary effect of moderate alcohol consumption was independent of other risk factors and held for nonatherosclerotic stroke subtypes.

Sacco and colleagues[8] carried out a population-based incident case-control study of racial-ethnic disparities on the impact of stroke risk factors that revealed the association of hypertension (HTN) and DM in blacks and Hispanics and atrial fibrillation and coronary artery disease (CAD) in white northern Manhattan residents. A weakness of the study was the lack of insight into physical activity. Gardener and colleagues[9] carried out a population-based prospective cohort study of Mediterranean style diet (MedDi) and risk of IS, myocardial infarction (MI), and vascular death demonstrating the inverse relation between MedDi score and composite outcome of IS, MI, or vascular death. A weakness of the study was the lack of relation to race-ethnicity despite MeDi in Hispanics. In a related study of dietary fat intake and IS risk more typical of a Western diet,[10] stroke-free community residents of northern Manhattan more than 40 years of age underwent evaluation of their medical history and had their diet assessed by a food-frequency survey. Cox proportional hazard models calculated the risk of incident IS. During a mean of 5.5 years of follow-up, 142 IS occurred. After adjusting for potential confounders, the risk of IS was higher in the upper quintile of total fat intake compared with the lowest quintile. Total fat intake greater than 65 g was associated with increased risk of IS. Risk was attenuated after controlling for caloric intake. The results suggested that increased daily total fat intake, especially greater than 65 g, characteristic of a Western-type diet significantly increased the risk of IS.

The impact of an underlying metabolic syndrome recognized by the constellation of vascular risk factors, including elevated blood pressure, elevated blood glucose, obesity, and dyslipidemia, on IS was later investigated by Boden-Albala and colleagues[11] in a prospective, population-based cohort study. Subjects aged 40 years or older, never diagnosed with IR, and residing in northern Manhattan were found to have an increased risk of IS and vascular events after adjustment for sociodemographic and risk factors. The effect of the metabolic syndrome on IS risk was greater among women than among Hispanics compared with blacks and whites. An analysis of the etiologic fraction estimate suggested that elimination of the metabolic syndrome would result in a 19% reduction in overall stroke, a 30% reduction of stroke in women, and a 35% reduction of stroke among Hispanics.

The population-attributable risks of HTN and diabetes for IS was studied by Willey and coworkers[12] using multivariable Cox models to calculate the hazard ratio (HR), population attributable risk (PAR), and 95% confidence intervals for the end point of stroke. The PARs resulting from HTN and diabetes were, respectively, 29.9% (95% confidence interval, 12.5–47.4) and 19.5% (95% confidence interval, 12.4–26.5) for stroke. The PAR resulting from HTN and diabetes for stroke differed by race-ethnicity and age (P for differences <.05). PAR for stroke resulting from HTN was greater among Hispanics (50.6%; 95% confidence interval, 29.2–71.9) than non-Hispanic whites (2.6%; 95% confidence interval, −33.2 to 38.6). The PAR for stroke resulting from HTN and diabetes was greater in those less than 80 years of age than in those 80 years of age and older. These results concluded that HTN and diabetes have important effects on the burden of stroke, particularly among those younger than 80 years and Hispanics.

There are guidelines for the primary prevention of IS.[13] Important nonmodifiable risk factors for IS include age, sex, ethnicity, and heredity. Modifiable risk factors include HTN, cardiovascular disease (CVD), DM, hyperlipidemia, asymptomatic carotid stenosis, cigarette smoking, and alcohol abuse. Data from NOMASS also provided new insights into these stroke risk factors.[14] Physical activity had a protective effect against stroke, with relatively low levels of exercise, such as regular walking, producing this effect.[15] High-density lipoproteins (HDLs) were protective against stroke, whereas lipoproteins increased stroke risk.[16,17] If stroke is subdivided into atherosclerotic, large-artery carotid disease, and intracranial atherosclerotic disease and nonatherosclerotic cryptogenic, lacunar, and cardio-embolic stroke categories, the protective effect of HDL was increased further in events of atherosclerotic origin. Drug treatment to lower low-density lipoprotein (LDL) and triglyceride levels and increase HDL reduces the risk for stroke as well as cardiovascular events.

There is evidence to suggest that blood vessel endothelial injury is involved in the atherosclerotic process and linked to increased incidence of stroke, mechanisms of which could include elevated homocysteine levels and infectious agents that infect the endothelium. Homocysteine, an important new risk factor for stroke, is both genetically and environmentally controlled.[18] Some individuals with homocysteinemia have a genetic defect in the enzyme cystathionine β synthetase. One-half of affected patients who are homozygous for the enzyme defect die at a young age of venous thrombosis and premature atherosclerosis, whereas heterozygous individuals are at risk for premature atherosclerosis. *Chlamydophila pneumoniae*, a common cause of community-acquired pneumonia, pharyngitis, and sinusitis and bacterial flora involved in periodontal disease, is theoretically capable of infecting the endothelium and inflicting injury and may provide useful predictors of IS. The sum total of these injurious events of the endothelium could stimulate platelet aggregation, adhesion, monocyte migration, and plaque formation, so as to begin the atherosclerotic process, increasing the risk of stroke. Periodontal disease, which affects up to 20% of those aged 60 years to 64 years, can be an important infectious agent and could theoretically elevate C-reactive protein levels, increasing the risk of CVD and stroke.

The Greater Cincinnati/Northern Kentucky Stroke Study[19] estimated that 37% to 42% of all IS in blacks and whites could be attributable to the effects of DM alone or in combination with HTN; however, those with IS and DM tended to be younger and black, with HTN, MI, and higher cholesterol levels than non-DM. Early population-based epidemiologic studies in elderly individuals revealed an association of carotid artery atherosclerosis with stroke risk with the assumption that increasing age, HTN, systolic blood pressure, DM, and smoking but not lipids and lipoproteins were consistently related.[20,21] Data on elderly patients studied by NOMASS[22] demonstrated that apolipoprotein A-1 and B were significant determinants of moderate to severe carotid artery atherosclerosis; HLD was protective, whereas total cholesterol, triglycerides, and LDL cholesterol showed no association.

Although a single most likely cause of CI is emphasized in leading stroke registries,[23,24] other investigators have emphasized the multiple potential causes of infarct.[25–27] The Lausanne,[25] Belsancon,[26] and Ege Stroke Registries[27] noted rates of multiple potential causes of CI of 7.0%, 4.7%, and 3.4%, respectively. This phenomenon has probably been underestimated in the literature, because several other stroke registries have sometimes included patients with 2 potential causes of infarct in "undetermined" subgroups.[23,24,28] In ascertaining the frequency of multiple potential causes of CI, the Lausanne Stroke Registry[25] distinguished subgroups of patients with large and small-artery disease and cardiac embolism as follows: Large-artery disease was diagnosed in those with 1 or more risk factors, including age greater than 50 years, arterial HTN, DM, cigarette smoking, hypercholesterolemia, stenosis of at least 50% of the lumen diameter in the appropriate large artery demonstrated by Doppler ultrasonography, 3-dimensional magnetic resonance imaging (MRA), and conventional cerebral angiography. Small-artery disease was presumed in those with long-standing arterial HTN or DM and a CI less than 15 mm in diameter limited to the territory of deep perforating vessels, in the absence of a cardiac or arterial source of embolism. Cardiac embolism was presumed in the presence of endocarditis, mitral stenosis, atrial fibrillation, sick sinus syndrome, intracardiac thrombus or tumor, prosthetic aortic or mitral values, left ventricular aneurysm or akinesia after MI, and global cardiac hypokinesia or dyskinesia. One particular type, pure motor stroke, so noted in 52% of patients, was the most common lacunar syndrome in the Lausanne Stroke Registry[25] followed by ataxic hemiparesis in 13% and dysarthria-clumsy hand syndrome in 3%. Pure motor stroke in 71% predominated in the patients with both large-artery and cardiac embolic disease, as did ataxic hemiparesis and pure motor stroke, which occurred in one-third each of patients with combined large and small-artery disease and cardiac embolism.

NEURORADIOLOGIC METHODS TO DETECT STROKE

It is noteworthy to describe the available methods to detect stroke used in routine care and clinical studies. Brain computed tomography (CT) and MRI using T1- and T2-weighted equally sensitive to the detection of ischemic stroke and hematoma.[29] The addition of diffusion-weighted imaging (DWI) to the latter, detects ischemic regions within minutes of symptom onset, as well as, relatively small cortical and subcortical lesions including those in the brainstem and cerebellum, and other valuable information about the vascular territory with a sensitivity and specificity that approaches 100%.[30] Additional available studies for stroke evaluation, including 3-dimensional MRA of arteries of the neck and cerebral circulation, extracranial and transcranial Doppler ultrasonography with frequency spectral analysis, and B-mode echo tomography of the carotid, vertebrobasilar, and selected intracranial arteries, are all readily available at most centers and can provide useful information in stroke classification and management.

Acute IS occurs when a cerebral vessel is occluded and a core of brain tissue dies; however, the surrounding area termed the *ischemic penumbra*, which is hypoperfused, remains at risk of further infarction. Deep brain ischemic leads to a cascade of Na^+/K^+ channels that results in cytotoxic edema with the net uptake of water in affected brain tissue and narrowing of the extracellular matrix due to reduction in Brownian molecular motion.[31] The categorization of subtypes of IS is more than an academic exercise because it is inextricably linked to further management, the goal of which is to accurately ascertain the site, size, age, and vascular territory of an ischemic lesion within hours of symptom onset by early brain neuroimaging and to consider one of the many treatment protocols, including intravenous recombinant tissue plasminogen activator (rt-PA), and other measures to restore or improve perfusion, without which the infarcted core may continue to enlarge and progressively replace ischemic tissue in the penumbra.

The categorization of subtypes of IS, previously based on risk factor profiles, clinical features of the stroke, and findings on brain imaging using CT and MRI, has shifted in the direction of etiopathogenesis recognizing the 5 essential types for purposes of acute management in clinical trials, including large-artery atherosclerotic embolic and thrombotic, moderate- and high-risk cardioembolic, small-vessel occlusive lacunar, and those due to other causes, undetermined, or with negative or incomplete evaluations.[24] Although noncontrast CT of the brain has been the standard for evaluation of patients with suspected stroke and to which all other brain imaging studies are compared, it is insensitive in detecting acute and small cortical or subcortical infarctions, especially in the posterior fossa. With the advent of rt-PA treatment there has been interest in refining CT to identify subtle early signs of ischemic brain injury and arterial occlusion that might impact on the decision to treat with rt-PA based on the more favorable outcome of the ischemic penumbra administered within 3 hours of symptom onset.[32] Such refinements in CT imaging include perfusion-CT using whole-brain perfusion and dynamic perfusion that allow differentiation of reversible and irreversible ischemia and identification of the ischemic penumbra and helical CT angiography to rapidly and noninvasively evaluate vascular stenosis ad occlusions, all with the benefit of rapid data acquisition and performance with conventional CT equipment but the disadvantage of the requirement for iodine contrast and additional radiation exposures.[30] The combination of perfusion-weighted imaging (PWI) to demonstrate areas of reduced cerebral perfusion along with DWI to depict areas of irreversible injury leads to mismatched areas, the PWI often being larger than DWI, representing the tissue at risk in the ischemic penumbra.[29] Prospective studies of patients studied with sequential neuroimaging for ACI that included DWI, PWI, T2-weighted MRI and MRA, 35 patients subjected to rt-PA with mismatch of PWI/DWI in the area of ischemic penumbra, and cerebral arterial occlusion shown by MRA showed significant reduction in infarct size and recanalization consistent with salvation of at-risk ischemic tissue.[33]

GENETIC BASIS OF STROKE

IS is considered to be a highly complex disease consisting of a group of heterogeneous disorders with multiple genetic and environmental risk factors and can, therefore, be viewed as a paradigm for late-onset, complex polygenic diseases.[34] Several lines of evidence support a role for genetic factors in the pathogenesis of stroke, including studies of twins[35] and familial aggregation.[36] Both environmental and genetic risk factors for IS have been well characterized.[37] Duggirala and co-workers[38] demonstrated high heritability, with 66.0% to 74.9% of the total variation being accounted for by genetic factors and the remainder being attributable to covariates, such as lipids, diabetes, HTN, and smoking. Catto and colleagues[39] reviewed evidence that stroke had a genetic basis and that the hemostatic system was an important risk factor.

The association between the stroke and a specific allele of a single nucleotide polymorphism (SNP) within functional candidate genes has been analyzed between patients and controls. Most such studies however use relatively small numbers of patients and controls, and their results may not be replicated. A disadvantage of the hypothesis-based approach to candidate gene studies is that the genes involved in the pathogenesis of the disease, such as stroke, through unknown pathways may be overlooked. The hypothesis-free approach used by GWAS allows stroke research to overcome this drawback because in these studies nearly all common variants in the entire genome can be tested for their associations.[40] There is a catalogue of published GWAS available online (http://www.genome.gov/26525384). In contrast to linkage studies, GWAS use readily available case-control data sets rather than multiplex family based sets, permitting collection of much larger data sets.[41] Early stroke studies that used GWAS examined the association with CVD. Two loci on chromosome 4q25 in *PITX2* and at 16q22 in *ZFHX3* associated with atrial fibrillation were found to be risk factors for cardioembolic stroke[42,43] similar to another on chromosome 9p21 originally associated with CAD and later found to be a risk factor for large-artery stroke.[44] It is now recognized that different genetic risk factors predispose to specific stroke subtypes. For example, the variant in the protein kinase C family of *PRKCH* associates with small-vessel stroke,[45] whereas variants associated with *PITX2* and *ZFHX3* predict cardioembolic stroke, while those associated with *HDAC9* and the 9p21 loci predispose to large-vessel stroke.[46]

Three loci, respectively, at 1q24.2 in Factor V (*F5*) encoding coagulation factor V, at 7q36.1 in nitric oxide synthase 3 encoding human endothelial nitric oxide synthase, and at 11p11.2 in Factor II encoding a 622-residue prepropeptide with a molecular mass of about 70 kD, are all associated with IS susceptibility; one at 13q12.3 in arachidonate 5-lipooxygenase activating protein (*ALOX5AP*) encoding 5-lipoxygenase-activating proteins associated with stroke susceptibility and another at 14q23.1 in *PRKCH* (protein kinase C) encoding *PRKCH* that is associated with susceptibility to CI.

Bersano and colleagues[47] reviewed genetic polymorphisms implicated in the development of stroke. Candidate genes included those involved in hemostasis (*F5*), the renin-angiotensin-aldosterone system (angiotensin-converting enzyme), homocysteine (methylenetetrahydrofolate reductase), and lipoprotein metabolism (apolipoprotein E). Campbell and colleagues[48] noted that increased serum levels of soluble vascular adhesion molecule-1 (vascular cell adhesion molecule 1) predicted recurrent IS in a study of 252 patients. A smaller but similar trend was noted for serum levels of N-terminal pro-B-type natriuretic peptide (natriuretic peptide precursor B).

In a GWAS of 4 large cohorts, including 19,602 Caucasians in whom 1544 incident strokes developed over an average follow-up of 11 years, Ikram and coworkers[49] found linkage to rs11833579 and rs12425791 on chromosome 12p13 near or within the *NINJ2* gene. Both SNPs showed significant associations with total stroke ($P = 4.8 \times 10[-9]$ and $P = 1.5 \times 10[-8]$, respectively) and IS ($P = 2.3 \times 10[-10]$ and $P = 2.6 \times 10[-9]$, respectively). A significant association with rs12425791 was replicated in 3 additional cohorts, yielding an overall HR of 1.29 ($P = 1.1 \times 10[-9]$). The International Stroke Genetics Consortium and Wellcome Trust Case-Control Consortium[50] were unable to replicate an association between IS and the rs11833579 and rs12425791 variants at 12p13 in a combined sample of 8637 cases and 8733 controls of European ancestry as well as in a population-based genome-wide cohort study of 278 IS among 22,054 participants.

GENETIC ANIMAL MODEL

Rubattu and colleagues[51] studied the stroke-prone spontaneously hypertensive rat as a model organism for a complex form of human stroke, mating it with the stroke-resistant spontaneously hypertensive rat. The investigators then performed a genome-wide screen in the resultant cohort whereby latency until stroke but not HTN (a major confounder) segregated identifying 3 major quantitative trait loci, *STR1-3*, with lod scores of 7.4, 4.7, and 3.0, respectively, that accounted for 28% of the overall phenotypic variance. *STR2* colocalized with the genes encoding atrial and brain natriuretic factor peptides with important vasoactive properties.

GENETICS OF STROKE IN YOUNG ADULTS

Terni and colleagues[52] reviewed the single-gene causes of IS in young adults noting that IS was a common cause of admission of young patients in stroke units. In particular, the yearly incidence of stroke increased from 2.4 per 100,000 in people aged 20 to 24 years, to 4.5 per 100,000 for those aged 30 to 34 years, and to 32.9 per 100,000 for people aged 45 to 49 years. Stroke was slightly more frequent in women aged 20 to 30 years and in men older than 35 years. Traditional risk factors for stroke, such HTN and DM, and large extracranial and intracranial atherosclerosis, small-vessel disease, and atrial fibrillation, which play an important role in older patients, occur less frequently in young adults. The main clinical challenge in management of a young adult with stroke is the identification of its cause, which may remain undetermined. Four monogenic disorders can manifest stroke as a prominent finding.

Mitochondrial encephalomyopathy with lactic acidosis and strokelike episode is a maternally inherited mitochondrial disease. Point mutations occur in polypeptide-encoding and transfer RNA (tRNA) genes, notably, A3243G and T3271C I tRNA Leu (UUR).[53] Familial hemiplegic migraine leads to strokelike episodes in childhood and teenage years with heterozygous mutations in the calcium ion channel gene (*CACNA1A*) at chromosome 19p13.13 encoding the alpha 1 subunit of the voltage-gated calcium channel in neurons.

Cerebral autosomal dominant (AD) arteriopathy with subcortical infarcts and leukoencephalopathy type 1 due to AD mutations in the *NOTCH3* gene on chromosome 19p13.12 is a progressive disorder of the small arterial vessels of the brain manifested by migraine, strokes, and white matter lesions, with resultant cognitive impairment in some patients.[54]

Cerebral small-vessel disease can be associated with mutations in the collagen type IV gene (*COL4A1*) at chromosome 13q34 encoding the α1 subunit of collagen type IV is an AD disorder that presents IS and to a lesser extent ICH with or without ocular anomalies. Shah and colleagues[55] described 5 affected children from 4 families with recurrent stroke, infantile hemiplegia/spastic quadriplegia, infantile spasms, and ocular anomalies identifying heterozygosity for 4 different missense mutations in the *COL4A1* gene, including the G755R substitution in 1 boy and a G773R substitution (120130.0021) in 2 sibs.

Fabry disease is an X-linked congenital lysosomal storage disorder due to a mutation in the *GLA* gene encoding alpha-galactosidase A on chromosome Xq22. The disorder is a systemic disease, manifest as progressive renal failure and cardiac disease with IS, small-fiber peripheral neuropathy, and skin lesions, among other abnormalities.[56]

GENETIC INFLUENCES OF WHITE MATTER LESION AND HYPERINTENSITY PROGRESSION

White matter hyperintensities (WMHs) or white matter lesions (WMLs) on T2-weighted MRI are associated with increasing age and cardiovascular risk factors, particularly HTN, and are predictive of both stroke and dementia in prospective community populations.[57] Severe confluent WMHs are often found in patients presenting with stroke and are more common in patients with the small-vessel stroke subtype.[58] The WMH burden is linked to poor clinical outcomes after stroke,[59] making it important to understand the possible heritable aspects.

Hofer and colleagues[60] estimated heritability of WML progression and sought common genetic variants associated with WML progression in elderly participants from the Cohorts for Heart and Aging Research in Genomic Epidemiology consortium. To assess the relative contribution of genetic factors to progression of WML, the investigators used cohort risk models that included demographics, vascular risk factors, plus SNPs that were known to be associated cross-sectionally with WMLs. Among 1085 subjects that showed WML progression, the heritability estimate for WML progression was 6.5%, and no SNPs achieved genome-wide significance ($P<5 \times 10[-8]$). SNP variants were previously related to WML explained only 0.8% to 11.7% more of the variance in WML progression than age, vascular risk factors, and baseline WML burden. Thus, common genetic factors contribute little to the progression of age-related WMLs in middle-aged and older adults. Although the contribution of genetic factors seems to be large during the initiating phase of white matter damage, the propagating phase of WMLs seems to be mainly influenced by nongenetic determinants. With the exception of HTN, these nongenetic risk factors for WML progression remain largely unknown.

Verhaaren and colleagues[61] conducted a meta-analysis of multiethnic GWAS influencing WMH burden among 21,079 middle-aged to elderly individuals from 29 population-based cohorts free of dementia and stroke and of European, African, Hispanic, or Asian descent. Four novel genetic loci that implicated inflammatory and glial proliferative pathways in the development of WMH were identified. A meta-analysis conducted for each ethnicity separately and for the combined sample confirmed a previously known locus on chromosome 17q25 ($P = 2.7 \times 10[-19]$) and identified novel loci on chromosome 10q24 ($P = 1.6 \times 10 [-9]$) and 2p21 ($P = 4.4 \times 10[-8]$) in those of European ancestry and 2 additional loci on chromosome 1q22 ($P = 2.0 \times 10[-8]$) and 2p16 ($P = 1.5 \times 10[-8]$) in multiethnic ancestry.

Traylor and colleagues[62] conducted GWAS of WMH volumes (WMHV) for 3670 patients with stroke from the United Kingdom, United States, Australia, Belgium, and Italy. Genetics associations were sought with WMHs in a stroke population and then examined as to whether genetic loci previously linked to WMHV in community populations also associated in patients with stroke. Having established that genetic associations were shared between the 2 populations, meta-analysis testing was performed. There were no associations at genome-wide significance with WMHV in patients with stroke concluding that genetic associations with WMHV are shared in otherwise healthy individuals and patients with stroke indicating a common genetic susceptibility in cerebral small-vessel disease.

GENETIC ASPECTS OF LACUNAR STROKES

Traylor and colleagues[63] studied the genetic aspects of lacunar strokes noting that they composed about 20% of all strokes, yet GWAS had not been informative. Pathologic and radiological studies suggested that there may be different pathologies underlying lacunar strokes leading to the differentiation into isolated lacunar infarcts and multiple lacunar infarcts and leukoaraiosis. The investigators performed GWAS in MRI-verified cohort of 1012 lacunar stroke cases and 964 controls. By the extent of leukoaraiosis grade, patients were subtyped into 2 groups: isolated lacunar infarct and single lacunar infarct with absent or mild leukoaraiosis multiple lacunar infarcts or lacunar infarct with moderate or severe confluent leukoaraiosis. An assessment of heritability of lacunar stroke was performed using a calculation of genetic relationships across 8,122,203 SNPs after discarding genotypes and SNPs with a probability less than 90%. Their results indicated a substantial heritable component to MRI-verified lacunar stroke in 20% to 25% and its 2 subtypes: isolated lacunar infarct in 15% to 18% and multiple lacunar infarcts/leukoaraiosis in 23% to 28%. This heritable component was significantly enriched for sites affecting expression of genes. The risk of the 2 subtypes of lacunar stroke in isolation, but not in combination, was associated with rare variation in the genome. Lacunar stroke, when defined by MRI, was a highly heritable complex disease. Because the investigators partitioned their choice of SNP data on regulatory regions, including all SNPs that overlapped a transcription factor–binding site and DNase peak, as well as either having a matched transcription factor motif or a matched DNase footprint, the SNPs represented regions where regulatory factors were thought to bind to the genome.

GENETIC BASIS FOR STROKE AND MIGRAINE

Migraine is a headache disorder characterized by recurrent attacks of severe, often throbbing, headache. Most patients have migraine without aura (MO); however, a third have headaches preceded by aura (MA) composed of transient neurologic disturbances.[64] Epidemiologic studies have shown a doubling of the risk of IS in people who have MA,[65] and one large meta-analysis of case-control and observational cohort studies reported that the risk of stroke is increased in people with migraine (relative risk [RR] 2.16, 95% confidence interval 1.89–2.48). This increase in risk was consistent in people who had MA (RR 2.27, 1.61–3.19) and MO (RR 1.83, 1.06–3.15) as well as in those taking oral contraceptives (RR 8.72, 5.05–15.05).[66] A meta-analyses of 9 studies that investigated the association between any migraine and IS revealed a significantly higher risk among people who had MA (RR 2.16, 1.53–3.03) compared with people who had MO (RR 1.23, 0.90–1.69; meta-regression for aura status $P = .02$).[67] Although the pathophysiology linking IS and MA or MO is poorly understood, suggested mechanisms include cortical spreading depression,[68] endothelial dysfunction,[69] enhanced platelet activation,[70] and vasoconstriction.[71] Malik and colleagues[72] investigated the shared genetic basis of migraine and IS noting shared genetic susceptibility to migraine and IS, with a particularly strong overlap between MO and large-artery IS.

REFERENCES

1. Feigin VL, Mensah GA, Norrving B, et al. GBD 2013 Stroke Panel Experts Group. Atlas of the Global Burden of Stroke (1990-2013): the GBD 2013 Study. Neuroepidemiology 2015;45:230–6.
2. Sacco RL, Boden-Albala B, Gan R, et al. Stroke incidence among white, black and Hispanic residents of an urban community. Am J Epidemiol 1998;147:259–68.
3. Bureau of the Census. 1990 census of population and housing. Washington, DC: Bureau of the Census; US Department of Commerce; 1990.
4. Community Health Profiles. Take care New York. Inwood and Washington Heights. 2nd edition. Manhattan (NY): New York City Department of Health and Mental Hygiene; 2006.

5. Jacobs BS, Boden-Albala B, Lin IF, et al. Stroke in the young in the northern Manhattan stroke Study. Stroke 2002;33:2789–93.
6. Sacco RL, Elkind M, Boden-Albala B, et al. The protective effect of moderate alcohol consumption on ischemic stroke. JAMA 1999;281:53–60.
7. Elkind MS, Sciacca R, Boden-Albala B, et al. Moderate alcohol consumption reduced risk of ischemic stroke: the Northern Manhattan Study. Stroke 2006;37: 13–9.
8. Sacco RL, Boden-Albala B, Abel G, et al. Race-ethnic disparities in the impact of stroke risk factors: the Northern Manhattan Stroke Study. Stroke 2011;32: 1725–31.
9. Gardener H, Wright CB, Gu Y, et al. Mediterranean style diet and risk of ischemic stroke, myocardial infarction, and vascular death: the Northern Manhattan Study. Am J Clin Nutr 2011;94:1458–64.
10. Boden-Albala B, Elkind MS, White H, et al. Dietary total fat intake and ischemic stroke risk: the Northern Manhattan Study. Neuroepidemiology 2009;32:296–301.
11. Boden-Albala B, Sacco RL, Lee HS, et al. Metabolic syndrome and ischemic stroke risk: Northern Manhattan Study. Stroke 2008;39:30–5.
12. Willey JZ, Moon YP, Kahn E, et al. Population attributable risks of hypertension and diabetes for cardiovascular disease and stroke in the Northern Manhattan Study. J Am Heart Assoc 2014;3:e00106.
13. Goldstein LB, Adams R, Alberts MJ, et al. Primary prevention of ischemic stroke. A guidelines from the American Heart Association/American Stroke Association Stroke Council: cosponsored by the Atherosclerotic Peripheral Vascular Disease Interdisciplinary Working Group; Cardiovascular Nursing Council; Clinical Cardiology Council; Nutrition, Physical Activity, and Metabolism Council; and the Quality of Care and Outcomes Research Interdisciplinary Working Group. Circulation 2006;113:e873–923.
14. Sacco RL. Newer risk factors for stroke. Neurology 2001;57(Suppl 2):S31–4.
15. Sacco RL, Gan R, Boden-Albala B, et al. Leisure-time physical activity and ischemic stroke risk: the Northern Manhattan Stroke Study. Stroke 1998;29:380–7.
16. Sacco RL, Benson RT, Kargman DE, et al. High-density lipoprotein cholesterol and ischemic stroke in the elderly: the Northern Manhattan Stroke Study. JAMA 2001;285:2729–35.
17. Kargman DE, Berglund LF, Boden-Albala B, et al. Increased stroke risk and lipoprotein (a) in a racially mixed area: the Northern Manhattan Stroke Study. Stroke 1999;30:251.
18. Sacco RL, Roberts JK, Jacobs BS. Homocysteine as a risk factor for ischemic stroke: an epidemiological story in evolution. Neuroepidemiology 1998;17: 167–73.
19. Kissela BM, Khoury J, Kleindorfer D, et al. Epidemiology of ischemic stroke in patients with diabetes: the greater Cincinnati/Northern Kentucky Stroke Study. Diabetes Care 2005;28:355–9.
20. Fine-Edelstein JS, Wolf PA, O'Leary DH, et al. Precursors of extracranial carotid atherosclerosis in the Framingham Study. Neurology 1994;44:1046–50.
21. Sutton-Tyrrell K, Alcorn HG, Wolfson SK Jr, et al. Predictors of carotid stenosis in older adults with and without systolic hypertension. Stroke 1993;24:355–61.
22. Jeng JS, Sacco RL, Kargman DE, et al. Apolipoproteins and carotid artery atherosclerosis in an elderly multiethnic population: the Northern Manhattan stroke study. Atherosclerosis 2002;165:317–25.
23. Foulkes MA, Wolf PA, Price TR, et al. The Stroke Data Bank: design, methods, and baseline characteristics. Stroke 1988;19:547–54.

24. Adams HP Jr, Bendixen BH, Kappelle LJ, et al. Classification of subtype of acute ischemic stroke. Definitions for use in multicenter clinical trial. TOAST. Trial of org 10172 in acute stroke treatment. Stroke 1993;24:35–41.

25. Moncayo J, Devuyst G, Van Melle G, et al. Coexisting causes of ischemic stroke. Arch Neurol 2000;57:1139–44.

26. Moulin T, Tatu L, Crépin-Leblond T, et al. The Besançon Stroke Registry: an acute stroke registry of 2,500 consecutive patients. Eur Neurol 1997;38:10–20.

27. Kumral E, Ozkaya B, Sagduyu A, et al. The Ege Stroke Registry: a hospital-based study in the Aegean region, Izmir, Turkey. Analysis of 2,000 stroke patients. Cerebrovasc Dis 1998;8:278–88.

28. Yip PK, Jeng JS, Lee TK, et al. Subtypes of ischemic stroke. A hospital-based stroke registry in Taiwan (SCAN-IV). Stroke 1997;28:2507–12.

29. Mohr JP, Biller J, Hilal SK, et al. Magnetic resonance versus computed tomographic imaging in acute stroke. Stroke 1995;26:807–12.

30. Adams HP Jr, del Zoppo G, Alberts MJ, et al. Guidelines for the early management of adults with ischemic stroke: a guideline from the American Heart Association/American Stroke Association Stroke Council, Clinical Cardiology Council, Cardiovascular Radiology and Intervention Council, and the Atherosclerotic Peripheral Vascular Disease and Quality of Care Outcomes in Research Interdisciplinary Working Groups: the American Academy of Neurology affirms the value of this guideline as an educational tool for neurologists. Circulation 2007;115: e478–534.

31. Wintermark M, Fiebach J. Imaging of brain parenchyma in stroke. Handb Clin Neurol 2009;94:1011–9.

32. Tissue plasminogen activator for acute ischemic stroke. The National Institute of Neurological Disorders and Stroke rtPA Stroke Study Group. N Engl J Med 1995; 333:1581–7.

33. Jansen O, Schellinger P, Fiebach J, et al. Early recanalization in acute ischaemic stroke saves tissue at risk defined by MRI. Lancet 1999;353:2036–7.

34. Dominiczak AF, McBride MW. Genetics of common polygenic stroke. Nat Genet 2003;35:116–7.

35. Brass LM, Isaacsohn JL, Merikangas KR, et al. A study of twins and stroke. Stroke 1992;23:221–3.

36. Brass LM, Shaker LA. Family history in patients with transient ischemic attacks. Stroke 1991;22:837–41.

37. Sacco RL, Benjamin EJ, Broderick JP, et al. American Heart Association Prevention Conference. IV. Prevention and rehabilitation of stroke. Risk factors. Stroke 1997;28:1507–17.

38. Duggirala R, Villalpando CG, O'Leary DH, et al. Genetic basis of variation in carotid artery wall thickness. Stroke 1996;27:833–7.

39. Catto AJ. Genetic aspects of the hemostatic system in cerebrovascular disease. Neurology 2001;57(Suppl 2):S24–30.

40. Hindorff LA, Sethupathy P, Junkins HA, et al. Potential etiologic and functional implications of genome-wide association loci for human diseases and traits. Proc Natl Acad Sci U S A 2009;106:9362–7.

41. Tan MS, Jiang T, Tan J, et al. Genome-wide association studies in neurology. Ann Transl Med 2014;2(12):124.

42. Gretarsdottir S, Thorleifsson G, Manolescu A, et al. Risk variants for atrial fibrillation on chromosome 4q25 associate with ischemic stroke. Ann Neurol 2008;64: 402–9.

43. Gudbjartsson DR, Holm H, Gretarsdottir S, et al. A sequence variant in ZFHX3 on 16q22 associated with atrial fibrillation and ischemic stroke. Nat Genet 2009;41: 876–8.
44. Gschwendtner A, Bevan S, Cole JW, et al. Sequence variants on chromosome 9p21.3 confer risk for atherosclerotic stroke. Ann Neurol 2009;65:531–9.
45. Kubo M, Hata J, Ninomiya T, et al. A nonsynonymous SNP in PRKCH (protein kinase C eta) increases the risk of cerebral infarction. Nat Genet 2007;39:212–7.
46. Traylor M, Farrall M, Holliday EG, et al. Genetic risk factors for ischaemic stroke and its subtypes (the METASTROKE collaboration): a meta-analysis of genome-wide association studies. Lancet Neurol 2012;11:951–62.
47. Bersano A, Ballabio E, Bresolin N, et al. Genetic polymorphisms for the study of multifactorial stroke. Hum Mutat 2008;29:776–95.
48. Campbell DJ, Woodward M, Chalmers JP, et al. Soluble vascular cell adhesion molecule 1 and N-terminal pro-B-type natriuretic peptide in predicting ischemic stroke in patients with cerebrovascular disease. Arch Neurol 2006;63:60–5.
49. Ikram MA, Seshadri S, Bis JC, et al. Genome-wide association studies of stroke. N Engl J Med 2009;360:1718–28.
50. International Stroke Genetics Consortium, Wellcome Trust Case-Control Consortium 2. Failure to validate association between 12p13 variants and ischemic stroke. N Engl J Med 2010;362:1547–50.
51. Rubattu S, Volpe M, Kreutz R, et al. Chromosomal mapping of quantitative trait loci contributing to stroke in a rat model of complex human disease. Nat Genet 1996;13:429–34.
52. Terni E, Giannini N, Brondi M, et al. Genetics of ischaemic stroke in young adults. BBA Clin 2014;3:96–106.
53. Sharma P, Yadav S, Meschia JF. Genetics of ischaemic stroke. J Neurol Neurosurg Psychiatry 2013;84:1302–8.
54. Kalimo H, Viitanen M, Amberla K, et al. CADASIL: hereditary disease of arteries causing brain infarcts and dementia. Neuropathol Appl Neurobiol 1999;25: 257–65.
55. Shah S, Ellard S, Kneen R, et al. Childhood presentation of COL4A1 mutations. Dev Med Child Neurol 2012;54:569–74.
56. Schiffmann R. Fabry disease. Pharmacol Ther 2009;122:65–77.
57. Debette S, Markus HS. The clinical importance of white matter hyperintensities on brain magnetic resonance imaging: systematic review and meta-analysis. BMJ 2010;341:c3666.
58. Rost NS, Rahman RM, Biffi A, et al. White matter hyperintensity volume is increased in small vessel stroke subtypes. Neurology 2010;75:1670–7.
59. Arsava EM, Rahman R, Rosand J, et al. Severity of leukoaraiosis correlates with clinical outcome after ischemic stroke. Neurology 2009;72:1403–10.
60. Hofer E, Cavalieri M, Bis JC, et al, Cohorts for Heart and Aging Research in Genomic Epidemiology Consortium. White matter lesion progression: genome-wide search for genetic influences. Stroke 2015;46:3048–57.
61. Verhaaren BF, Debette S, Bis JC, et al. Multiethnic genome-wide association study of cerebral white matter hyperintensities on MRI. Circ Cardiovasc Genet 2015;8:398–409.
62. Traylor M, Zhang CR, Adib-Samil P, et al, International Stroke Genetics Consortium. Genome-wide meta-analysis of cerebral white matter hyperintensities in patients with stroke. Neurology 2016;86:146–53.
63. Traylor M, Bevan S, Baron JC, et al. Genetic architecture of lacunar stroke. Stroke 2015;46:2407–12.

64. Launer LJ, Terwindt GM, Ferrari MD. The prevalence and characteristics of migraine in a population-based cohort: the GEM study. Neurology 1999;53: 537–42.
65. Kurth T, Chabriat H, Bousser MG. Migraine and stroke: a complex association with clinical implications. Lancet Neurol 2012;11:92–100.
66. Etminan M, Takkouche B, Isorna FC, et al. Risk of ischaemic stroke in people with migraine: systematic review and meta-analysis of observational studies. BMJ 2005;330:63.
67. Schurks M, Rist PM, Bigal ME, et al. Migraine and cardiovascular disease: systematic review and meta-analysis. BMJ 2009;339:b3914.
68. Nozari A, Dilekoz E, Sukhotinsky I, et al. Microemboli may link spreading depression, migraine aura, and patent foramen ovale. Ann Neurol 2010;67:221–9.
69. Stam AH, Haan J, van den Maagdenberg AM, et al. Migraine and genetic and acquired vasculopathies. Cephalalgia 2009;29:1006–17.
70. Zeller JA, Frahm K, Baron R, et al. Platelet-leukocyte interaction and platelet activation in migraine: a link to ischemic stroke? J Neurol Neurosurg Psychiatry 2004; 75:984–7.
71. Friberg L, Olesen J, Lassen NA, et al. Cerebral oxygen extraction, oxygen consumption, and regional cerebral blood flow during the aura phase of migraine. Stroke 1994;25:974–9.
72. Malik R, Freilinger T, Winsvold BS, et al. Shared genetic basis for migraine and ischemic stroke. A genome-wide analysis of common variants. Neurology 2015; 84:2132–45.

Epidemiology of Brain Tumors

Katharine A. McNeill, MD

KEYWORDS

- Glioma • Meningioma • Pituitary adenoma • Medulloblastoma • Ionizing radiation
- Neurofibromatosis

KEY POINTS

- Although central nervous system (CNS) tumors are rare in adults, they are a significant cause of morbidity and mortality in young adults and are the most common solid tumors in infants and children.
- The most common tumors in children are pilocytic astrocytomas and medulloblastomas compared with meningiomas, pituitary tumors, and glioblastomas in adults.
- Ionizing radiation increases the risk for brain tumors, whereas cell phones that are nonionizing do not.
- Although several hereditary CNS syndromes may be associated with an increased risk of brain tumors, 95% of brain tumors are nonfamilial.

EPIDEMIOLOGY OF PRIMARY BRAIN TUMORS

Although CNS tumors are rare, they are a significant cause of cancer morbidity and mortality, especially in children and young adults where they respectively account for approximately 30% and 20% of cancer deaths (**Figs. 1** and **2**). They are also a cause of excessive mortality relative to other cancers. CNS tumors are predicted to represent 1.4% of new cancer diagnoses in 2015 and will cause 2.6% of cancer deaths.[1] The commonest CNS tumors in children are pilocytic astrocytoma, embryonal tumors, and malignant gliomas (**Fig. 3**) whereas meningiomas, pituitary tumors, and malignant gliomas are most common adult brain tumor types (**Fig. 4**). The most common histology by age group and their median age at diagnosis among the various types of brain tumors are summarized in **Tables 1** and **2**.

This review addresses the incidences and prevalences of the commest types of childhood and adulthood brain tumors as well as their recurrence and survival rates. It reviews common genetic and environmental risk factors causally associated with brain tumors and temporal incidence trends.

Disclosure Statement: The author has nothing to disclose.
Division of Neuroepidemiology, Department of Neurology, New York University School of Medicine, and the Laura and Isaac Perlmutter Cancer Center, 240 East 38th Street, 19th Floor, New York, NY 10016, USA
E-mail address: Katharine.McNeill@nyumc.org

Neurol Clin 34 (2016) 981–998
http://dx.doi.org/10.1016/j.ncl.2016.06.014
0733-8619/16/$ – see front matter © 2016 Elsevier Inc. All rights reserved.

neurologic.theclinics.com

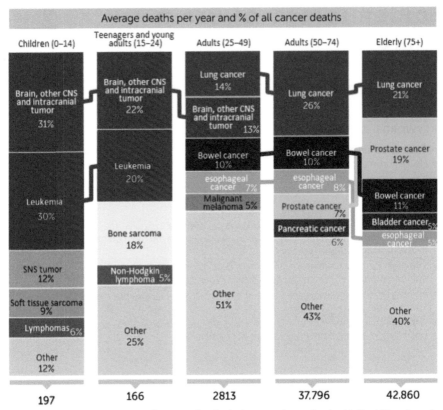

Fig. 1. Most common causes of cancer deaths in boys and men in the United Kingdom, by age, 2010 to 2012. (*From* Cancer Research UK. Available at: http://www.cancerresearchuk.org/health-professional/cancer-statistics/mortality/age. Accessed August 1, 2015.)

Meningiomas

Meningiomas are the commonest brain tumors in adults accounting for 36% of all brain tumors in the Central Brain Tumor Registry of the United States (CBTRUS).[2] The CBTRUS estimates that there will be approximately 24,000 new meningiomas diagnosed in the United States in 2015, with an estimated incidence of 7.61 per 100,000.[2] The prevalence is difficult to measure because the lesions are often asymptomatic and incidentally diagnosed. Several large autopsy studies from the pre-MRI era reported a prevalence ranging from 1.0% to 2.7%.[3–5] Overall, 85% were diagnosed incidentally and 15% were symptomatic in 1 large autopsy study.[4] The prevalence estimate of 0.3% to 0.9% in the modern era of MRI was somewhat lower,[6,7] likely owing to the younger population studied and the threshold for detection of small lesions on imaging.

The incidence of meningioma steadily increases with age (**Fig. 5**) being twice as common in women as in men and 20% more common in blacks than in whites.[2,8] A majority of meningiomas are benign (grade I), with 5% to 20% atypical (grade II) and 1% to 3% malignant in type (grade III).[9] Benign meningiomas are an insignificant cause of mortality although skull-based tumors can cause significant morbidity. By contrast, atypical and malignant meningiomas can be associated with significant morbidity and mortality and high rates of recurrence. Approximately one-half of

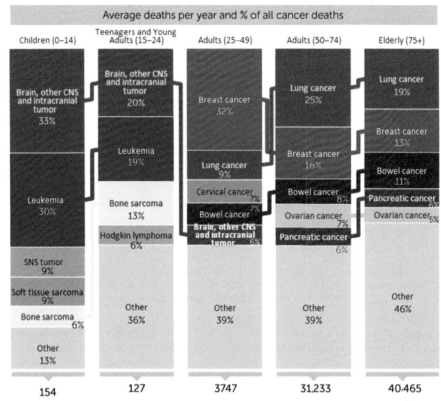

Fig. 2. Most common causes of cancer deaths in girls and women in the United Kingdom, by age, 2010 to 2012. (*From* Cancer Research UK. Available at: http://www.cancerresearchuk.org/health-professional/cancer-statistics/mortality/age. Accessed August 1, 2015.)

atypical meningiomas recur over a decade and late recurrences are common, with a majority of malignant meningiomas recurring at a median interval of 2 years. Survival and recurrence rates for atypical and malignant meningiomas are summarized in **Table 3**.

Gliomas

Gliomas account for 24% of brain tumors in adults (see **Fig. 4**) and as a group are the second most common brain tumors in adults. The CBTRUS estimates that approximately 20,000 new gliomas will be diagnosed in the United States in 2015.[2] These tumors vary widely in histology from benign and potentially surgically curable grade I tumors (pilocytic astrocytoma) to locally aggressive grade IV tumors with a high risk of recurrence or progression (glioblastoma). Survival varies by histology, with pilocytic astrocytoma having a 10-year survival of greater than 90%, whereas only 5% of patients with glioblastoma survive to 5 years. Survival rate by histology is summarized in **Fig. 6**.

Approximately one-half of gliomas are glioblastomas, the commonest malignant primary brain tumor in adults.[2] Glioblastomas and other malignant gliomas represent approximately 75% of malignant brain tumors.[2] The age-adjusted incidence rates of gliomas that vary by histology and country are summarized in **Table 2**. Their

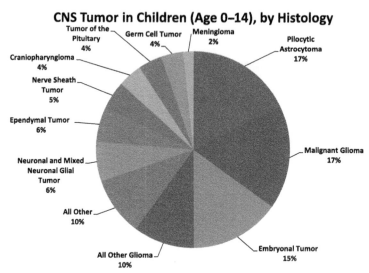

Fig. 3. CNS tumor histology in children. (*Adapted from* Ostrom QT, Gittleman H, Liao P, et al. CBTRUS statistical report: primary brain and central nervous system tumors diagnosed in the United States in 2007–2011. Neuro Oncol 2014;16 Suppl 4:iv1–iv63.)

respective incidences also vary significantly with geographic region (**Table 4**); however, it is not certain whether this is due to either lack of consistent definitions of histologic subtypes, differences in data collection, surveillances methods between countries, or true differences in incidence.[10,11] The CBTRUS estimates the incidence of gliomas and glioblastomas to be 6.61 and 3.19 per 100,000, respectively, in the United States.

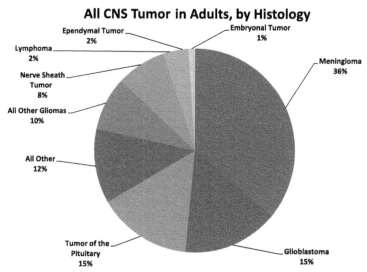

Fig. 4. CNS tumor histology in adults. (*Adapted from* Ostrom QT, Gittleman H, Liao P, et al. CBTRUS statistical report: primary brain and central nervous system tumors diagnosed in the United States in 2007–2011. Neuro Oncol 2014;16 Suppl 4:iv1–iv63.)

Table 1
Most common histology by age group

Age (Y)	Most Common Histology	Second Most Common Histology	Third Most Common Histology
0–4	Embryonal tumors	Pilocytic astrocytoma	Malignant glioma
5–9	Pilocytic astrocytoma	Malignant glioma	Embryonal tumors
10–14	Pilocytic astrocytoma	Malignant glioma	Neuronal and glioneuronal tumors
15–19	Tumors of the pituitary	Pilocytic astrocytoma	Neuronal and glioneuronal tumors
20–34	Tumors of the pituitary	Meningioma	Nerve sheath tumors
35–44	Meningioma	Tumors of the pituitary	Nerve sheath tumors
45–54	Meningioma	Tumors of the pituitary	Glioblastoma
55–64	Meningioma	Glioblastoma	Tumors of the pituitary
65–74	Meningioma	Glioblastoma	Tumors of the pituitary
75–85	Meningioma	Glioblastoma	Tumors of the pituitary
85+	Meningioma	Glioblastoma	Tumors of the pituitary
Overall	Meningioma (7.61 per 100,000)	Tumors of the pituitary (3.29 per 100,000)	Glioblastoma (3.19 per 100,000)

Adapted from Ostrom QT, Gittleman H, Liao P, et al. CBTRUS statistical report: primary brain and central nervous system tumors diagnosed in the United States in 2007–2011. Neuro Oncol 2014;16 Suppl 4:iv1–iv63.

Gliomas have a slight male preponderance, with 55% occurring in men. Those in the United States more commonly affect non-Hispanic white than Hispanic, black, or Asian ethnic groups.[2] The incidence of gliomas over the life span of an individual varies by tumor histology. Grade I (pilocytic astrocytoma) tumors occurs predominantly in children and young adults, whereas grade II (oligodendroglial) tumors peak in the 3rd to 4th decades, with the incidence of malignant gliomas increasing in older age to a maximum in the 6th to 7th decades. The age-adjusted incidence rates by histology are summarized in **Figs. 5** and **7**.

Table 2
Median age at tumor diagnosis, by histology

Histology, Non-Neuroepithelial	Median Age (Y)	Histology, Neuroepithelial	Median Age
Embryonal tumors	9	Pilocytic astrocytoma	13
Germ cell tumors	17	Mixed glioneuronal tumors	27
Choroid plexus tumors	19	Oligodendroglioma	43
Tumors of the pineal region	33	Ependymal tumors	44
Craniopharyngioma	42	Diffuse astrocytoma	48
Tumors of the pituitary	51	Anaplastic Oligodendroglioma	49
Meningioma	65	Anaplastic astrocytoma	53
Lymphoma	65	Glioblastoma	64

Adapted from Ostrom QT, Gittleman H, Liao P, et al. CBTRUS statistical report: primary brain and central nervous system tumors diagnosed in the United States in 2007–2011. Neuro Oncol 2014;16 Suppl 4:iv1–iv63.

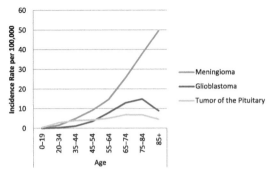

Fig. 5. Age-adjusted incidence rate of the most common CNS tumors by histology and age, CBTRUS, 2007 to 2011. (*Adapted from* Ostrom QT, Gittleman H, Liao P, et al. CBTRUS statistical report: primary brain and central nervous system tumors diagnosed in the United States in 2007–2011. Neuro Oncol 2014;16 Suppl 4:iv1–iv63.)

Pituitary Tumors

Pituitary tumors are the third most common brain tumor in adults, accounting for 15% of adult tumors. The CBTRUS estimates that 11,000 new pituitary tumors will be diagnosed in the United States in 2015, with an incidence of 3.47 per 100,000. A majority of pituitary tumors are benign adenomas, although craniopharyngiomas and other types of histology comprise a minority of pituitary tumors. Like meningiomas, they are often asymptomatic and incidentally diagnosed, especially microadenomas and non–hormone-secreting tumors, making estimates of the prevalence difficult to ascertain. In 1 large meta-analysis of radiographic and autopsy studies of pituitary tumors, it was estimated that pituitary tumors occurred in 14% of patients in autopsy series and 23% of neuroradiographic series, suggesting that many tumors were undiagnosed.[12]

Pituitary tumors are more common in women than in men and relatively more common in blacks and Hispanics than whites and Asians (**Table 5**). The incidence of such tumors increase with age, peaking in the 7th decade (see **Fig. 5**). Although pituitary adenomas are generally benign, there does seem to be excess associated mortality; however, it is unclear whether that is due to morbidity of surgery, perioperative medical complications, related endocrinopathy, or tumor recurrence and progression. One large series from a Swedish Cancer Registry[13] found a standardized mortality ratio of observed to expected deaths of 2.0 (95% CI, 1.9–2.2) with a median survival was 18 years for men and 25 years for women and estimated respective 10-year survival of 69% and 76%. A recent retrospective cohort of patients from the United Kingdom noted a standardized mortality ratio of 3.6 (95% CI, 2.9–4.5).[14] Although pituitary adenomas are often cured by surgical resection, recurrences occur in 7% to 12%, and

Table 3					
Survival and recurrence rates for atypical and malignant meningiomas					
	Median Survival (y)	5-Year Survival Rate (%)	Median Recurrence-Free Survival (y)	Recurrence Rate at 5 Years (%)	Recurrence Rate at 10 Years (%)
Atypical meningioma[69,70]	11–19	80–95	12	23	45
Malignant meningioma[70–72]	2–7	28–64	2	55	85

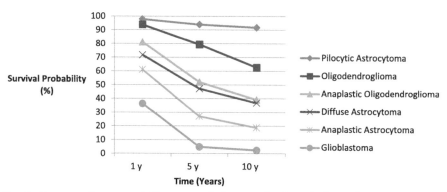

Fig. 6. One-year, 5-year, and 10-year survival rates of selected glioma histology, CBTRUS 2007 to 2011. (*Adapted from* Ostrom QT, Gittleman H, Liao P, et al. CBTRUS statistical report: primary brain and central nervous system tumors diagnosed in the United States in 2007–2011. Neuro Oncol 2014;16 Suppl 4:iv1–iv63.)

60% to 65% of patients progress after subtotal resection[15,16]; however, recurrences can be treated effectively with repeat resection or radiotherapy.

Pediatric Brain Tumors

Approximately 1 in 2000 children are diagnosed with a brain tumor by the age of 14 in the United States according to the CBTRUS. Brain tumors are the commonest solid

Table 4
Age-adjusted incidence rates per 100,000 by histology and country

Histology	Country/Region	Years	Incidence Rate
Pilocytic astrocytoma	Austria	2005	0.57
	Korea	2005	0.18
	US	2006–2010	0.33
Oligodendroglioma	Austria	2005	0.20
	England	1999–2003	0.21
	Korea	2005	0.10
	US	2006–2010	0.27
Anaplastic astrocytoma	Austria	2005	0.44
	Korea	2005	0.13
	US	2006–2010	0.37
Glioblastoma	Australia	2000–2008	3.40
	England	1999–2003	2.05
	Korea	2005	0.59
	US	2006–2010	3.19
	Greece	2005–2007	3.69
All astrocytic tumors	Austria	2005	5.33
	England	1999–2003	3.48
	Europe	1995–2002	4.80
All oligodendroglial rumors	Austria	2005	0.70
	Europe	1995–2002	0.40
All fliomas	Finland	2000–2002	4.67
	Greece	2005–2007	5.73

Adapted from Ostrom QT, Bauchet L, Davis FG, et al. The epidemiology of glioma in adults: a "state of the science" review. Neuro Oncol 2014;16(7):896–913.

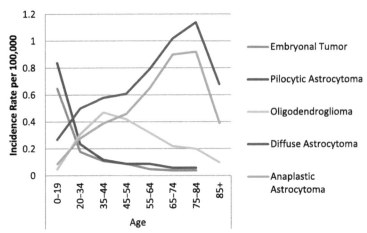

Fig. 7. Age-adjusted incidence rate of selected CNS tumors by histology and age, CBTRUS, 2007 to 2011. (*Adapted from* Ostrom QT, Gittleman H, Liao P, et al. CBTRUS statistical report: primary brain and central nervous system tumors diagnosed in the United States in 2007–2011. Neuro Oncol 2014;16 Suppl 4:iv1–iv63.)

tumor in infants and children, and the most common cause of cancer death in children.[17] The CBTRUS estimates that 3420 new CNS tumors will be diagnosed in infants and children in the United States in 2015.[17] Approximately one-half of brain tumors in infants and children are gliomas, of which the majority are pilocytic astrocytoma or other low-grade gliomas. Embryonal tumors that accounted for 15% and rare histologic types comprising another one-third of pediatric brain tumors were similarly noted in large cohorts treated in Germany, Canada, Egypt, Brazil, and Morocco.[18–22] The median age at diagnosis and incidence rates of pediatric brain tumors are summarized in **Table 6**. One-year, 5-year, and 10-year survival rates by histology are summarized in **Table 7**.

Embryonal tumors are the most common malignant brain tumors of childhood. Medulloblastomas and primitive neuroectodermal tumors (PNETs) share common

Table 5 Age-adjusted incidence rates of pituitary tumors by age and race, per 100,000 in the United States	
Overall	2.87
Gender	
Male	2.71
Female	3.11
Race	
White	2.59
Black	4.76
American Indian/Alaskan Natives	2.28
Asian or Pacific Islanders	2.13
Non-Spanish Hispanic	2.79
Spanish Hispanic	3.55

Adapted from Gittleman H, Ostrom QT, Farah PD, et al. Descriptive epidemiology of pituitary tumors in the United States, 2004-2009. J Neurosurg 2014;121(3):527–35.

Table 6
Average annual age-adjusted incidence rates of pediatric brain and central nervous system tumors by histology in the United States

Histology	N	All Tumors (%)	Median Age	Incidence Rate
Gliomas	8487	52.9	6.0	2.78
Pilocytic astrocytoma	2821	17.6	7.0	0.93
Other low-grade gliomas	2296	14.3	6.0	0.75
High-grade glioma	1784	11.1	7.0	0.59
Ependymal tumors	879	5.5	4.0	0.29
Other glioma	707	4.4	7.0	0.23
Embryonal tumors	2413	15.0	4.0	0.79
Medulloblastoma	1494	9.3	6.0	0.49
PNET	360	2.2	3.5	0.12
AT/RT	363	2.3	1.0	0.12
Other embryonal tumors	196	1.2	1.0	0.06
Tumors of cranial and spinal nerves	758	4.7	7.0	0.25
Tumors of the pineal region	701	4.4	6.5	0.23
Craniopharyngioma	648	4.0	8.0	0.21
Tumors of the pituitary	625	3.9	12.0	0.20
Germ cell tumors	590	3.7	9.0	0.15
Tumors of meninges	458	2.9	9.0	0.15
Choroid plexus tumors	362	2.3	1.0	0.12
Neuronal and mixed neuronal-glial tumors	140	0.9	9.0	0.05
Lymphomas and hematopoietic neoplasms	70	0.4	6.0	0.02
Other/unclassified tumors	792	4.9	9.0	0.26
Total	16,044	100	7.0	5.26 per 100,000

Adapted from Ostrom QT, de Blank PM, Kruchko C et al. Alex's Lemonade Stand Foundation Infant and childhood primary brain and central nervous system tumors diagnosed in the United States in 2007-2011. Neuro Oncol 2015;16 Suppl 10:x1–x36.

histologic features but vary by location, with medulloblastomas arising within the posterior fossa and PNETs supratentorially. Medulloblastomas have a bimodal distribution peaking at 3 to 4 years of age or between 8 and 9 years of age. Boys are 1.7 times more likely to develop them compared with girls[23] and they occur 4 times more often than supratentorial tumors. PNETs and atypical teratoid/rhabdoid tumors (AT/RTs) tend to occur in younger patients, with most diagnosed before age 5 years; however, like medulloblastomas, they affect boys more often than girls[23,24]; the survival in this tumor type is summarized in **Table 7**.

RISK FACTORS FOR BRAIN TUMORS

Many possible contributory environmental risk factors for the development of brain tumors have been proposed and studied, but few are well established. **Table 4** summarizes those for which no clear association has been established. The number of cases studied among large cohorts has been small.[25] An association has been described for several industrial and occupational exposures and brain tumors (**Box 1**), although

Table 7
One-year, 5-year, and 10-year survival rates for selected histology of pediatric central nervous system tumors

Histology	1-Year (%)	5-Year (%)	10-Year (%)
Gliomas	87	77	73
Pilocytic astrocytoma	99	98	96
Other low-grade gliomas	95	90	85
High-grade glioma	56	30	26
Ependymal tumors	93	80	64
Other glioma	97	93	91
Embryonal tumors	80	62	56
Medulloblastoma	87	70	63
PNET	77	56	49
AT/RT	48	28	26
Other embryonal tumors	80	65	63
Tumors of the pineal region	98	89	89
Germ cell tumors	93	87	80
Tumors of meninges	77	56	48
Choroid plexus tumors	81	61	58
Neuronal and mixed neuronal-glial tumors	85	55	43
Lymphomas and hematopoietic neoplasms	87	81	76
Other/unclassified tumors	60	50	43
Total	86	73	69

Adapted from Ostrom, QT, de Blank PM, Kruchko C, et al. Alex's Lemonade Stand Foundation Infant and childhood primary brain and central nervous system tumors diagnosed in the United States in 2007-2011. Neuro Oncol 2015;16 Suppl 10:x1–x36.

none have been well established. There are several risk factors for which an association with brain tumors has been established, including ionizing radiation, genetic susceptibility, and allergic aspects.

Ionizing Radiation

Ionizing radiation is well established as an environmental risk factor for brain tumors. Exposures include radiation for benign medical conditions, such as tinea capitis,[26,27] skin hemangiomas,[28,29] and adenoid hypertrophy[30] as well as prophylactic cranial irradiation for childhood leukemia, lymphoma, or irradiation of brain tumors in children.[31–33] Brain tumors were cited among atomic bomb survivors,[34,35] in Chernobyl clean-up workers,[36] and among US nuclear workers.[37] A variety of CNS tumors have been described, including hemangioblastomas, lymphomas, and embryonal tumors,[26,30,31,33] but the commonest radiation-induced tumors were meningiomas, gliomas, and schwannomas.[26,31,33] The median interval between radiation and diagnosis of a radiation-induced glioma was 9 to 18 years although generally longer for radiation-induced meningiomas, where it ranged from 17 to 23 years.[31,33,38] The risk of developing a radiation-induced tumor was highest in exposed infants and those initially exposed in infancy, decreasing as the age at the time of radiation exposure increased. There is evidence of a dose-response relationship with a greater risk of developing a radiation-induced tumor after higher radiation doses.[39] A large meta-analysis of patients exposed to 0.07 Gy to 10 Gy of cranial irradiation reported an excess relative

---

Box 1
Environmental risk factors investigated in epidemiologic studies for association with brain tumors

Minimal to No Evidence of Association

Head trauma

Dietary calcium intake

Dietary N-nitroso compound intake

Dietary antioxidant intake

Dietary maternal N-nitroso compound intake

Dietary maternal and early life antioxidant intake

Maternal folate supplementation

Tobacco smoking

Alcohol consumption

Electromagnetic fields

Air pollution

Inconclusive Evidence of Association

Pesticides

Fertilizers

Formaldehyde

Synthetic rubber

Vinyl chloride

Petrochemicals and petroleum

Adapted from Wrensch M, Minn Y, Chew T, et al. Epidemiology of primary brain tumors: current concepts and review of the literature. Neuro Oncol 2002;4(4):278–99; and Fisher JL, Schwartzbaum JA, Wrensch M, et al. Epidemiology of brain tumors. Neurol Clin 2007;25(4):867–90, vii.

---

risk of 0.079 per Gy to 0.56 per Gy of radiation for gliomas, and 0.64 per Gy to 5.1 per Gy for meningiomas.[39] The risk of developing meningiomas seemed greater than the risk of developing gliomas across studies.[39]

Nonionizing Radiation

Since the advent of cellular telephones in the 1980s, there has been concern regarding the risk of exposure to radiofrequency electromagnetic fields and a possible relationship between cell phone use and incidence of brain tumors. Some studies suggested such an association,[40,41] but those studies were tainted by selection and recall bias. The differential use of proxy interviews also introduced bias. One large case-control study,[42] for instance, performed proxy interviews in 13% of glioma patients compared with 1% of controls. The INTERPHONE Study[42] provides an excellent review of these possible sources of bias.

Several cohort studies of cell phone use found no evidence of a relationship to brain tumors,[43,44] and the largest case-control study to date, the INTERPHONE Study, which included more than 5000 cases of meningioma and glioma from 13 countries, found no evidence for an increased risk of glioma or meningioma associated with cell phone use. There was a reduced odds ratio (OR) of ever having been a regular cell phone user in both glioma (OR 0.81; 95% CI, 0.70–0.94) and meningioma (OR 0.79; 95% CI, 0.68–0.91), although those findings were likely due to participation bias. There was also a suggestion of an increased risk of glioma at the top decile of exposure (OR 1.40, 95% CI, 1.03–1.89), but several of these cases reported implausible phone use (≥12 h/d). There was evidence that cases overestimated cell phone use relative to controls, calling this finding into question.[42] Because there was some suggestion of concordance between brain tumor side and preferred side of phone use, and higher OR for tumors located in the temporal lobe where field strength was highest, there is continuing interest in this issue.[42] A large prospective cohort study that aims to study 250,000 cell phone users in 5 European countries and follow them for 25 years, is ongoing,[45] but at present, the weight of the evidence does not suggest a relationship between cell phone use and brain tumors.

Genetic Susceptibility and Hereditary Syndromes

Although there are several genetic syndromes associated with an increased risk of brain tumors, a majority of brain tumors are sporadic. In 1 study of 500 patients with glioma,[46] for instance, less than 1% had a known hereditary syndrome. In contrast, approximately 5% of glioma cases are familial, defined as 2 or more gliomas among first–degree or second-degree relatives,[47] suggesting that there may be other genetic predispositions outside of these known hereditary syndromes. Familial aggregation was reported in gliomas[48,49] and meningioma,[50] with 1 such report of a low penetrance at the 15q23-26.3 gene locus in patients with familial glioma in Finland,[51] but the genetic basis of familial aggregation remains not well understood in most cases.

A complete review of familial syndromes associated with brain tumors is outside the scope of this review, although several excellent reviews are available for interested readers.[52,53] Neurofibromatosis type I is the commonest familial syndrome associated with brain tumors, present in approximately 1 in 3000 live births[54] and a hallmark feature of the syndrome with optic pathway gliomas present in approximately 15% of patients, and hemispheric and brainstem gliomas so noted in about 3% of patients.[53] Although inheritance is autosomal dominant, approximately 30% to 50% of patients have de novo mutations in the NF1 gene, located on the 17q11.2 chromosomal locus.[54] Neurofibromatosis type II is less frequent, occurring in 1 in 33,000 to 40,000 live births. Its hallmark feature is bilateral vestibular schwannomas with up to 50% developing multiple meningiomas. Schwannomas can occur in other cranial and spinal nerves and approximately 2% to 5% of patients develop ependymomas.[53] Other hereditary syndromes associated with brain tumors are summarized in **Table 8**.

Allergic and Immune-Related Conditions

There is mounting evidence that allergies and autoimmune conditions are inversely correlated with glioma risk. Several groups have reported a reduced risk of glioma in patients with allergy or a variety of autoimmune conditions.[55–58] One large population-based study in the United Kingdom found a reduced risk of glioma in patients with asthma (OR 0.71; 95% CI, 0.54–0.92), hay fever (OR 0.73; 95% CI, 0.59–0.90), and eczema (OR 0.74; 95% CI, 0.56–0.97).[57] Another international study from France, Germany, Sweden, Australia, Canada, and the United States[59] showed an inverse correlation between allergic diseases and glioma (OR 0.6; 95% CI, 0.5–0.7) but not with meningioma. Other investigators[60] found a decreased total IgE level in glioma cases compared with controls. The

Table 8
Genetic syndromes associated with brain tumors

	Central Nervous System Tumors	Chromosome	Gene	Associated Tumors
Neurofibromatosis type 1	Optic pathway glioma Gliomas	17q11.2	NF1	Pheochromocytoma, gastrointestinal stromal tumors, Juvenile chronic myelogenous leukemia, rhabdomyosarcoma
Neurofibromatosis type 2	Vestibular schwannoma Ependymoma Meningioma	22q12	NF2	None
Tuberous sclerosis	Subependymal giant cell astrocytoma	9q34, 16p13.3	TSC1 TSC2	Cardiac rhabdomyoma, renal angiomyolipoma
Li-Fraumeni syndrome	Gliomas PNET/ medulloblastoma Choroid plexus carcinoma	17p13.1	TP53	Breast carcinoma, sarcomas, leukemia, adrenocortical carcinoma
Cowden disease	Dysplastic gangliocytoma of the cerebellum	10q23	PTEN	Colon polyps, breast and thyroid carcinomas
Turcot syndrome				
Type 1	Medulloblastoma	5q21	APC	Colon carcinoma
Type 2	Glioblastoma	3p21 7p22	MLH1 PMS2	
von Hippel-Lindau	Hemangioblastoma	3p25	VHL	Renal cell carcinomas, pheochromocytomas, tumors of the endolymphatic sac
Nevoid basal cell carcinoma syndrome (Gorlin syndrome)	Medulloblastoma Meningioma	9q31	PTCH	Basal cell carcinoma

Adapted from Hottinger AF, Khakoo Y. Neurooncology of familial cancer syndromes. J Child Neurol 2009;24(12):1526–35.

exact mechanism is unclear but may be due to increased tumor and immune surveillance in those with allergies and tumor-related immune suppression.[61]

TEMPORAL TRENDS

Although there was an apparent increase in brain tumor incidence in the decades between 1970 and the 2000, this was deemed due to improvements in detection concomitant with the introduction of MRI in the 1980s.[62] Although some groups have reported increased[63,64] or decreased[65,66] incidence rates of brain tumors, others have reported stable incidence.[67,68] It is thought, therefore, that any change in incidence rates noted during that period is likely to be due to changing classifications of tumors, improved diagnostic accuracy, better reporting, and access to health care.[20]

SUMMARY

Brain tumors are uncommon in adults and an important cause of mortality in children and young adults. An understanding of their epidemiology is essential for clinical and academic neurologists alike who are involved in the care of patients or investigating the cause of primary brain tumors. Although there are several well known risk factors and heritable syndromes, most tumors arise outside the settings of these exposures or genetic predispositions.

Unrecognized and, therefore, untreated, it is essential for practicing neurologists to be aware of the importance of evaluating suspected mass lesions based on suggestive symptoms and sign. The age at presentation may be a clue to a particular histologic diagnosis because many of these tumors present in distinct age groups, although significant overlap can occur, making it important to obtain pathologic confirmation of the tumor type and grade. The heterogeneity of the different types of brain tumors is underscored by the relative lack of impact on survival in benign lesions to median survival of 1 to 2 years in malignant lesions. Epidemiologically sound clinical investigative studies are imperative to the understanding of the genetic changes and risk factors associated with the propensity to develop primary brain tumors. Comparative clinicopathologic and immune cytologic studies will continue to be useful in refining approaches to classifications within and among the major categories of primary CNS tumors.

REFERENCES

1. Howlader N, Noone AM, Krapcho M, et al. SEER Cancer Statistics Review, 1975-2012. 2015. Available at: http://seer.cancer.gov/csr/1975_2012/.
2. Ostrom QT, Gittleman H, Liao P, et al. CBTRUS statistical report: primary brain and central nervous system tumors diagnosed in the United States in 2007-2011. Neuro Oncol 2014;16(Suppl 4):iv1–63.
3. Bellur SN, Chandra V. Meningioma size. Its relationship to other diseases. Arch Neurol 1981;38(7):458–9.
4. Nakasu S, Hirano A, Shimura T, et al. Incidental meningiomas in autopsy study. Surg Neurol 1987;27(4):319–22.
5. Rausing A, Ybo W, Stenflo J. Intracranial meningioma–a population study of ten years. Acta Neurol Scand 1970;46(1):102–10.
6. Morris Z, Whiteley WN, Longstreth WT Jr, et al. Incidental findings on brain magnetic resonance imaging: systematic review and meta-analysis. BMJ 2009;339: b3016.
7. Vernooij MW, Ikram MA, Tanghe HL, et al. Incidental findings on brain MRI in the general population. N Engl J Med 2007;357(18):1821–8.
8. Dolecek TA, Dressler EV, Thakkar JP, et al. Epidemiology of meningiomas post-public law 107-206: the benign brain tumor cancer registries amendment act. Cancer 2015;121(14):2400–10.
9. Louis DN, Ongaki H, Wiestler OD, et al, editors. WHO classification of tumours of the central nervous system. 4th edition. Lyon (France): International Agency for Research on Cancer (IARC); 2007.
10. Ostrom QT, Bauchet L, Davis FG, et al. The epidemiology of glioma in adults: a "state of the science" review. Neuro Oncol 2014;16(7):896–913.
11. Ostrom QT, Gittleman H, Stetson L, et al. Epidemiology of gliomas. Cancer Treat Res 2015;163:1–14.
12. Ezzat S, Asa SL, Couldwell WT, et al. The prevalence of pituitary adenomas: a systematic review. Cancer 2004;101(3):613–9.

13. Nilsson B, Gustavasson-Kadaka E, Bengtsson BA, et al. Pituitary adenomas in Sweden between 1958 and 1991: incidence, survival, and mortality. J Clin Endocrinol Metab 2000;85(4):1420–5.
14. Ntali G, Capatina C, Fazal-Sanderson V, et al. Mortality in patients with nonfunctioning pituitary adenoma is increased: systematic analysis of 546 cases with long follow-up. Eur J Endocrinol 2016;174(2):137–45.
15. Dallapiazza RF, Grober Y, Starke RM, et al. Long-term results of endonasal endoscopic transsphenoidal resection of nonfunctioning pituitary macroadenomas. Neurosurgery 2015;76(1):42–52 [discussion: 52–3].
16. Berkmann S, Schlaffer S, Nimsky C, et al. Follow-up and long-term outcome of nonfunctioning pituitary adenoma operated by transsphenoidal surgery with intraoperative high-field magnetic resonance imaging. Acta Neurochir (Wien) 2014;156(12):2233–43 [discussion: 2243].
17. Ostrom QT, de Blank PM, Kruchko C, et al. Alex's Lemonade Stand Foundation Infant and childhood primary brain and central nervous system tumors diagnosed in the United States in 2007-2011. Neuro Oncol 2015;16(Suppl 10):x1–36.
18. Ezzat S, Kamal M, El-Khateeb N, et al. Pediatric brain tumors in a low/middle income country: does it differ from that in developed world? J Neurooncol 2016; 126(2):371–6.
19. Harmouch A, Taleb M, Lasseini A, et al. Epidemiology of pediatric primary tumors of the nervous system: a retrospective study of 633 cases from a single Moroccan institution. Neurochirurgie 2012;58(1):14–8.
20. Kaderali Z, Lamberti-Pasculli M, Rutka JT. The changing epidemiology of paediatric brain tumours: a review from the Hospital for Sick Children. Childs Nerv Syst 2009;25(7):787–93.
21. Rickert CH, Paulus W. Epidemiology of central nervous system tumors in childhood and adolescence based on the new WHO classification. Childs Nerv Syst 2001;17(9):503–11.
22. Rosemberg S, Fujiwara D. Epidemiology of pediatric tumors of the nervous system according to the WHO 2000 classification: a report of 1,195 cases from a single institution. Childs Nerv Syst 2005;21(11):940–4.
23. Packer RJ, Macdonald T, Vezina G, et al. Medulloblastoma and primitive neuroectodermal tumors. Handb Clin Neurol 2012;105:529–48.
24. Strother D. Atypical teratoid rhabdoid tumors of childhood: diagnosis, treatment and challenges. Expert Rev Anticancer Ther 2005;5(5):907–15.
25. Wrensch M, Minn Y, Chew T, et al. Epidemiology of primary brain tumors: current concepts and review of the literature. Neuro Oncol 2002;4(4):278–99.
26. Shore RE, Moseson M, Harley N, et al. Tumors and other diseases following childhood x-ray treatment for ringworm of the scalp (Tinea capitis). Health Phys 2003; 85(4):404–8.
27. Sadetzki S, Chetrit A, Freedman L, et al. Long-term follow-up for brain tumor development after childhood exposure to ionizing radiation for tinea capitis. Radiat Res 2005;163(4):424–32.
28. Karlsson P, Holmberg E, Lundberg LM, et al. Intracranial tumors after radium treatment for skin hemangioma during infancy–a cohort and case-control study. Radiat Res 1997;148(2):161–7.
29. Lindberg S, Karlsson P, Arvidsson B, et al. Cancer incidence after radiotherapy for skin haemangioma during infancy. Acta Oncol 1995;34(6):735–40.
30. Yeh H, Matanoski GM, Wang Ny, et al. Cancer incidence after childhood nasopharyngeal radium irradiation: a follow-up study in Washington County, Maryland. Am J Epidemiol 2001;153(8):749–56.

31. Neglia JP, Robison LL, Stovall M, et al. New primary neoplasms of the central nervous system in survivors of childhood cancer: a report from the Childhood Cancer Survivor Study. J Natl Cancer Inst 2006;98(21):1528–37.
32. Little MP, de Vathaire F, Shamsaldin A, et al. Risks of brain tumour following treatment for cancer in childhood: modification by genetic factors, radiotherapy and chemotherapy. Int J Cancer 1998;78(3):269–75.
33. Taylor A, Little MP, Winter DL, et al. Population-based risks of CNS tumors in survivors of childhood cancer: the British Childhood Cancer Survivor Study. J Clin Oncol 2010;28(36):5287–93.
34. Thompson DE, Mabuchi K, Ron E, et al. Cancer incidence in atomic bomb survivors. Part II: solid tumors, 1958-1987. Radiat Res 1994;137(2 Suppl):S17–67.
35. Preston DL, Ron E, Tokuoka S, et al. Solid cancer incidence in atomic bomb survivors: 1958-1998. Radiat Res 2007;168(1):1–64.
36. Rahu M, Rahu K, Auvinen A, et al. Cancer risk among Chernobyl cleanup workers in Estonia and Latvia, 1986-1998. Int J Cancer 2006;119(1):162–8.
37. Alexander V, DiMarco JH. Reappraisal of brain tumor risk among U.S. nuclear workers: a 10-year review. Occup Med 2001;16(2):289–315.
38. Walter AW, Hancock ML, Pui CH, et al. Secondary brain tumors in children treated for acute lymphoblastic leukemia at St Jude Children's Research Hospital. J Clin Oncol 1998;16(12):3761–7.
39. Braganza MZ, Kitahara CM, Berrington de González A, et al. Ionizing radiation and the risk of brain and central nervous system tumors: a systematic review. Neuro Oncol 2012;14(11):1316–24.
40. Schuz J, Böhler E, Berg G, et al. Cellular phones, cordless phones, and the risks of glioma and meningioma (Interphone Study Group, Germany). Am J Epidemiol 2006;163(6):512–20.
41. Hardell L, Carlberg M, Hansson Mild K. Pooled analysis of two case-control studies on use of cellular and cordless telephones and the risk for malignant brain tumours diagnosed in 1997-2003. Int Arch Occup Environ Health 2006; 79(8):630–9.
42. Group IS. Brain tumour risk in relation to mobile telephone use: results of the INTERPHONE international case-control study. Int J Epidemiol 2010;39(3):675–94.
43. Ahlbom A, Green A, Kheifets L, et al. Epidemiology of health effects of radiofrequency exposure. Environ Health Perspect 2004;112(17):1741–54.
44. Schuz J, Jacobsen R, Olsen JH, et al. Cellular telephone use and cancer risk: update of a nationwide Danish cohort. J Natl Cancer Inst 2006;98(23):1707–13.
45. Schuz J, Elliott P, Auvinen A, et al. An international prospective cohort study of mobile phone users and health (Cosmos): design considerations and enrolment. Cancer Epidemiol 2011;35(1):37–43.
46. Wrensch M, Lee M, Miike R, et al. Familial and personal medical history of cancer and nervous system conditions among adults with glioma and controls. Am J Epidemiol 1997;145(7):581–93.
47. Malmer B, Iselius L, Holmberg E, et al. Genetic epidemiology of glioma. Br J Cancer 2001;84(3):429–34.
48. Thuwe I, Lundstrom B, Walinder J. Familial brain tumour. Lancet 1979;1(8114): 504.
49. Malmer B, Haraldsson S, Einarsdottir E, et al. Homozygosity mapping of familial glioma in Northern Sweden. Acta Oncol 2005;44(2):114–9.
50. Hemminki K, Li X. Familial risks in nervous system tumors. Cancer Epidemiol Biomarkers Prev 2003;12(11 Pt 1):1137–42.

51. Paunu N, Lahermo P, Onkamo P, et al. A novel low-penetrance locus for familial glioma at 15q23-q26.3. Cancer Res 2002;62(13):3798–802.
52. Ranger AM, Patel YK, Chaudhary N, et al. Familial syndromes associated with intracranial tumours: a review. Childs Nerv Syst 2014;30(1):47–64.
53. Hottinger AF, Khakoo Y. Neurooncology of familial cancer syndromes. J Child Neurol 2009;24(12):1526–35.
54. Walker L, Thompson D, Easton D, et al. A prospective study of neurofibromatosis type 1 cancer incidence in the UK. Br J Cancer 2006;95(2):233–8.
55. Brenner AV, Linet MS, Fine HA, et al. History of allergies and autoimmune diseases and risk of brain tumors in adults. Int J Cancer 2002;99(2):252–9.
56. Wiemels JL, Wiencke JK, Sison JD, et al. History of allergies among adults with glioma and controls. Int J Cancer 2002;98(4):609–15.
57. Schoemaker MJ, Swerdlow AJ, Hepworth SJ, et al. History of allergies and risk of glioma in adults. Int J Cancer 2006;119(9):2165–72.
58. Schwartzbaum J, Jonsson F, Ahlbom A, et al. Cohort studies of association between self-reported allergic conditions, immune-related diagnoses and glioma and meningioma risk. Int J Cancer 2003;106(3):423–8.
59. Schlehofer B, Blettner M, Preston-Martin S, et al. Role of medical history in brain tumour development. Results from the international adult brain tumour study. Int J Cancer 1999;82(2):155–60.
60. Wiemels JL, Wiencke JK, Patoka J, et al. Reduced immunoglobulin E and allergy among adults with glioma compared with controls. Cancer Res 2004;64(22):8468–73.
61. Fisher JL, Schwartzbaum JA, Wrensch M, et al. Epidemiology of brain tumors. Neurol Clin 2007;25(4):867–90, vii.
62. Smith MA, Freidlin B, Ries LA, et al. Trends in reported incidence of primary malignant brain tumors in children in the United States. J Natl Cancer Inst 1998;90(17):1269–77.
63. Gurney JG, Davis S, Severson RK, et al. Trends in cancer incidence among children in the U.S. Cancer 1996;78(3):532–41.
64. Dobes M, Khurana VG, Shadbolt B, et al. Increasing incidence of glioblastoma multiforme and meningioma, and decreasing incidence of Schwannoma (2000-2008): findings of a multicenter Australian study. Surg Neurol Int 2011;2:176.
65. Gittleman HR, Ostrom QT, Rouse CD, et al. Trends in central nervous system tumor incidence relative to other common cancers in adults, adolescents, and children in the United States, 2000 to 2010. Cancer 2015;121(1):102–12.
66. Barchana M, Margaliot M, Liphshitz I. Changes in brain glioma incidence and laterality correlates with use of mobile phones–a nationwide population based study in Israel. Asian Pac J Cancer Prev 2012;13(11):5857–63.
67. Little MP, Rajaraman P, Curtis RE, et al. Mobile phone use and glioma risk: comparison of epidemiological study results with incidence trends in the United States. BMJ 2012;344:e1147.
68. Deltour I, Auvinen A, Feychting M, et al. Mobile phone use and incidence of glioma in the Nordic countries 1979-2008: consistency check. Epidemiology 2012;23(2):301–7.
69. Hammouche S, Clark S, Wong AH, et al. Long-term survival analysis of atypical meningiomas: survival rates, prognostic factors, operative and radiotherapy treatment. Acta Neurochir (Wien) 2014;156(8):1475–81.
70. Palma L, Celli P, Franco C, et al. Long-term prognosis for atypical and malignant meningiomas: a study of 71 surgical cases. J Neurosurg 1997;86(5):793–800.

71. Moliterno J, Cope WP, Vartanian ED, et al. Survival in patients treated for anaplastic meningioma. J Neurosurg 2015;123(1):23–30.
72. Perry A, Scheithauer BW, Stafford SL, et al. "Malignancy" in meningiomas: a clinicopathologic study of 116 patients, with grading implications. Cancer 1999; 85(9):2046–56.

The Epidemiology of Neuromuscular Diseases

Jaydeep M. Bhatt, MD

KEYWORDS

- Neuromuscular disease • Epidemiology • Global health • Burden of disease
- Public health

KEY POINTS

- The goal of this article is to examine current understanding of the epidemiology and burden of neuromuscular diseases in different global regions, focusing on the neuromuscular diseases listed in Box 1, divided by anatomic origin.
- Neuromuscular diseases are a relatively rare heterogeneous group of disorders that affect the function of various components of the peripheral nervous system.
- Rapid advances in genome sequencing have elucidated the pathogenetic mechanisms of several neuromuscular diseases and permitted recognition of therapeutic targets for interventional clinical trials.
- Understanding epidemiologic trends across global regions can aid governments, nongovernmental organizations, and international institutions formulate policies focused on prevention and surveillance.

 Video content accompanies this article at http://www.neurologic.theclinics. com.

ANTERIOR HORN
Spinal Muscular Atrophy

Spinal muscular atrophy (SMA) is a genetic disease involving degeneration of anterior horn cells in the spinal cord and motor neurons in the nuclei of the lower brainstem (**Box 1**).[1] The causative genetic mutation is usually inherited in an autosomal-recessive (AR) pattern, disrupting production of the survival motor neuron protein.[2] Although first described clinically and pathologically in infants with motor paralysis,[3] SMA disorders have a heterogeneous age of onset and clinical course, which provide the basis for its classification. SMA type I is the most common and severe form, affecting infants at birth or after a few months, resulting in severe weakness and ultimately death from respiratory failure by age 2. SMA type II is an intermediate form with onset of symptoms between 6

The author has nothing to disclose.
Department of Neurology, New York University School of Medicine, 240 East 38th Street, 20th Floor, New York, NY 10016, USA
E-mail address: jaydeep.bhatt@nyumc.org

Box 1
Neuroanatomical classification of neuromuscular diseases

Anterior horn

- Spinal muscular atrophy (SMA)
- Amyotrophic lateral sclerosis (ALS)
- Post polio syndrome (PPS)

Nerve

- Guillain-Barre syndrome (GBS)
- Chronic inflammatory demyelinating polyneuropathy (CIDP)

Neuromuscular junction

- Myasthenia gravis (MG)

Muscle

- Duchenne muscular dystrophy (DMD)
- Becker muscular dystrophy (BMD)
- Polymyositis (PM)
- Dermatomyositis (DM)
- Inclusion body myositis (IBM)

---

and 18 months of age; patients can sit independently but rarely can ambulate. With appropriate respiratory care, patients may survive into the third or fourth decade. SMA type III is a mild form with variable onset between late adolescence and childhood with ability to ambulate into the fifth decade and may live a life expectancy seen in a normal population.[4] SMA type IV is the rarest form of the disorder with onset in adulthood and slower rates of disability progression. All presentations of SMA have decreased or absent reflexes, weakness of proximal muscles, and progressive respiratory decompensation as shared clinical features.[5,6] Select global incidence and prevalence rates of SMA are summarized in **Table 1**.

Type I has the highest incidence of the SMA types, but because of early mortality, type II and type III are more prevalent.[16] The highest incidence and prevalence rates of SMA in the studies examined were reported by Burd and colleagues[8] in North Dakota, which included only type I patients. The investigators included 14 patients from retrospective review of birth and death certificates and a coded diagnosis; medical records were not found for 6 patients. Possibility of misclassification and heterogeneity may account for the high estimates. Ludvigsson and coworkers[11] studied the incidence of all SMA types from a national registry in Iceland during a 15-year period, with a combined incidence of 13.7 per 100,000 live births, which did not differ significantly from other studied populations.

SMA prevalence rates from UK,[7] Swedish,[9] Irish,[10] and English[13] populations show similar rates across Western Europe. MacMillan and Harper[7] retrospectively searched hospital inpatient records, genetic outpatient records, and electrodiagnostic testing records for their districts in South Wales and noted rates were likely underestimated because of ascertainment methods used to maximize diagnostic accuracy as well as possible variation in gene frequency between populations.[7] In contrast, Ludvigsson and colleagues[11] examined several neuromuscular diseases and used district and health insurance registries, communications with

Table 1
Select global incidence and prevalence rates of spinal muscular atrophy

Country	Study Period	Incidence per 100,000	Prevalence per 100,000	Authors, References
UK	1968–1990	4.4[a]	1.3	MacMillan & Harper,[7] 1991
US	1980–1987	14.9	11.5	Burd et al,[8] 1991
Sweden	1988	—	1.9	Ahlström et al,[9] 1993
Ireland	1993–1994	—	1.4	Hughes et al,[10] 1996
Iceland	1982–1996	13.7	—	Ludvigsson et al,[11] 1999
Cuba	1996–2002	3.53[a]	—	Zaldívar et al,[12] 2005
England	2007	—	1.87	Norwood et al,[13] 2009
Germany	1974–1987	9.8[a]	0.17[a]	Thieme et al,[14] 1993
Poland	1976–1985	10.26	1.26[b]	Spiegler et al,[15] 1990

[a] Includes SMA type I only.
[b] Includes SMA type II and type III only.

general practitioners, and postal surveys and concluded their reported higher prevalence was due to the large number of data sources and well-established national health care system. In addition, the investigators noted that calculation of prevalence rates from registry information was enhanced by medical record validation by a neurologist for accuracy.[11] Prevalence rates for SMA type I were observed to be higher in Central[14] and Eastern[15] Europe compared with Western Europe, but more populations require accurate ascertainment before establishing this hypothesis.

Higher prevalence rates have been reported in other populations experiencing relative religious and social isolation[17] and from founder effect.[18] Studies examining the prenatal diagnosis of SMA type 1 in global regions with high rates of consanguinity such as Iran demonstrate risk rates corresponding to the increased prevalence in such populations and AR mode of disease inheritance.[19]

Amyotrophic Lateral Sclerosis

Amyotrophic lateral sclerosis (ALS) is a progressive neuromuscular disease characterized by degeneration of motor neurons in the brain, brainstem, and spinal cord that control voluntary and involuntary muscles.[20] Most ALS cases occur in patients without any family history; in 5% to 10% of patients, there is an inheritance pattern, and several genetic mutations have been identified. Limb weakness is the most common presenting symptom, but there are several other presenting symptoms, including weakness of speaking, swallowing, and breathing muscles; muscle spasticity; loss of dexterity; hyperactive reflexes; and difficulty walking. Recent clinical evidence also suggests a link between ALS and cognitive dysfunction in some patients.[21] Clinical progression is typically rapid and leads to mortality, because there is no current reversible treatment. There are several other degenerative motor neuron diseases along a clinical spectrum.

This article focuses on ALS and its global incidence and prevalence rates (**Table 2**). Cronin and colleagues[47] reviewed global literature for ALS incidence and determined rates may be lower in African, Asian, and Hispanic patients compared with those obtained in Caucasian populations. Definite conclusions regarding epidemiologic variation among ethnic groups were not possible because of methodological differences in non-Caucasian reports. North American and European studies report a consistent

Table 2
Select global incidence and prevalence rates of amyotrophic lateral sclerosis

Country (state or region)	Study Period	Incidence per 100,000	Prevalence per 100,000	Reference
US (Texas)	1985–1988	1.1	3.04	Annegers et al,[22] 1991
Estonia	1985–1995	1.3–1.98	N/A	Gross-Paju et al,[23] 1998
Japan	1989–1993	1.43	47.7	Yoshida et al,[24] 1998
France	1994–1995	2.5	N/A	Preux et al,[25] 2000
England	2002–2006	1.06	4.91	Abhinav et al,[26] 2007
Nova Scotia	2003	2.24	N/A	Bonaparte et al,[27] 2007
Scotland	1989–1998	2.4	N/A	Forbes et al,[28] 2007
Ireland	1995–2004	2	6.2	O'Toole et al,[29] 2008
New Zealand	1985–2006	1.6 (1985)–3.3 (2006)	N/A	Murphy et al,[30] 2008
US (Missouri)	1998–2002	3.9	4.2	Turabelidze et al,[31] 2008
Uruguay	2002–2003	1.37	1.9	Vazquez et al,[32] 1998
Italy	1995–2004	2.9	7.89	Chiò et al,[33] 2009
Sweden	1991–2005	2.32 (1991-1993)– 2.98 (2003-2005)	N/A	Fang et al,[34] 2009
Europe	1998–1999	2.16	N/A	Logroscino et al,[35] 2010
Iran (Isfahan)	2002–2006	0.42	1.57	Sajjadi et al,[36] 2010
Norway (More and Romsdal County)	1988–2007	2.17	4.06	Gundersen et al,[37] 2011
Netherlands	2006–2009	2.77	10.32	Huisman et al,[38] 2011
Faroe Islands	1987–2009	2.6	8.2	Joensen[39] 2012
Argentina (Buenos Aires)	—	3.17	8.86	Bettini et al,[40] 2013
Brazil (Porto Alegre)	2010	N/A	5	Linden Junior et al,[41] 2013
Italy (Piedmont)	1995–2004	3.41	N/A	Migliaretti et al,[42] 2013
US (Georgia)	2001–2005	N/A	38.5[a]	Wittie et al,[43] 2013
Japan	2009–2010	2.2	9.9	Doi et al,[44] 2014
US	2010–2011	N/A	3.9	Mehta et al,[45] 2014
Germany	2009–2010	2.6	N/A	Uenal et al,[46] 2014

[a] Reported figure is period prevalence.

incidence between 1 and 3 patients per 100,000 per year and prevalence rates between 2 and 8 per 100,000. Independent analyses have found an increase in ALS incidence over several time periods[30,48] that may be attributed to longer lifespans.[49] Studies of a Missouri county in the United States[31] and Piedmont and Aosta Valley, Italy[42] noted higher than average incidence that may be explained by relatively smaller population samples, age distribution, and clustering of cases. Wittie and colleagues[43] used a capture-recapture analysis from multiple sources to maximize ascertainment in the state of Georgia in the United States and reported a 5-year period prevalence of 38.5 per 100,000.[43] Missing databases, incomplete demographic data, coding variation, and population growth in the studied region complicated methodology. Yoshida and coworkers[24] obtained a point prevalence of 47.7 per 100,000 examining a single prefecture in Japan without the current established diagnostic criteria and focusing on a single town within the prefecture.

Despite extensive global research, risk factors for ALS other than male sex, age, and family history have not been established. Associations between certain genes, increased physical fitness, occupations with electric field and heavy metal exposure, military duty, and head trauma among several others and an increased risk of ALS have been studied without any definite established risk.[50] Smoking is a probable risk factor.[51]

Postpolio Syndrome

Epidemic polio affected populations in several global regions for more than one hundred years before the vaccine era in the mid 20th century. Poliovirus is transmitted from person to person through the fecal-oral route and replicates in the gastrointestinal tract before spreading to the central nervous system, where it manifests in several possible forms. Paralytic polio is a form of polio causing flaccid weakness from replication of the virus in anterior horn cells of the spinal cord and/or motor nuclei of the brainstem and accounts for 0.1% to 2% of epidemic polio infections. The paralysis may occur in the limbs, facial muscles, and muscles involving swallowing or speech alone or in combination and typically spreads over 5 to 6 days.[52] Postpolio syndrome (PPS) is a neuromuscular disorder that produces new weakness and fatigue in individuals with a history of paralytic polio and was first described in the late nineteenth century. PPS may occur 8 to 71 years after initial paralysis, with an average interim of 35 years, with severity of the initial infection leading to earlier onset of new symptoms. There have been several proposed causes of PPS, including loss of motor neurons with normal aging coupled with prior depletion from acute polio infection.[53]

Takemura and colleagues[54] performed a cross-sectional survey in Kitakyushu, Japan of possible polio survivors showing a prevalence of 18 per 100,000 population using Halstead's criteria.[55] More than 60% of studied patients required an assistive device for activities of daily living because of motor debility. By comparison, a higher prevalence rate of 92 per 100,000, conducted by survey, was reported in Örebro, Sweden in 1988. The higher prevalence was attributed to search methodology and adequate time to develop the disease since the last Swedish epidemic of 1953 to 1954, along with a reporting rate of PPS symptoms in 80% of patients affected by the epidemic. Identified risk factors for PPS include severity of acute paralytic polio, greater degree of recovery after initial infection, age of onset of acute illness, longer interval after acute illness, older age at clinical presentation, and female gender. The high frequency of new weakness as a symptom combined with a relatively large number of polio survivors makes PPS the most prevalent motor neuron disease in North America.[56]

PERIPHERAL NERVE
Guillain-Barre Syndrome

Guillain-Barre syndrome (GBS) is an eponym that refers to diverse acute peripheral neuropathic disorders, named after investigators of the early 1900s who first described 3 patients with progressive sensorimotor dysfunction, absent reflexes, and specific biochemical abnormalities in cerebrospinal fluid (CSF).[57,58] The disease typically occurs after a gastrointestinal or respiratory infection, which is thought to trigger an immune response that causes damage to components of peripheral nerves. There is a possible association of certain vaccines and increased occurrence of GBS, but this is controversial, and a definite causal link is unproven.[59] GBS usually follows a single time course and does not recur. There are heterogeneous forms of GBS with varying clinical presentations depending on distribution of symptoms and peripheral nerve components involved. Common clinical features include dysfunction of the autonomic nervous system, abnormal sensations, pain, and severe weakness that may involve limb, facial, breathing, and swallowing muscles. Diagnosis is aided by specific electrodiagnostic test findings, and the disease is treatable with therapies that suppress the immune system with different mechanisms of action. Select global incidence and prevalence rates of GBS are summarized in **Table 3**.

McGrogan and colleagues[74] reviewed worldwide literature on the epidemiology of GBS identifying 63 prospective and retrospective studies for global trends. The reported incidence rates were consistent; children showed 0.34 to 1.34 per 100,000, and the overall range was 0.84 to 1.91 per 100,000. Of note, a decreased incidence was found between the 1980s and 1990s and increased incidence with age greater than 50 years. A criteria-based meta-analysis of population-based studies in North America and Europe with at least 20 subjects identified and cases confirmed by neurologists prospectively found GBS incidence increased by 20% for every decade in age and higher risk in men.[75] Other geographic regions were not included, because incidence was not known well and because of possible regional variation in epidemiology.

Table 3
Select global incidence and prevalence rates of Guillain-Barre syndrome

Country	Study Period	Incidence per 100,000	Prevalence	Reference
Tanzania	1984–1992	0.83	N/A	Howlett et al,[60] 1996
Sweden	1978–1993	1.77	N/A	Jiang et al,[61] 1997
US	1995–1991	3.0	N/A	Prevots & Sutter,[62] 1997
England	1993–1994	1.2	N/A	Rees et al,[63] 1998
Italy	1995–1996	1.36	N/A	Chio et al,[64] 2003
Spain (Cantabria)	1998–1999	1.26	N/A	Cuadrado et al,[65] 2004
Brazil (Sao Paulo)	1995–2002	0.6	N/A	Rocha et al,[66] 2004
Iran	2003	2.11	N/A	Arami et al,[67] 2006
Germany	2003–2005	1.75	N/A	Lehmann et al,[68] 2007
Greece	1996–2005	1.22	N/A	Markoula et al,[69] 2007
Canada (Alberta)	1994–2004	1.6	N/A	Hauck et al,[70] 2008
Netherlands	1996–2008	1.14	N/A	van der Maas et al,[71] 2011
US	2000–2009	1.72	N/A	Shui et al,[72] 2012
China (Jiangsu)	2008–2010	0.59	N/A	Chen et al,[73] 2014

Prevots and Sutter[62] reported a higher than average rate in a 6-year retrospective review of a national discharge and death certificate database. Limitations may have included specificity of GBS classification, limitation to participating hospitals, and 60% to 79% positive predictive value of GBS-coded discharges. Analysis of discharges from a hospital in São Paulo, Brazil reported a lower than average incidence of 0.6 per 100,000 without a bimodal distribution and with increased frequency during hotter months.[66] Chen and colleagues[73] also obtained a lower incidence of 0.59 from a large population in Jiangsu province, China, identifying cases retrospectively in hospitals that may have treated GBS. Accordingly, Cheng and colleagues[76] reported a lower adult incidence of 0.66 per 100,000 in China, although pediatric incidence was consistent with global literature.

Chronic Inflammatory Demyelinating Polyneuropathy

In contrast to GBS, chronic inflammatory demyelinating polyneuropathy (CIDP) is a relapsing or progressive peripheral nerve disease with duration of at least 8 to 12 weeks. Similar to GBS, it is clinically heterogeneous and treatable with immunosuppressant therapies, with comparable findings on neurologic examination, CSF biochemistry, and electrodiagnostic testing.[77] Preceding infections, vaccinations, and surgeries are not as common in CIDP as they are in GBS. Select global incidence and prevalence rates of CIDP are summarized in **Table 4**.

In a retrospective review of CIDP in a Minnesota county classified as "definite or probable" based on core clinical criteria and electrodiagnostic testing, Laughlin and colleagues[81] noted high prevalence and incidence rates matching GBS incidence in the same population.[84] A prospective study of 192 registered polyneuropathy patients in a Norwegian county showed 7.7 per 100,000 prevalence rate, occurring in a relatively smaller population compared with other studies. Rajabelly[82] and coworkers noted a significant difference in CIDP incidence when using the European Federation of Neurological Societies/Peripheral Nerve Society (EFNS/PNS) criteria compared with those developed by the Ad Hoc Subcommittee of the American Academy of Neurology (AAN). The EFNS/PNS incidence rate was 50% higher, attributed to the strict electrodiagnostic and muscle biopsy requirements of the AAN criteria, which lower its sensitivity for CIDP case ascertainment[85] (**Figs. 1–3**, Video 1). The investigators corroborated age-related figures with prior findings, noting low pediatric

Table 4				
Select global incidence and prevalence rates of chronic inflammatory demyelinating polyneuropathy				
Country	Study Period	Incidence per 100,000	Prevalence per 100,000	Reference
Japan	1988–1992	N/A	0.81	Kusumi et al,[78] 1995
Norway	1999	N/A	7.7	Mygland & Monstad,[79] 2001
Italy	2001	0.36	3.58	Chiò et al,[80] 2007
US	2000	1.6	8.9	Laughlin et al,[81] 2009
UK	2008	0.7 per EFNS/PNS criteria/0.35 per AAN criteria	4.77	Rajabally et al,[82] 2009
England	2008	N/A	2.84	Mahdi-Rogers & Hughes,[83] 2014

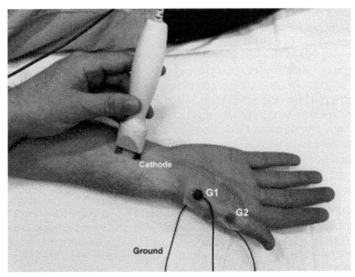

Fig. 1. Motor conduction study setup. Median motor study, recording the abductor pollicis brevis muscle, stimulating the median nerve at the wrist. In motor studies, the "belly-tendon" method is used for recording. The active recording electrode (G1) is placed on the center of the muscle, with the reference electrode (G2) placed distally over the tendon. (*From* Preston DC, Shapiro BE. Electromyography and neuromuscular disorders. 3rd edition. Elsevier; 2013. p. 19–35; with permission.)

prevalence rate, higher rate in older adults, and male predominance. No specific risk factors for CIDP have been identified in the global literature.

NEUROMUSCULAR JUNCTION
Myasthenia Gravis

Myasthenia gravis (MG) is the most common neuromuscular junction disorder (NMJ). The NMJ is a space between a motor nerve and a muscle in which biochemical signaling occurs. MG has a well-characterized pathophysiology due to immune-mediated NMJ block are of critical receptors on the muscle membrane, the subtypes of which are classified by the involved receptor.[86] A milder manifestation of the illness results in only eye muscles weakness alone, which can foreshadow more severe generalized weakness and morbidity. MG once a potentially fatal disease, is currently treated with combination immune-modulating therapies to control symptoms and influence its natural history. Select global incidence and prevalence rates of MG are summarized in **Table 5**.

Carr and colleagues[101] examined all population-based studies in global literature and included 55 for analysis of epidemiologic trends, noting marked variation in pooled incidence and prevalence rates between populations in similar areas using analogous methodologies, which limited the validity of the estimates. The pooled incidence of all subtypes ranged from 1.7 to 21.3 million person-years and prevalence ranged from 15 to 179 per million persons. An increasing trend in incidence and prevalence was observed, likely corresponding to advances in diagnostic means as well as methodology to optimize ascertainment. Murai and coworkers[94] reported a high annual incidence of 11.8 per 100,000 persons from a nationwide questionnaire based survey of randomly selected hospitals throughout Japan. The

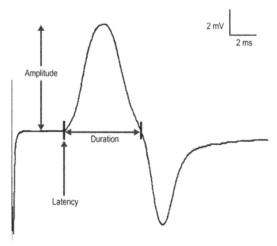

Fig. 2. Compound muscle action potential (CMAP). The CMAP represents the summation of all the underlying muscle fiber action potentials. With recording electrodes properly placed, the CMAP is a biphasic potential with an initial negative deflection. Latency is the time from the stimulus to the initial negative deflection from baseline. Amplitude is most commonly measured from baseline to negative peak but also can be measured from peak to peak. Duration is measured from the initial deflection from baseline to the first baseline crossing (ie, negative peak duration). In addition, negative CMAP area (ie, the area above the baseline) is calculated by most modern computerized electromyographic machines. Latency reflects only the fastest conducting motor fibers. All fibers contribute to amplitude and area. Duration is primarily a measure of synchrony. (*From* Preston DC, Shapiro BE. Electromyography and neuromuscular disorders. 3rd edition. Elsevier; 2013. p. 19–35; with permission.)

highest reported prevalence of 35 per 100,000 occurred in Sardinia, Italy; the investigators studied the databases of 21 general practitioners for MG codes over a decade, with diagnosis made by a specialist physician and without specific diagnostic criteria identified.[99]

MUSCLE
Duchenne Muscular Dystrophy and Becker Muscular Dystrophy

Muscular dystrophies are a group of inherited disorders resulting in progressive weakness and loss of muscle mass secondary to defects in genes needed for normal muscle function. There is a diverse clinical spectrum in this group with differences in distribution and degree of motor impairment, age of onset, rate of progression, and inheritance pattern. Both Duchenne muscular dystrophy (*DMD*) and Becker muscular dystrophy (BMD) are caused by X-linked mutations in the gene at Xp 21.2 - p21.1 that produces dystrophin, a critical protein component of the cytoskeleton in human muscle membranes. Because of its X-linked transmission, fully affected individuals are invariably male patients. DMD is the more severe form with the least dystrophin production and greater extent of DNA alteration, whereas BMD has a milder clinical presentation because of relative preservation of DNA sequences in the affected gene. DMD typically occurs between ages 2 and 3 with preferential weakness of legs more than arms, involving muscles closer to the shoulder and hip girdles. The progression of weakness in DMD significantly affects ambulation, and affected patients are usually confined to a wheelchair by age 12,[102] with only few patients surviving past

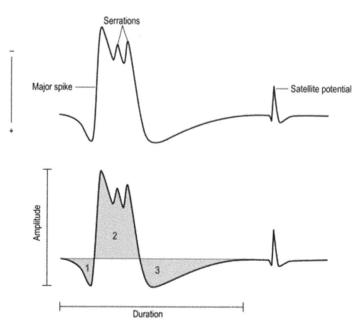

Fig. 3. Motor unit action potential (MUAP) measurements. Duration is measured as the time from the initial deflection of the MUAP from baseline to its final return to baseline. It is the parameter that best reflects the number of muscle fibers in the motor unit. Amplitude reflects only muscle fibers very close to the needle and is measured peak to peak. Phases (*shaded areas*) can be determined by counting the number of baseline crossings and adding one. MUAPs are generally triphasic. Serrations (also called turns) are changes in direction of the potential that do not cross the baseline. The major spike is the largest positive-to-negative deflection, usually occurring after the first positive peak. Satellite, or linked, potentials occur after the main potential and usually represent early reinnervation of muscle fibers. (*From* Preston DC, Shapiro BE. Electromyography and neuromuscular disorders. 3rd edition. Elsevier; 2013. p. 19–35; with permission.)

the third decade.[103] BMD patients ambulate until at least 15 years of age and may survive a normal life span. Both DMD and BMD may affect cardiac muscle adversely, leading to further morbidity and mortality. Of note, there an overall female predominance of 3:2, and recent study showed incidence peaks in women at a younger age than in men with rates equalizing with increased life expectancy.[104] Select global incidence and prevalence rates of DMD and BMD are summarized in **Tables 6** and **7**.

The highest known incidence and prevalence of DMD were reported by MacMillan and Harper[7] in South Wales, with differences likely due to ascertainment methods and/or truly higher disease frequency. The highest reported prevalence of BMD was 7.29 per 100,000 male patients by Norwood and colleagues[13] in Northern England, obtained by examining muscle biopsy and/or dystrophin gene mutations of patients with genetic muscle disease in an established neuromuscular center. Siciliano and colleagues[107] noted a marked reduction in the incidence of DMD in northwest Tuscany, attributed to carrier testing and genetic counseling, limiting DMD recurrence. An increase in BMD incidence in the same region was ascribed to advances in molecular genetic testing, allowing for a more specific diagnosis in those BMD patients formerly misdiagnosed due to atypical clinical presentation. A population-based assessment from 4 states in the United States reported a combined DMD/BMD point

Table 5
Select global incidence and prevalence rates of myasthenia gravis

Country (Region)	Study Period	Incidence per 100,000	Prevalence per 100,000	Reference
Norway	2008	1.6	13.1	Andersen et al,[87] 2014
Spain	1991–2000	2.127	N/A	Aragones et al,[88] 2003
Austria	1992–2009	N/A	15.69	Cetin et al,[89] 2012
Australia	2009	2.49	11.71	Gattellari et al,[90] 2012
Taiwan	2000–2007	2.1	8.4 (2000)–>14 (2007)	Lai & Tseng,[91] 2010
Trinidad	2010	N/A	7.8	Maharaj et al,[92] 2013
Tanzania (Dar Es Salaam)	1988–1998	0.3	N/A	Matuja et al,[93] 2001
Japan (Nagano Prefecture)	2007	11.8	N/A	Murai et al,[94] 2011
Italy (Trento)	2005–2009	1.48	12.96	Pallaver et al,[95] 2011
Denmark	1996–2009	Early onset 0.42, late onset 1.89	N/A	Pedersen et al,[96] 2013
US (Virginia)	1970–1984	0.91	13.4 (1980)–14.2 (1984)	Phillips et al,[97] 1992
England (Cambridgeshire)	1965–1992	1.1	15	Robertson et al,[98] 1998
Italy (Sardinia)	2009	N/A	35	Sardu et al,[99] 2012
Hong Kong	1975–1987	0.4	5.35 (adults), 6.22 (kids)	Yu et al,[100] 1992

prevalence range of 13 to 18 per 100,000 male patients in 2007.[113] A recent meta-analysis of global literature for DMD and BMD showed a pooled prevalence of 4.78 and 1.53 per 100,000 male patients, respectively. The incidence of DMD ranged from 10.71 to 27.78 per 100,000.[114]

Table 6
Select global incidence and prevalence rates of Duchenne muscular dystrophy

Country	Study Period	Incidence per 10^5 Males	Prevalence per 10^5 Males	Reference
UK	1968–1990	34.7	9.6	MacMillan & Harper,[7] 1991
Sweden	1988	—	0.7	Ahlström et al,[9] 1993
Ireland	1993–1994	—	4.2	Hughes et al,[10] 1996
England	2007	—	8.29	Norwood et al,[13] 2009
Japan	1957–1985	15.41	7.13	Nakagawa et al,[105] 1991
Netherlands	1961–1982	N/A	23.7	van Essen et al,[106] 1992
Italy	1965–1976 1977–1994	23.12 10.71	N/A	Siciliano et al,[107] 1999
Denmark	1977–2001	2.0	3.1 (1977), 5.5 (2002)	Jeppesen et al,[108] 2003

Table 7
Select global incidence and prevalence rates of Becker muscular dystrophy

Country	Study Period	Incidence per 10^5 Males	Prevalence per 10^5 Males	Reference
UK	1968–1990	—	5.0	MacMillan et al,[7] 1991
Ireland	1993–1994	—	4.2	Hughes et al,[10] 1996
England	2007	—	7.29	Norwood et al,[13] 2009
Japan	1957–1985	3.21	1.82	Nakagawa et al,[105] 1991
Italy	1965–1976 1977–1994	1.06 2.42	N/A	Siciliano et al,[107] 1999
UK	1940–1965	5.43 (minimum)/5.83 (probable including unconfirmed cases)	2.38 (minimum)/ 2.61 (probable)	Bushby et al,[109] 1991
Italy	1959–1968	7.2	2.01	Mostacciuolo et al,[110] 1993
South Africa	1987–1992	N/A	0.00001 (minimum)	Ballo et al,[111] 1994
Slovenia	1969–1984	5.7	1.2	Peterlin et al,[112] 1997

Myotonic Dystrophy

Myotonic dystrophy (MD) is an autosomal dominant (AD) disorder caused by heterozygous trinucleotide repeat expansion (CAG) in the dystrophia myotonica. Protein Kinase gene (DMPK) at chromosome 19 of 13. It affects multiple organ systems and is the most common form of adult muscular dystrophy.[115] In addition to muscle weakness, patients have protracted muscle contraction (myotonia) as well as cataracts, cardiac abnormalities, infertility, endocrine abnormalities, and cognitive impairment. There are 2 forms, type 1 and type 2, each caused by abnormal repetitions of DNA; type 2 tends to have a milder clinical presentation and preferentially affects muscles closer to the shoulder and hip girdles. Select global incidence and prevalence rates of MD are summarized in **Table 8**.

There is a wide variation in reported prevalence in different global regions, in addition to marked known differences among ethnic populations.[120] López de Munain and colleagues[116] studied a population of 689,836 in a Spanish region with a high prevalence of MD type 1, with observed differences from prior studies likely due to methodological differences, population growth, and genetic isolation. Ford and coworkers[119] noted their prevalence in Otago, New Zealand was among patients of European descent only and concluded this may have been due to population effect and cultural differences. Recent studies in Germany and Finland determining the frequency of MD type 1 and type 2 mutations and molecular diagnosis found the prevalence of type 2 mutations is higher than previously considered and may be near equal to type 1, with likely underestimation in prior type 2 prevalence rates due to incomplete or uncharacteristic phenotypic expression.[121,122]

Polymyositis

Polymyositis (PM) is an idiopathic immune-mediated inflammatory muscle disease with a complex diversity of causes producing progressive limb weakness occurring

Table 8
Select global incidence and prevalence rates of myotonic dystrophy

Country	Study Period	Incidence per 100,000	Prevalence per 100,000	Reference
Spain	1989–1991	N/A	26.5	López de Munain et al,[116] 1993
Croatia	1980–1994	N/A	18.1	Medica et al,[117] 1997
Israel	1994	N/A	9.4	Segel et al,[118] 2003
New Zealand	2001	N/A	11.6	Ford et al,[119] 2006

over weeks to months without evidence of a family member similarly affected.[123] Other diagnostic features may include involvement of swallowing muscles, multiorgan damage, high serum creatine kinase (CK) enzyme levels, and noted absence of a skin rash, eye weakness, and facial weakness. PM has been associated with systemic autoimmune disease, systemic connective tissue disease, parasites, viruses, bacteria, and certain drugs. Despite additional diagnostic tools such as electromyography and muscle biopsy, diagnosis of PM is challenging and often delayed because of slow onset and lack of a specific clinical sign for identification. Select global incidence and prevalence rates of PM are summarized in **Table 9**.

The highest incidence was reported by Oddis and colleagues[124] among 2 counties in Pennsylvania; the true PM incidence is likely lower than 5.5 per million because this included dermatomyositis (DM) patients. Wilson and coworkers[126] reported a high prevalence in a single county in Minnesota, which may not be comparable to a general nationwide sample. Retrospective analysis of a large US-based health plan with a national membership for standardized diagnostic codes showed PM incidence and prevalence rates higher than the US country studies.[125] The investigators note that wide variations in population characteristics, such as age and gender, and inherent limitations to diagnosis codes limits comparison of their figures to previous reports from other global populations. In addition, many epidemiologic studies calculated pooled rates for more than one inflammatory myopathy, including PM, making it difficult to discern PM alone.

Dermatomyositis

Compared with PM, DM presents with a similar pattern of weakness, shares certain immune-mediated features on muscle biopsy analysis, and may also affect multiple

Table 9
Select global incidence and prevalence rates of polymyositis

Country (state or region)	Study Period	Incidence per 10^6	Prevalence per 10^5	Reference
US (Pennsylvania)	1963–1982	5.5[a]	N/A	Oddis et al,[124] 1990
US	2003–2008	38.0[b]	9.7	Furst et al,[125] 2012
US (Minnesota)	1981–2000	4.1[b]	3.45[b]	Wilson et al,[126] 2008
Spain (Buenos Aires)	1999–2009	7.5	7.2	Rosa et al,[127] 2013
China	2005–2009	6.0	2.4–3.6	See et al,[128] 2013
South Australia	1980–2009	4.1	N/A	Tan et al,[129] 2013

[a] Includes DM patients.
[b] Age and gender adjusted rate.

organ systems. Unlike PM, DM is also a skin disease that may precede, occur with, or occur after muscle disease and which may occur in childhood.[130] Both PM and DM have a greater risk of associated cancers, with a higher risk in DM, and when possible, screening for malignancy should be performed.[131] Select global incidence and prevalence rates of DM are summarized in **Table 10**.

Bendewald and coworkers[132] conducted a retrospective population-based study of DM in a Minnesota county, with an adjusted incidence of 9.63 per million and prevalence of 21.42 per 100,000 persons. Of interest, the investigators note a rising incidence of DM over 3 decades, consistent with trends reported by Oddis and colleagues.[124] Several studies showed prevalence to be higher in women and with older age for both PM and DM. Bernatsky and colleagues[133] used 3 different case definitions to retrospectively estimate prevalence of PM and DM from population-based data, with highest rates in older urban women and lowest in young urban men.

Inclusion Body Myositis

In contrast to PM and DM, inclusion body myositis (IBM) has distinct demographic, clinical, and muscle biopsy features. The nonfamilial sporadic form is the most common muscle disease in men over the age of 50, and asymmetric weakness typically involves muscles near the hands and feet early in the clinical course and at a younger age. Facial weakness and difficulty swallowing are more common in IBM than PM and DM. Because of relatively recent recognition as an independent disorder, earlier public health studies of PM and DM likely included misclassified IBM cases, and it is likely still underdiagnosed.[134] Select global incidence and prevalence rates of IBM are summarized in **Table 11**.

Suzuki and colleagues[138] identified IBM patients diagnosed on clinical grounds with muscle biopsy confirmation at a national center in Japan and reported increasing numbers of cases yearly from 1989 to 2005, and a high prevalence of 9.83 compared with 4.9 per million reported by Badrising and coworkers[136] in the Netherlands. The different estimations may be due to varying degrees of referral and ascertainment bias, different microscopic criteria for verification, or a truly higher incidence in the Japanese population. A markedly low prevalence was observed in Turkey, which was a muscle biopsy–based study with no confirmation of reported clinical findings and inclusion of "most suggestive" cases based on light microscope findings and history on request form.[137] Data on the incidence of IBM are sparse, with a wide range of 0.9 to 7.9 per million, with the latter rate adjusted for age and gender.[126,135] Precise risk factors are unknown, but recent reports suggest a combination of environmental triggers, aging, and genetic susceptibility.[139]

Table 10
Select global incidence and prevalence rates of dermatomyositis

Country (state or region)	Study Period	Incidence per 10^6	Prevalence per 10^5	Reference
US	2003–2008	14.0[a]	5.9	Furst et al,[125] 2012
Spain (Buenos Aires)	1999–2009	3.2	10.22	Rosa et al,[127] 2013
China	2005–2009	7.0	2.4–3.6	See et al,[128] 2013
South Australia	1980–2009	1.0	N/A	Tan et al,[129] 2013
US (Minnesota)	1976–2007	9.63[a]	21.42	Bendewald et al,[132] 2010

[a] Age and gender adjusted rate.

Table 11
Select global incidence and prevalence rates of inclusion body myositis

Country (state)	Study Period	Incidence per 10^6	Prevalence per 10^6	Reference
Finland	1990	0.9	N/A	Kaipiainen-Seppänen & Aho,[135] 1996
Netherlands	1982–1999	N/A	4.9	Badrising et al,[136] 2000
Istanbul/Turkey	1993–2011	N/A	0.679	Oflazer et al,[137] 2011
Japan	1999–2007	N/A	9.83	Suzuki et al,[138] 2012
US (Minnesota)	1981–2000	7.9[a]	70.6[a]	Wilson et al,[126] 2008

[a] Age and gender adjusted rate.

THE GLOBAL BURDEN OF NEUROMUSCULAR DISEASE

Currently, there are no established metrics of the global burden of the neuromuscular disorders described in this article, either individually or collectively. Endeavors to ascertain the global burden of diseases have not measured years of life lost, years lived with disability, and disability-adjusted life years (DALY) for any neuromuscular disorders. The Global Burden of Disease Study 2013 sponsored by the Institute for Health Metrics and Evaluation at the University of Washington estimates the burden of diseases for 21 regions and 188 countries from 1990 to 2013.[140] Under the neurologic disorders category, there are several noncommunicable diseases, including Alzheimer disease and other dementias, Parkinson disease, epilepsy, multiple sclerosis, headache disorders, and "other neurologic disorders." The "other neurologic disorders" category shows a 15% increase in DALYs across all ages and a 3% reduction in age standardized DALYs. Examination of neurologic diagnosis codes represented by "other neurologic disorders" shows grouping of every other neurologic subcategory; it is not possible to discern the contribution of neuromuscular diseases.

A recent commissioned US study reported the direct and indirect medical costs of SMA and ALS for affected individuals by examining claims data from public and private insurers.[141] Examination of the economic impact of ALS in Canada shows significant unreimbursed out-of-pocket expenses.[142] Similar studies measure the substantial economic cost of DMD in 4 developed countries[143] and CIDP in southeast England.[144]

Paralytic polio is estimated to result in 13 to 14 DALYs lost in low- and middle-income countries[145]; however, there are no available data on the global impact of PPS. There are several important studies examining the social and economic burden affecting polio survivors, mainly in developed countries.[146] Almost all polio survivors in developed countries are 50 years or older, with certain populations having a higher proportion working part-time rather than full time[147] and increased requirements for disability benefits.[148] Although robust global health initiatives are underway to eradicate acute polio in the developing world, underreporting of PPS and diversion of resources from other diseases and socioeconomic conditions have led to insufficient attention to PPS. Studies in China,[149] Lebanon,[150] and Nigeria[151] have demonstrated disproportionate decreases in income, employment, marriage rates, and quality-of-life measurements in specific PPS populations.

ACKNOWLEDGMENTS

The author thanks Susanna Nguy at NYU School of Medicine for her significant contributions in the preparation of this article. This includes acquisition of references from various sources as well as data extraction for compilation and tabulation in a timely manner.

SUPPLEMENTARY DATA

Supplementary data related to this article can be found at http://dx.doi.org/10.1016/j. ncl.2016.06.017.

REFERENCES

1. Deenen JCW, Horlings CGC, Jan JGM, et al. The epidemiology of neuromuscular disorders: a comprehensive overview of the literature. Neuromuscul Disord 2015;2:73–85.
2. Schmalbruch H, Haase G. Spinal muscular atrophy: present state. Brain Pathol 2001;11(2):231–47.
3. Iannaccone ST, Caneris O, Hoffmann J. In: Ashwal S, editor. Founders of child neurology. San Francisco (CA): Norman Publishing; 1990. p. 278–84.
4. Zerres K, Rudnik-Schöneborn S, Forrest E, et al. A collaborative study on the natural history of childhood and juvenile onset proximal spinal muscular atrophy (type II and III SMA): 569 patients. J Neurol Sci 1997;146(1):67–72.
5. Arnold WD, Kassar D, Kissel JT. Spinal muscular atrophy: diagnosis and management in a new therapeutic era. Muscle Nerve 2015;51(2):157–67.
6. Ioos C, Mrad S, Barois A, et al. Respiratory capacity course in patients with infantile spinal muscular atrophy. Chest 2014;126(3):831–7.
7. MacMillan JC, Harper PS. Single-gene neurological disorders in South Wales: an epidemiological study. Ann Neurol 1991;30:411–4.
8. Burd L, Short SK, Martsolf JT, et al. Prevalence of type I spinal muscular atrophy in North Dakota. Am J Med Genet 1991;41(2):212–5.
9. Ahlström G, Gunnarsson LG, Leissner P, et al. Epidemiology of neuromuscular diseases, including the post polio sequelae, in a Swedish county. Neuroepidemiology 1993;12(5):262–9.
10. Hughes MI, Hicks EM, Nevin NC, et al. The prevalence of inherited neuromuscular disease in Northern Ireland. Neuromuscul Disord 1996;6(1):69–73.
11. Ludvigsson P, Olafsson E, Hauser WA. Spinal muscular atrophy. Neuroepidemiology 1999;18(5):265–9.
12. Zaldívar T, Montejo Y, Acevedo AM, et al. Evidence of reduced frequency of spinal muscular atrophy type I in the Cuban population. Neurology 2005;65(4): 636–8.
13. Norwood FL, Harling C, Chinnery PF, et al. Prevalence of genetic muscle disease in Northern England: in-depth analysis of a muscle clinic population. Brain 2009;132:3175–86.
14. Thieme A, Mitulla B, Schulze F, et al. Epidemiological data on Werdnig-Hoffmann disease in Germany (West-Thüringen). Hum Genet 1993;91(3):295–7.
15. Spiegler AW, Hausmanowa-Petrusewicz I, Borkowska J, et al. Population data on acute infantile and chronic childhood spinal muscular atrophy in Warsaw. Hum Genet 1990;85:211–4.
16. Byers RK, Banker BQ. Infantile muscular atrophy. Arch Neurol 1961;5:140–64.
17. Fried K, Mundel G. High incidence of spinal muscular atrophy type I (Werdnig-Hoffmann disease) in the Karaite community in Israel. Clin Genet 1977;12(4): 250–1.
18. Schaap T. Werdnig-Hoffmann disease on Reunion Island: a founder effect? Clin Genet 1985;27(6):617–9.

19. Khaniani MS, Derakhshan SM, Abasalizadeh S. Prenatal diagnosis of spinal muscular atrophy: clinical experience and molecular genetics of SMN gene analysis in 36 cases. J Prenat Med 2013;7(3):32–4.
20. Mitsumoto H, Chad DA, Pioro EP. Contemporary neurology series. In: Amyotrophic lateral sclerosis. Philadelphia: Davis Company; 1998. p. 164–76.
21. Ringholz GM, Appel SH, Bradshaw M, et al. Prevalence and patterns of cognitive impairment in sporadic ALS. Neurology 2005;65(4):586–90.
22. Annegers JF, Appel S, Lee JRJ, et al. Incidence and prevalence of amyotrophic lateral sclerosis in Harris County, Texas, 1985-1988. Arch Neurol 1991;48(6): 589–93.
23. Gross-Paju K, Ööpik M, Lüüs SM, et al. Motor neurone disease in South Estonia diagnosis and incidence rate. Acta Neurol Scand 1998;98(1):22–8.
24. Yoshida S, Uebayashi Y, Kihira T, et al. Epidemiology of motor neuron disease in the Kii Peninsula of Japan, 1989–1993: active or disappearing focus? J Neurol Sci 1998;155(2):146–55.
25. Preux PM, Druet-Cabanac M, Couratier P, et al. Estimation of the amyotrophic lateral sclerosis incidence by capture-recapture method in the Limousin region of France. J Clin Epidemiol 2000;53(10):1025–9.
26. Abhinav K, Stanton B, Johnston C, et al. Amyotrophic lateral sclerosis in South-East England: a population-based study. TheSouth-East England register for amyotrophic lateral sclerosis (SEALS Registry). Neuroepidemiology 2007; 29(1–2):44–8.
27. Bonaparte JP, Grant IA, Benstead TJ, et al. ALS incidence in Nova Scotia over a 20-year-period: a prospective study. Can J Neurol Sci 2007;34(1):69–73.
28. Forbes RB, Colville S, Parratt J, et al. The incidence of motor neuron disease in Scotland. J Neurol 2007;254(7):866–9.
29. O'Toole O, Traynor BJ, Brennan P, et al. Epidemiology and clinical features of amyotrophic lateral sclerosis in Ireland between 1995 and 2004. J Neurol Neurosurg Psychiatry 2008;79:30–2.
30. Murphy M, Quinn S, Young J, et al. Increasing incidence of ALS in Canterbury, New Zealand: a 22-year study. Neurology 2008;71(23):1889–95.
31. Turabelidze G, Zhu BP, Schootman M, et al. An epidemiologic investigation of amyotrophic lateral sclerosis in Jefferson County, Missouri, 1998–2002. Neurotoxicology 2008;29(1):81–6.
32. Vazquez MC, Ketzoian C, Legnani C, et al. Incidence and prevalence of amyotrophic lateral sclerosis in Uruguay: a population-based study. Neuroepidemiology 1998;30(2):105–11.
33. Chiò A, Mora G, Calvo A, et al. Epidemiology of ALS in Italy: a 10-year prospective population-based study. Neurology 2009;72(8):725–31.
34. Fang F, Valdimarsdóttir U, Bellocco R, et al. Amyotrophic lateral sclerosis in Sweden, 1991-2005. Arch Neurol 2009;66(4):515–9.
35. Logroscino G, Traynor BJ, Hardiman O, et al. Incidence of amyotrophic lateral sclerosis in Europe. J Neurol Neurosurg Psychiatry 2010;81(4):385–90.
36. Sajjadi M, Etemadifar M, Nemati A, et al. Epidemiology of amyotrophic lateral sclerosis in Isfahan, Iran. Eur J Neurol 2010;17(7):984–9.
37. Gundersen MD, Yaseen R, Midgard R. Incidence and clinical features of amyotrophic lateral sclerosis in Møre and Romsdal County, Norway. Neuroepidemiology 2011;37(1):58–63.
38. Huisman MH, de Jong SW, van Doormaal PT, et al. Population based epidemiology of amyotrophic lateral sclerosis using capture–recapture methodology. J Neurol Neurosurg Psychiatry 2011;82(10):1165–70.

39. Joensen P. Incidence of amyotrophic lateral sclerosis in the Faroe Islands. Acta Neurol Scand 2012;126(1):62–6.

40. Bettini M, Vicens J, Giunta DH, et al. Incidence and prevalence of amyotrophic lateral sclerosis in an HMO of Buenos Aires, Argentina. Amyotroph Lateral Scler Frontotemporal Degener 2013;14(7–8):598–603.

41. Linden Junior E, Becker J, Schestatsky P, et al. Prevalence of amyotrophic lateral sclerosis in the city of Porto Alegre, in Southern Brazil. Arq Neuropsiquiatr 2013;71(12):959–62.

42. Migliaretti G, Berchialla P, Dalmasso P, et al. Amyotrophic lateral sclerosis in Piedmont (Italy): a Bayesian spatial analysis of the incident cases. Amyotroph Lateral Scler Frontotemporal Degener 2013;14(1):58–65.

43. Wittie M, Nelson LM, Usher S, et al. Utility of capture-recapture methodology to assess completeness of amyotrophic lateral sclerosis case ascertainment. Neuroepidemiology 2013;40(2):133–41.

44. Doi Y, Atsuta N, Sobue G, et al. Prevalence and incidence of amyotrophic lateral sclerosis in Japan. J Epidemiol 2014;24(6):494.

45. Mehta P, Antao V, Kaye W, et al. Prevalence of amyotrophic lateral sclerosis—United States, 2010-2011. MMWR Surveill Summ 2014;63(Suppl 7):1–14.

46. Uenal H, Rosenbohm A, Kufeldt J, et al. Incidence and geographical variation of amyotrophic lateral sclerosis (ALS) in Southern Germany–completeness of the ALS registry Swabia. PLoS One 2014;9(4):e93932.

47. Cronin S, Hardiman O, Traynor BJ. Ethnic variation in the incidence of ALS: a systematic review. Neurology 2007;68(13):1002–7.

48. Noonan CW, White MC, Thurman D, et al. Temporal and geographic variation in United States motor neuron disease mortality, 1969–1998. Neurology 2005; 64(7):1215–21.

49. Chio A, Magnani C, Schiffer D. Gompertzian analysis of amyotrophic lateral sclerosis mortality in Italy, 1957–1987; application to birth cohorts. Neuroepidemiology 1995;14(6):269–77.

50. Ingre C, Roos PM, Piehl F, et al. Risk factors for amyotrophic lateral sclerosis. Clin Epidemiol 2015;7:181.

51. Armon C. Smoking may be considered an established risk factor for sporadic ALS. Neurology 2009;73(20):1693–8.

52. Jubelt B, Simionescu L. Poliomyelitis and the post-polio syndrome. Motor disorders. 3rd edition. Rochester (MN): The American Association of Neuromuscular and Electrodiagnostic Medicine; 2013. p. 781–91.

53. Jubelt B, Cashman NR. Neurological manifestations of the post-polio syndrome. Crit Rev Neurobiol 1986;3(3):199–220.

54. Takemura J, Saeki S, Hachisuka K, et al. Prevalence of post-polio syndrome based on a cross-sectional survey in Kitakyushu, Japan. J Rehabil Med 2004; 36(1):1–3.

55. Halstead LS. Post-polio sequelae: assessment and differential diagnosis for post-polio syndrome. Orthopedics 1991;14(11):1209–17.

56. Trojan DA, Cashman NR. Post-poliomyelitis syndrome. Muscle Nerve 2005; 31(1):6–19.

57. Guillain G, Barré JA, Strohl A. Sur un syndrome de radilcu lonévrite avec hyperalbuminose du liquid céphalo-rachidien sans reaction cellulaire. Remarques sur les catactères cliniques et graphiques de reflexes tendineux. Bull Mem Soc Med Hop Paris 1916;40:1462–70.

58. Dimachkie MM, Barohn RJ. Acute inflammatory demyelinating polyneuropathy. Motor disorders. 3rd edition. Rochester (MN): The American Association of Neuromuscular and Electrodiagnostic Medicine; 2013. p. 385–400.
59. Baxter R, Bakshi N, Fireman B, et al. Lack of association of Guillain-Barré syndrome with vaccinations. Clin Infect Dis 2013;57(2):197–204.
60. Howlett WP, Vedeler CA, Nyland H, et al. Guillain-Barré syndrome in northern Tanzania: a comparison of epidemiological and clinical findings with western Norway. Acta Neurol Scand 1996;93(1):44–9.
61. Jiang GX, Cheng Q, Link H, et al. Epidemiological features of Guillain-Barré syndrome in Sweden, 1978-93. J Neurol Neurosurg Psychiatry 1997;62(5):447–53.
62. Prevots DR, Sutter RW. Assessment of Guillain-Barré syndrome mortality and morbidity in the United States: implications for acute flaccid paralysis surveillance. J Infect Dis 1997;175(Suppl 1):S151–5.
63. Rees JH, Thompson RD, Smeeton NC, et al. Epidemiological study of Guillain-Barré syndrome in south east England. J Neurol Neurosurg Psychiatry 1998; 64(1):74–7.
64. Chio A, Cocito D, Leone M, et al. Guillain-Barré syndrome: a prospective, population-based incidence and outcome survey. Neurology 2003;60(7): 1146–50.
65. Cuadrado JI, de Pedro-Cuesta J, Ara JR, et al. Public health surveillance and incidence of adulthood Guillain-Barre syndrome in Spain, 1998–1999: the view from a sentinel network of neurologists. Neurol Sci 2004;25(2):57–65.
66. Rocha MS, Brucki SM, Carvalho AA, et al. Epidemiologic features of Guillain-Barré syndrome in São Paulo, Brazil. Arquivos de neuro-psiquiatria 2004; 62(1):33–7.
67. Arami MA, Yazdchi M, Khandaghi R. Epidemiology and characteristics of Guillain-Barre syndrome in the northwest of Iran. Ann Saudi Med 2006;26(1): 22–7.
68. Lehmann HC, Köhne A, Meyer zu Hörste G, et al. Incidence of Guillain-Barre syndrome in Germany. J Peripher Nerv Syst 2007;12(4):285.
69. Markoula S, Giannopoulos S, Sarmas I, et al. Guillain-Barré syndrome in northwest Greece. Acta Neurol Scand 2007;115(3):167–73.
70. Hauck LJ, White C, Feasby TE, et al. Incidence of Guillain–Barré syndrome in Alberta, Canada: an administrative data study. J Neurol Neurosurg Psychiatry 2008;79(3):318–20.
71. van der Maas NA, Kramer MA, Jacobs BC, et al. Guillain-Barré syndrome: background incidence rates in The Netherlands. J Peripher Nerv Syst 2011;16(3): 243–9.
72. Shui IM, Rett MD, Weintraub E, et al. Vaccine Safety Datalink Research Team. Guillain-Barré syndrome incidence in a large United States cohort (2000–2009). Neuroepidemiology 2012;39(2):109–15.
73. Chen Y, Ma F, Zhang J, et al. Population incidence of Guillain–Barré syndrome in parts of China: three large populations in Jiangsu province, 2008–2010. Eur J Neurol 2014;21(1):124–9.
74. McGrogan A, Madle GC, Seaman HE, et al. The epidemiology of Guillain-Barré syndrome worldwide: a systematic literature review. Neuroepidemiology 2009; 32(2):150–63.
75. Sejvar JJ, Baughman AL, Wise M, et al. Population incidence of Guillain-Barré syndrome: a systematic review and meta-analysis. Neuroepidemiology 2011; 36(2):123–33.

76. Cheng Q, Wang DS, Jiang GX, et al. Distinct pattern of age-specific incidence of Guillain-Barre syndrome in Harbin, China. J Peripher Nerv Syst 2002;7(3):208–9.

77. Köller H, Kieseier BC, Jander S, et al. Chronic inflammatory demyelinating polyneuropathy. N Engl J Med 2005;352(13):1343–56.

78. Kusumi M, Nakashima K, Nakayama H, et al. Epidemiology of inflammatory neurological and inflammatory neuromuscular diseases in Tottori Prefecture, Japan. Psychiatry Clin Neurosci 1995;49(3):169–74.

79. Mygland Å, Monstad P. Chronic polyneuropathies in Vest-Agder, Norway. Eur J Neurol 2001;8(2):157–65.

80. Chiò A, Cocito D, Bottacchi E, et al. Idiopathic chronic inflammatory demyelinating polyneuropathy: an epidemiological study in Italy. J Neurol Neurosurg Psychiatry 2007;78(12):1349–53.

81. Laughlin RS, Dyck PJ, Melton LJ, et al. Incidence and prevalence of CIDP and the association of diabetes mellitus. Neurology 2009;73(1):39–45.

82. Rajabally YA, Simpson BS, Beri S, et al. Epidemiologic variability of chronic inflammatory demyelinating polyneuropathy with different diagnostic criteria: study of a UK population. Muscle nerve 2009;39(4):432–8.

83. Mahdi-Rogers M, Hughes RA. Epidemiology of chronic inflammatory neuropathies in southeast England. Eur J Neurol 2014;21(1):28–33.

84. Kennedy RH, Danielson MA, Mulder DW, et al. Guillain-Barré syndrome: a 42-year epidemiologic and clinical study. Mayo Clin Proc 1978;53(2):93–9.

85. Magda P, Latov N, Brannagan TH, et al. Comparison of electrodiagnostic abnormalities and criteria in a cohort of patients with chronic inflammatory demyelinating polyneuropathy. Arch Neurol 2003;60(12):1755–9.

86. Keesey JC. Clinical evaluation and management of myasthenia gravis. Muscle Nerve 2004;29(4):484–505.

87. Andersen JB, Heldal AT, Engeland A, et al. Myasthenia gravis epidemiology in a national cohort; combining multiple disease registries. Acta Neurol Scand 2014; 129(s198):26–31.

88. Aragones JM, Bolibar I, Bonfill X, et al. Myasthenia gravis a higher than expected incidence in the elderly. Neurology 2003;60(6):1024–6.

89. Cetin H, Fülöp G, Zach H, et al. Epidemiology of myasthenia gravis in Austria: rising prevalence in an ageing society. Wien klin Wochenschr 2012;124(21–22): 763–8.

90. Gattellari M, Goumas C, Worthington JM. A national epidemiological study of myasthenia gravis in Australia. Eur J Neurol 2012;19(11):1413–20.

91. Lai CH, Tseng HF. Nationwide population-based epidemiological study of myasthenia gravis in Taiwan. Neuroepidemiology 2010;35(1):66–71.

92. Maharaj J, Bahadursingh S, Ramcharan K. Myasthenia gravis in South Trinidad. West Indian Med J 2013;62(6):510–4.

93. Matuja WBP, Aris EA, Gabone J, et al. Incidence and characteristics of myasthenia gravis in Dar Es Salaam, Tanzania. East Afr Med J 2001;78(9):473–7.

94. Murai H, Yamashita N, Watanabe M, et al. Characteristics of myasthenia gravis according to onset-age: Japanese nationwide survey. J Neurol Sci 2011;305(1): 97–102.

95. Pallaver F, Riviera AP, Piffer S, et al. Change in myasthenia gravis epidemiology in Trento, Italy, after twenty years. Neuroepidemiology 2011;36(4):282–7.

96. Pedersen EG, Hallas J, Hansen K, et al. Late-onset myasthenia not on the increase: a nationwide register study in Denmark, 1996–2009. Eur J Neurol 2013;20(2):309–14.

97. Phillips LH, Torner JC, Anderson MS, et al. The epidemiology of myasthenia gravis in central and western Virginia. Neurology 1992;42(10):1888–93.
98. Robertson NP, Deans J, Compston DA. Myasthenia gravis: a population-based epidemiological study in Cambridgeshire, England. J Neurol Neurosurg Psychiatry 1998;65(4):492–6.
99. Sardu C, Cocco E, Mereu A, et al. Population based study of 12 autoimmune diseases in Sardinia, Italy: prevalence and comorbidity. PLoS One 2012;7(3): e32487.
100. Yu YL, Hawkins BR, Ip MS, et al. Myasthenia gravis in Hong Kong Chinese. Acta Neurol Scand 1992;86(2):113–9.
101. Carr AS, Cardwell CR, McCarron PO, et al. A systematic review of population based epidemiological studies in Myasthenia Gravis. BMC Neurol 2010; 10(1):46.
102. Younger DS. Childhood muscular dystrophies. Motor disorders. 3rd edition. Rochester (MN): The American Association of Neuromuscular and Electrodiagnostic Medicine; 2013. p. 547–56.
103. Passamano L, Taglia A, Palladino A, et al. Improvement of survival in Duchenne muscular dystrophy: retrospective analysis of 835 patients. Acta Myol 2012; 31(2):121.
104. Grob D, Brunner N, Namba T, et al. Lifetime course of myasthenia gravis. Muscle nerve 2008;37(2):141–9.
105. Nakagawa M, Nakahara K, Yoshidome H, et al. Epidemiology of progressive muscular dystrophy in Okinawa, Japan. Neuroepidemiology 1991;10(4):185–91.
106. van Essen AJ, Busch HF, te Meerman GJ, et al. Birth and population prevalence of Duchenne muscular dystrophy in The Netherlands. Hum Genet 1992;88(3): 258–66.
107. Siciliano G, Tessa A, Renna M, et al. Epidemiology of dystrophinopathies in North-West Tuscany: a molecular genetics-based revisitation. Clin Genet 1999;56(1):51–8.
108. Jeppesen J, Green A, Steffensen BF, et al. The Duchenne muscular dystrophy population in Denmark, 1977–2001: prevalence, incidence and survival in relation to the introduction of ventilator use. Neuromuscul Disord 2003;13(10): 804–12.
109. Bushby KM, Thambyayah M, Gardner-Medwin D. Prevalence and incidence of Becker muscular dystrophy. Lancet 1991;337(8748):1022–4.
110. Mostacciuolo ML, Miorin M, Pegoraro E, et al. Reappraisal of the incidence rate of Duchenne and Becker muscular dystrophies on the basis of molecular diagnosis. Neuroepidemiology 1993;12(6):326–30.
111. Ballo R, Viljoen D, Beighton P. Duchenne and Becker muscular dystrophy prevalence in South Africa and molecular findings in 128 persons affected. S Afr Med J 1994;84(8):494–6.
112. Peterlin B, Zidar J, Meznarič-Petruša M, et al. Genetic epidemiology of Duchenne and Becker muscular dystrophy in Slovenia. Clin Genet 1997;51(2): 94–7.
113. Prevalence of Duchenne/Becker muscular dystrophy among males aged 5-24 years—Four States, 2007. 2009. Available at: http://www.cdc.gov/mmwr/preview/mmwrhtml/mm5840a1.htm. Accessed November 30, 2015.
114. Mah JK, Korngut L, Dykeman J, et al. A systematic review and meta-analysis on the epidemiology of Duchenne and Becker muscular dystrophy. Neuromuscul Disord 2014;24(6):482–91.

115. Harper P. Myotonic dystrophy. Oxford (United Kingdom): Oxford University Press; 2009.
116. López de Munain A, Blanco A, Emparanza JI, et al. Prevalence of myotonic dystrophy in Guipuzcoa (Basque country, Spain). Neurology 1993;43(8):1573.
117. Medica I, Markovi D, Peterlin B. Genetic epidemiology of myotonic dystrophy in Istria, Croatia. Acta Neurol Scand 1997;95(3):164–6.
118. Segel R, Silverstein S, Lerer I, et al. Prevalence of myotonic dystrophy in Israeli Jewish communities: inter-community variation and founder premutations. Am J Med Genet A 2003;119(3):273–8.
119. Ford C, Kidd A, Hammond-Tooke G. Myotonic dystrophy in Otago, New Zealand. N Z Med J 2006;119(1241):U2145.
120. Tishkoff SA, Goldman A, Calafell F, et al. A global haplotype analysis of the myotonic dystrophy locus: implications for the evolution of modern humans and for the origin of myotonic dystrophy mutations. Am J Hum Genet 1998;62(6): 1389–402.
121. Udd B, Meola G, Krahe R, et al. 140th ENMC International Workshop: myotonic dystrophy DM2/PROMM and other myotonic dystrophies with guidelines on management. Neuromuscul Disord 2006;16:403–13.
122. Suominen T, Bachinski LL, Auvinen S, et al. Population frequency of myotonic dystrophy: higher than expected frequency of myotonic dystrophy type 2 (DM2) mutation in Finland. Eur J Hum Genet 2011;19(7):776–82.
123. Younger DS, Dalakas NS. Inflammatory myopathies. Motor disorders. 3rd edition. Rochester (MN): The American Association of Neuromuscular and Electrodiagnostic Medicine; 2013. p. 339–58.
124. Oddis CV, Conte CG, Steen VD, et al. Incidence of polymyositis-dermatomyositis: a 20-year study of hospital diagnosed cases in Allegheny County, PA 1963-1982. J Rheumatol 1990;17(10):1329–34.
125. Furst DE, Amato AA, Iorga ŞR, et al. Epidemiology of adult idiopathic inflammatory myopathies in a US managed care plan. Muscle Nerve 2012;45(5):676–83.
126. Wilson FC, Ytterberg SR, St Sauver JL, et al. Epidemiology of sporadic inclusion body myositis and polymyositis in Olmsted County, Minnesota. J Rheumatol 2008;35(3):445–7.
127. Rosa J, Garrot LF, Navarta DA, et al. Incidence and prevalence of polymyositis and dermatomyositis in a health management organization in Buenos Aires. J Clin Rheumatol 2013;19(6):303–7.
128. See LC, Kuo CF, Chou IJ, et al. Sex-and age-specific incidence of autoimmune rheumatic diseases in the Chinese population: a Taiwan population-based study. Semin Arthritis Rheum 2013;43(3):381–6.
129. Tan JA, Roberts-Thomson PJ, Blumbergs P, et al. Incidence and prevalence of idiopathic inflammatory myopathies in South Australia: a 30-year epidemiologic study of histology-proven cases. Int J Rheum Dis 2013;16(3):331–8.
130. Callen JP. Dermatomyositis. Lancet 2000;355(9197):53–7.
131. Hill CL, Zhang Y, Sigurgeirsson B, et al. Frequency of specific cancer types in dermatomyositis and polymyositis: a population-based study. Lancet 2001; 357(9250):96–100.
132. Bendewald MJ, Wetter DA, Li X, et al. Incidence of dermatomyositis and clinically amyopathic dermatomyositis: a population-based study in Olmsted County, Minnesota. Arch Dermatol 2010;146(1):26–30.
133. Bernatsky S, Joseph L, Pineau CA, et al. Estimating the prevalence of polymyositis and dermatomyositis from administrative data: age, sex and regional differences. Ann Rheum Dis 2009;68(7):1192–6.

134. Hopkinson ND, Hunt C, Powell RJ, et al. Inclusion body myositis: an underdiagnosed condition? Ann Rheum Dis 1993;52(2):147–51.

135. Kaipiainen-Seppänen O, Aho K. Incidence of rare systemic rheumatic and connective tissue diseases in Finland. J Intern Med 1996;240(2):81–4.

136. Badrising UA, Maat-Schieman M, Van Duinen SG, et al. Epidemiology of inclusion body myositis in the Netherlands: a nationwide study. Neurology 2000; 55(9):1385–8.

137. Oflazer PS, Deymeer F, Parman Y. Sporadic-inclusion body myositis (s-IBM) is not so prevalent in Istanbul/Turkey: a muscle biopsy based survey. Acta Myol 2011;30(1):34–6.

138. Suzuki N, Aoki M, Mori-Yoshimura M, et al. Increase in number of sporadic inclusion body myositis (sIBM) in Japan. J Neurol 2012;259(3):554–6.

139. Gang Q, Bettencourt C, Machado P, et al. Sporadic inclusion body myositis: the genetic contributions to the pathogenesis. Orphanet J Rare Dis 2014;9:88.

140. Murray CJ, Barber RM, Foreman KJ, et al. Global, regional, and national disability-adjusted life years (DALYs) for 306 diseases and injuries and healthy life expectancy (HALE) for 188 countries, 1990–2013: quantifying the epidemiological transition. Lancet 2015;386(10009):2145–91.

141. Cost of amyotrophic lateral sclerosis muscular dystrophy, and spinal muscular atrophy in the United States. 2012. Available at: http://staging2.mda.org/sites/default/files/Cost_Illness_Report.pdf. Accessed November 30, 2015.

142. Gladman M, Dharamshi C, Zinman L. Economic burden of amyotrophic lateral sclerosis: a Canadian study of out-of-pocket expenses. Amyotroph Lateral Scler Frontotemporal Degener 2014;15(5–6):426–32.

143. Landfeldt E, Lindgren P, Bell CF, et al. The burden of Duchenne muscular dystrophy: an international, cross-sectional study. Neurology 2014;83(6):529–36.

144. Mahdi-Rogers M, McCrone P, Hughes RA. Economic costs and quality of life in chronic inflammatory neuropathies in southeast England. Eur J Neurol 2014; 21(1):34–9.

145. Duintjer Tebbens RJ, Pallansch MA, Cochi SL, et al. Economic analysis of the global polio eradication initiative. Vaccine 2010;29(2):334–43.

146. Groce NE, Banks LM, Stein MA. Surviving polio in a post-polio world. Soc Sci Med 2014;107:171–8.

147. Farbu E, Gilhus NE. Poliomyelitis: long-time consequences for social life. Acta Neurol Scand 1997;96(6):353–8.

148. Rekand T, Kõrv J, Farbu E, et al. Long term outcome after poliomyelitis in different health and social conditions. J Epidemiol Community Health 2003; 57(5):368–72.

149. Dai F, Zhang RZ. Economic burden of poliomyelitis. Zhonghua Liu Xing Bing Xue Za Zhi 1996;17(3):169.

150. Shaar KH, McCarthy M. Disadvantage as a measure of handicap: a paired sibling study of disabled adults in Lebanon. Int J Epidemiol 1992;21(1):101–7.

151. Adegoke BO, Oni AA, Gbiri CA, et al. Paralytic poliomyelitis: quality of life of adolescent survivors. Hong Kong Physiother J 2012;30(20):93–8.

Epidemiology of Childhood and Adult Mental Illness

David S. Younger, MD, MPH, MS[a,b,*]

KEYWORDS

- Vaccination • Neuro-epidemiology • Public health

KEY POINTS

- Mental illness in adults accounts for a greater proportion of disability in developed countries than any other group of illnesses, including cancer and heart disease.
- Population-based surveys and surveillance provide much of the evidence needed to understand mental health promotion, mental illness prevention, and treatment programs in the United States.
- Childhood mental health disorders present serious deviations from expected cognitive, social, and emotional development are an important public health issue in the United States.
- Suicide is among the most important manifestation of mental illness in children, interacting with other factors resulting in an overall suicide rate of 4.5 per 100,000 in 2010.
- Mental illness can be managed effectively with increased access to mental health treatment services to reduced associated morbidity.

INTRODUCTION

The *term mental* illness refers to all diagnosable mental disorders and is characterized by sustained, abnormal alterations in thinking, mood, or behavior associated with distress and impaired functioning.[1] Mental illness is an important domestic and global public health problem because the condition it is associated with other chronic diseases, further increasing their morbidity and mortality. According to the World Health Organization (WHO), mental illness accounts for more disability in developed countries than any other group of illnesses, including cancer and heart disease.[2] Kessler and colleagues[3–5] noted that up to one-fourth of adults in the United States (US) reported symptoms of mental illness with one-half developing at least 1 mental illness during their lifetime, the commonest of which were anxiety and mood disorders. The impact of mental illness in children ranges from minor to severe disruptions in daily

The author has nothing to disclose.
[a] Division of Neuroepidemiology, Department of Neurology, New York University School of Medicine, New York, NY, USA; [b] College of Global Public Health, New York University, New York, NY, USA
* Corresponding author. 333 East 34th Street, 1J, New York, NY 10016.
E-mail address: david.younger@nyumc.org

Neurol Clin 34 (2016) 1023–1033
http://dx.doi.org/10.1016/j.ncl.2016.06.010
0733-8619/16/$ – see front matter © 2016 Elsevier Inc. All rights reserved.

neurologic.theclinics.com

functioning, with serious deviations from expected cognitive, social, and emotional development to incapacitating personal and social impairments. Mental illness in children is further associated with a life-long risk of anxiety, depression, and suicide.[6] In adults, mental illness leads to significant occupational impairments,[7–9] heightened morbidity, and premature mortality from concurrent chronic diseases. Mental illness may further increase the risk for adverse health outcomes associated with cardiovascular disease, diabetes, obesity, asthma, epilepsy, and cancer[10–12] owing to lesser use of medical care and treatment adherence[13,14] and concomitant abuse of tobacco and alcohol products.[15] Moreover, the rates for injuries, both intentional (homicide and suicide) and unintentional (motor vehicle) increased by 2- to 4-fold in those with mental illness compared with the general population.[16,17]

This paper reviews data from selected Centers for Disease Control and Prevention (CDC) surveillance and information systems that measured mental illness and the associated effects in US children[6] and adults,[7] and the global impact of mental illness.

METHODOLOGY OF SURVEILLANCE

Reeves and colleagues[7] provide an overview of public health surveillance in adult mental illness. Perou and colleagues[6] describe mental health surveillance in children. Surveillance in both reports involves the ongoing and systematic collection, analysis, interpretation, and dissemination of data used to develop public health interventions to reduce morbidity and mortality and improve health in their respective populations. The derived data are essential to the public health goals of reducing the incidence, prevalence, severity, and economic impact of mental illnesses. That information is used by public health officials, academicians, health care providers, and advocacy groups to track trends in mental illness prevalence and severity. It is also used to assess associations between mental illness and other chronic medical conditions in adults such as obesity, diabetes, heart disease, and alcohol and substance abuse; to identify populations at high risk for mental illness and target interventions, and prevention measures; and to provide outcome measures for evaluating mental illness interventions.

National Population Surveys and Reporting Systems

Adults and children
The National Health Interview Survey The National Health Intervention Survey (NHIS) is a national survey administered by the National Center for Health Statistics on the health of the civilian noninstitutionalized US population. Its main objective is to monitor the health of the US population through the collection and analysis of data on a broad range of health topics by in-person household interviews. Approximately 40,000 households per year were interviewed as of 2010.

The National Health and Nutrition Examination Survey The National Health and Nutrition Examination Survey (NHANES), administered by the National Center for Health Statistics, is designed to assess the health and nutritional status of adults and children in the US. It collects information derived from interviews, physical examinations, laboratory tests, nutritional assessment, and DNA repositories. As of 2008, approximately 5000 persons per year were interviewed.

National Vital Statistics System The National Vital Statistics System assembles mortality statistics from death certificates filed in the US and is processed by the CDC.

National Violent Death Reporting System The National Violent Death Reporting System (NVDRS) is a population-based active surveillance system among participating states administered by the CDC to provide a census of violent deaths that occur within participating states, including child maltreatment deaths, intimate partner homicides, and suicides, and legal intervention deaths such as when a decedent is killed by a police officer authorized to use deadly force.

National Survey on Drug Use and Health The National Survey on Drug Use and Health (NSDUH) is the primary source of statistical information on the use of alcohol, tobacco, illicit drugs, and nonmedical use of prescription drugs in the US. It collects data through in-person interviews with a representative sample of the noninstitutionalized population.

Adults
National Ambulatory Medical Care and the National Hospital Ambulatory Medical Care Surveys Two ambulatory surveillance surveys, the National Ambulatory Medical Care Survey and the National Hospital Ambulatory Medical Care Survey administered by the National Center for Health Statistics, collect sample data on the provision of ambulatory medical care services respectively in nonfederal, employed, office-based physician offices, and emergency room and outpatient departments of noninstitutionalized general and short-stay hospitals. In 2007, data were provided to the National Ambulatory Medical Care Survey on 32,778 visits. Survey data for the National Hospital Ambulatory Medical Care Survey is based on a nationally representative sample of 500 nonfederal short-stay (<30 days) hospitals.

Two other surveys, the National Hospital Discharge Survey and the National Nursing Home Survey, both administered by the National Centers for Health Statistics, provide national survey sample characteristics of inpatients discharged from nonfederal short-stay hospitals and Medicare or Medicaid licensed nursing homes.

Children alone
Autism and Developmental Disability Monitoring Network The Autism and Developmental Disabilities Monitoring network is a surveillance system conducted by the CDC to estimate the prevalence of autism spectrum disorders in 14 population-based sites. It uses health and educational records from health providers and schools.

National Survey of Children's Health The National Survey of Children's Health (NSCH) is a cross-sectional, random-digit, population-based telephone survey that collects information on the physical and emotional health of noninstitutionalized children age 17 years or younger to produce state and national estimates of child health and well-being.

School-Associated Violent Death Surveillance Study The School-Associated Violent Death Surveillance Study, conducted by the CDC in collaboration with the US Department of Education and the Department of Justice, describes the epidemiology of school-associated violent deaths and the potential risk factors for the deaths.

National Youth Risk Behavior Survey The National Youth Risk Behavior Survey (YRBS) monitors health risk behaviors that contribute substantially to the leading causes of death, disability, and social problems among children and young adults in the US using a 3-stage cluster design to produce a representative sample of public and private high school students in grades 9 through 12.

State-Based Surveys

Adults
The Behavioral Risk Factor Surveillance System The Behavioral Risk Factor Surveillance System (BRFSS) is a state-based system of health surveys administered by

the Public Health Surveillance Program Office. It collects information on health risk behaviors, preventive health practices, and health care access primarily related to chronic disease and injury through telephone interviews of 1 person (aged ≥18 years) from each household.

DIAGNOSTIC CLASSIFICATION OF MENTAL ILLNESS

Surveillance survey tools estimate the prevalence and trends in adult mental illness relying on symptom patterns. The diagnostic terminology used to describe mental illness diagnostic categories may vary. For example, depression could include major and minor depression, psychotic depression, depression not otherwise specified, bipolar disorder, dysthymia, moderate to severe depression, and mild depression. The American Psychiatric Association recognizes diagnostic categories based on symptoms observed by a health care professional or reported by the patient and classified mental disorders that are published in the *Diagnostic and Statistical Manual of Mental Disorders, Fourth Edition, Text Revision* (DSM-IV-TR).[18] The WHO *International Classification of Diseases, 10th Revision, Clinical Modification*[19] has defined mental illness categories that are congruent with but not identical to those in the DSM-IV-TR.

Childhood mental disorders include several categories that can be defined by the DSM-IV-TR,[18] some of which are primary mental illnesses and others of which have a close association with a mental disorder. Attention deficit hyperactivity disorder, oppositional defiant disorder, and conduct disorder are behavioral disorders that frequently occur together characterized by developmentally inappropriate levels of inattention, hyperactivity, impulsivity, or a combination thereof that impairs functioning in multiple settings. The autism spectrum disorders are a group of neurodevelopmental disorders characterized by impairments in social interactions and communications, as well as restricted repetitive and stereotypes patterns of behavior that emerge in the first few years of life. Mood and anxiety disorders include a range of conditions commonly characterized by feelings of depression, exaggerated anxiety or fear, low self-esteem, or all of them that persist or repeat over period of months or years. Substance use disorders and substance use refers to the use of alcohol and illicit drugs such as marijuana and inhalants, which among children have social, financial, and health consequences. Tic disorders include chronic motor or chronic vocal tics, transient tic disorder, and Tourette syndrome, the latter characterized by persistent motor and vocal tics that least for a least a year. Although not a primary mental disorder, Tourette syndrome may have mental illness as an associated feature.

RESULTS
Adults

Population surveys
Among 10,279 adults in the NHANES the prevalence of depression was 6.8% (95% confidence interval, 5.8–7.8), higher in women (8.4%) than men (4.9%), age 40 to 59 years (8.4%) compared with those age 18 to 39 years (6.2%) or 60 years (5.1%). Non-Hispanic blacks showed higher prevalence of depression (9.7%) than Mexican Americans (7.2%) or non-Hispanics white (6.2%), with a preponderance in Southeastern states (>10%). Among 198,678 adults in the BRFSS, the prevalence of depression was 8.2% (95% confidence interval, 7.8–8.6), higher in women (9.8%) than men (6.6%) age 40 to 59 years and 18 to 24 years (both 10.2%) than those 25 to 34 and 35 to 44 years (both 8.3%), or others greater than 55 years (6.1%) with a similar preponderance in Southeastern states. Psychological distress registered by the NHIS and the BRFSS 30 days before the survey was noted respectively in 3.2%

and 3.9% of respondents during 2009, with a preponderance in Southeastern states. An average of 3.5 mentally unhealthy days were reported in the BRFSS during the preceding 30 days; a lifetime diagnosis of anxiety was noted in 12.3% of adults in 2008. The NHIS reported a lifetime diagnosis of bipolar disorder and schizophrenia in 1.7% and 0.6% of adults in 2007, respectively.

Among 29,212 adults surveyed by the BRFSS for adverse childhood experiences during 2009 in 5 Southeastern states, 59.4% of respondents had at least 1 adverse childhood experience, and 8.7% reported 5 or more adverse childhood experiences, among them verbal, physical, sexual, and family dysfunction owing to incarceration, mental illness, substance abusing family member, domestic violence, or absence of a parent owing to divorce or separation.[20]

National Health Care Surveys

According to the National Ambulatory Medical Care Survey and National Hospital Ambulatory Medical Care Survey, during 2007 to 2008 an estimated 47.8 million ambulatory care visits were made by patients with primary mental illness, constituting 5% of all ambulatory care services in the US during that time period, of which the greatest proportion (31%) were for depression, followed by schizophrenia and other psychotic disorders (23%). According to the National Hospital Discharge Survey, mental illness was a primary diagnosis in 97.9 per 10,000 patients discharged from nonfederal short-stay hospitals in adults age 18 to 64 years. Mood disorders were the most common diagnosis followed by alcohol and drug use disorders so noted in 46.0 per 10,000 population age 18 to 44 years and 19.2 per 10,000 population in persons 65 years or older. Dementia and Alzheimer disease were the commonest diagnoses among nursing home residents with a primary diagnosis of mental illness, each increasing with age, mood disorders, and dementia in residents age 65 to 84 years.

Children

Data from the most recent NSCH estimated the prevalence of depression among children age 3 to 17 years as 3% in 2007. NSDUH and NHANES estimated the prevalence of lifetime and past year major depressive episode from 2010 to 2012 to be 12.8% and 8.1%, respectively, among adolescents age 12 to 17 years, with a prevalence of depression in the preceding 2 weeks of 6.7%. According to the NHIS, 7.1% of children age 12 to 17 years ever had a diagnosis of depression, 3.5% had current depression, and 5.1% for had a diagnosis of depression in the past year. In 2011, the YRBS reported that during the past year, 28.5% of high school students age 14 to 18 years reported feeling so sad or hopeless every day for 2 weeks or more in a row that they stopped doing usual activities. This feeling was higher among girls (35.9%) than boys (21.5%), and higher among Hispanic students (32.6%) than white non-Hispanic (27.2%) or black non-Hispanic students (24.7%). The overall estimate of 28.5% of children feeling sad or hopeless was much higher than NSDUH for lifetime or past year MDA estimates of 12.8%, a finding that could have been related to differences in survey methodologies, including the setting and mode of completing the YRBS at school through a paper survey compared with a household member completing the NSDUH, as well as the assessment by YRBS of only a single symptom of depression, whereas NSDUH assessed whether individuals met criteria for an major depressive episode using formal criteria.

Parent-reported anxiety among children in the US estimated by the NSCH, focusing primarily on phobias in children age 2 to 17 years noted a prevalence of 4.7% ever having anxiety and 3% prevalence of current anxiety disorders. NHANES noted that the prevalence of self-reported generalized anxiety disorder in 0.7% and phobias and fears in 2.6% of respondents. NHANES estimated that a prevalence of 8.3% of adolescents age 12 to 17 years who self-reported 14 or more mentally unhealthy days in the past month as a marker of mental distress.

Data on suicide gathered from the National Vital Statistics System and NVDRS in 16 states reported an overall suicide rate for children age 10 to 19 years of 4.5 per 100,000 in 2010 (National Vital Statistics System), and 4.2 suicides per 100,000 between 2005and to 2009 (NVDRS). White non-Hispanic children and non-Hispanic children of other races had higher rates of suicide than black non-Hispanic and Hispanic children, with the commonest modes of injury being hanging, suffocation, and firearms. Among those who died of suicide reported by the NVDRS, 29.5% disclosed an intent to die by suicide before the act, 35.5% had a diagnosed mental disorder at the time of death, and 26.4% were under treatment for a current mental disorder at the time of death with 21% overall having made a previous attempt.

DISCUSSION

The CDC national surveys such as the NHANES and NHIS and numerous other national tracking systems are useful for developing national policies and tracking progress toward national health goals for children and adults. The CDC BRFSS survey provides data at the state and substate and local levels that can be used for both national and state-level planning. Mental health disorders are substantial public health concerns because of their prevalence, early onset, impact, and associated costs to the child, family, and community. A total of 13% to 20% of children living in the US experienced a mental disorder in a given year and surveillance during 1994 to 2011.[6] The findings of this new report from the CDC are the first to describe the number of US children age 3 to 17 years who have specific mental disorders where there is recent or ongoing monitoring. There were, however, notable variations depending on whether the children or parents self-reported as well as the mental health descriptor that was used, notably in depression and anxiety disorders. For example, based on self-reporting in the NSDUH, the prevalence of lifetime and past year major depressive episode among adolescents from 2010 to 2011 was 12.8% and 8.1%, respectively. Parent reporting data from NSCH and NHIS noted a prevalence of ever having a diagnosed depression of 7.1% among adolescents age 12 to 17 years. The prevalence of unhealthy days for 2 or more weeks in the past month was 6.7% according to NHANES, with 28.5% of high school students age 14 to 18 years self-reporting sadness or hopelessness almost every day for 2 weeks or more causing them to stop usual activities (YRBS). Depression was higher among adolescent girls, and higher among Hispanic than white non-Hispanic or black non-Hispanic students.

The prevalence of parent-reported anxiety among children age 2 to 17 years was 4.7% for ever being anxious and 3% for a current anxiety disorder. The prevalence of self-reported mentally unhealthy days dichotomized at 2 or more weeks in the past month as an indicator of the severity of depression and anxiety disorders was 8.3% overall. The overall suicide rate for persons aged 10 to 19 years was 4.5 suicides per 100,000 persons in 2010. Adolescent boys age 12 to 17 years were more likely than girls to die by suicide, as were white non-Hispanic children and non-Hispanic children of other races than black non-Hispanic and Hispanic children. The commonest modes of suicide were hanging, suffocation, and firearm-related injury.

An estimated 25% of adults in the US had a mental illness in the previous year, and 6.8% of adults reported moderate to severe depression in the 2 weeks before completing a survey according the NHANES. Although the present surveys focused on depression, the National Epidemiologic Survey on Alcohol and Related conditions and the National Comorbidity Survey Replication estimates 14% and 18%, respectively, suffered from an anxiety disorder.[5,21] Anxiety disorders were as common in the population as depression and, like depression and severe psychological distress, they can result in high levels of impairment. The pathophysiologic characteristics of anxiety disorders are similar to those of depression and often are associated with the same chronic medical conditions.[22,23]

It was of interest that Southeastern states reported higher rates of depression in most categories. Future national and state-level mental illness surveillance should measure a wider range of psychiatric conditions and include anxiety disorders. Many mental illnesses can be managed successfully and increasing access to and use of mental health treatment services could reduce substantially the associated morbidity to the individual and society.

MENTAL ILLNESS AND THE MILLENNIUM DEVELOPMENT GOALS

There is compelling evidence that in developing countries mental illness is among the most important causes of sickness, disability, and in certain age groups, premature mortality.[15] It has been suggested that addressing mental health may be an integral part of health system interventions aimed at achieving some of the Millennium Development Goals (MDGs).[24] Population-based studies of the risk factors for depression and anxiety show that poor and marginalized people were at greater risk for preventing attainment of MDG 1, the eradication of extreme poverty and hunger.[25] A major reason why children may not be able to enroll or complete primary education, preventing attainment of MDG 2—the achievement of universal primary education, may be related to developmental and mental disorder, and learning disability.[26] MDG 4, the reduction in child mortality, may be associated with mental illness in pregnancy. Early childhood failure to thrive in babies less than 1 year was independently associated with depression in pregnancy among South Asian mothers.[27] A cohort study of depressed Pakistani mothers were at 5-fold greater risk to give birth to an underweight baby compared with nondepressed mothers, even after adjustment for confounders including socioeconomic status.[28] The association of low birth weight with depression during pregnancy was replicated in an India-based study.[29] Up to 30% of mothers suffer from postpartum depression in rural India,[30] urban South Africa,[31] and Vietnam,[32] impacting on MDG 5, and improving maternal health. Moreover, suicide is a leading cause of maternal death in developed countries.[33]

GLOBAL BURDEN OF MENTAL ILLNESS

In a given year, about 30% of the population worldwide is affected by a mental disorder and more than two-thirds of those affected do not receive the care they need. With 14% of the global disease burden attributed to neuropsychiatric disorders, 1 in 17 people have a serious mental health condition.[4] The projected burden of mental health disorders is expected to reach 15% by 2020, when common mental disorders will disable more people than complications arising from AIDS, heart disease, traffic accidents, and wars combined. Almost 28% of disability-adjusted life-years were globally attributed to neuropsychiatric disorders in 2005.[34]

Roughly 10% to 20% of children are affected by 1 or more mental or behavioral problems,[35] with estimates from the Western Cape region of South Africa of 17% that have a mental disorder.[36] In conflict areas such as Mosul, Iraq, the prevalence of mental illness can be 35%.[37] Only 15% to 30% of children worldwide receive the treatment they need.[38]

GLOBAL INEQUALITIES IN MENTAL HEALTH

According to the WHO, health inequalities are defined as 'differences in health status or in the distribution of health determinants between different population groups'.[38] They deter access to care, use, and outcomes of care, affecting all geographic regions whether rural or suburban, as well as both genders, racial and ethnic background, and sexual orientation. In almost all nations the poor are at a higher risk of developing mental disorders compared with the nonpoor. Poverty is both a determinant and consequence of poor mental health in that mental illness may increase the likelihood of living in poverty, because of its influence on functionality and ability to get or sustain employment.[39,40] In many developing nations, resources and infrastructure are scarce, and the advocacy and political is deficient limiting effective mental health legislations and interventions.[38] Families of people with mental health problems are often marginalized and are limited in their ability to champion for mental health issues owing to the stigma associated with these disorders. Although some progress is being made[41] to address the challenges posed by mental health problems, the burden of mental disorders in developing countries is compounded by high rates of stigma and discrimination.[42,43]

Stigma, myths, and misconceptions surrounding mental illness contribute to the discrimination and human rights violations experienced by people with mental illness in many developing countries,[44] with the result that they may be judged inaccurately by community and family members, and unnecessary restricted in the rights to work, go to school, marry, and participate in community and family functions. The stigma of mental illness may pervade the medical establishment and trainees, many of whom in Spain,[45] Saudi Arabia,[46] and Romania[47] voiced negative attitudes and a reluctance to specialize in psychiatry. In developing nations and communities with limited availability of modern mental health services and providers, there may be a reliance on nontraditional health and healing practices.[48,49]

There may be unmet medical needs in patients with mental illness in developing nations. Patients may leave the hospital without knowing their diagnosis or what medications they are taking, wait too long for referrals, appointments, and treatment, or may not be respected or given adequate emotional support.[50] In many communities, the burden of caring for the sick may be placed on women and children because of the high adult morbidity and mortality owing to human immunodeficiency virus/AIDS and other infectious diseases. This has resulted in age and gender inequities in primary caregiver's responsibilities for people living with mental illness. The increased international migration of health workers from developing to the developed nations and internal migration from rural poorer communities to wealthier urban communities in the developing nations has led to shortages of mental health care workers[51–53] a majority of people with mental illness in developing nations go untreated despite the availability of effective treatment. These large treatment gaps are not surprising, given that in many developing countries there is no budget for mental health services.

INTEGRATING MENTAL HEALTH INTO PRIMARY CARE

With a mismatch of mental health resources to those in need varying from 1 psychiatrist for every 100,000 people in much of Southeast Asia, to less than 1 for every 1 million people in sub-Saharan Africa,[38] there is a scarcity of psychiatric hospitals that are typically located in urban settings and away from family members. A key strategy for addressing inequalities in mental health care has been to integrate mental health within other primary care services.[54,55] The reasons for integrating mental health into primary care would generally make it affordable and cost effective, promoting access and respect. Community mental health services can help to reduce social stigma and discrimination by reducing the social isolation, neglect, and institutionalization of people living with mental health problems.

REFERENCES

1. US Department of Health and Human Services. Mental health: a report of the surgeon general. Rockville (MD): US Department of Health and Human Services; Substance Abuse and Mental Health Services Administration; Center for Mental Health Services; National Institutes of Health; National Institute of Mental Health; 1999.
2. World Health Organization (WHO). Promoting mental health: concepts, emerging evidence, practice (summary report). Geneva (Switzerland): World Health Organization; 2004.
3. Kessler RC, Berglund P, Demler O, et al. Lifetime prevalence and age-of-onset distributions of DSM-IV disorders in the National Comorbidity Survey Replication. Arch Gen Psychiatry 2005;62:593–602.
4. Kessler RC, Chiu WT, Demler O, et al. Prevalence, severity, and comorbidity of 12-month DSM-IV disorders in the National Comorbidity Survey Replication. Arch Gen Psychiatry 2005;62:617–709.
5. Kessler RC, Chiu WT, Colpe L, et al. The prevalence and correlates of serious mental illness (SMI) in the National Comorbidity Survey Replication (NCS-R) [Chapter 15]. In: Manderscheid RW, Berry JT, editors. Mental health, United States, 2004. Rockville (MD): Substance Abuse and Mental Health Services Administration; 2006. p. 1–20. DHHS Publication no. (SMA)-06-4195.
6. Perou R, Bitsko RH, Blumberg SJ, et al, Centers for Disease Control and Prevention (CDC). Mental health surveillance among children–United States, 2005-2011. MMWR Suppl 2013;62(Suppl 2):1–3.
7. Reeves WC, Strine TW, Pratt LA, et al, Centers for Disease Control and Prevention (CDC). Mental illness surveillance among adults in the United States. MMWR Surveill Summ 2011;60(Suppl 3):1–29.
8. Mathers CD, Loncar D. Projections of global mortality and burden of disease from 2002 to 2030. PLoS Med 2006;3:e442.
9. Murray CJ, Lopez AD. Global mortality, disability, and the contribution of risk factors: Global Burden of Disease Study. Lancet 1997;349:1436–42.
10. Kessler RC, Heeringa S, Lakoma MD, et al. Individual and societal effects of mental disorders on earnings in the United States: results from the National Comorbidity Survey Replication. Am J Psychiatry 2008;165:703–11.
11. Evans DL, Charney DS, Lewis L, et al. Mood disorders in the medically ill: scientific review and recommendations. Biol Psychiatry 2005;58:175–89.
12. El-Gabalawy R, Katz LY, Sareen J. Comorbidity and associated severity of borderline personality disorder and physical health conditions in a nationally representative sample. Psychosom Med 2010;72:641–7.
13. Broadbent E, Kydd R, Sanders D, et al. Unmet needs and treatment seeking in high users of mental health services: role of illness perceptions. Aust N Z J Psychiatry 2008;42:147–53.
14. Levinson D, Karger CJ, Haklai Z. Chronic physical conditions and use of health services among persons with mental disorders: results from the Israel National Health Survey. Gen Hosp Psychiatry 2008;30:226–32.
15. Miranda JJ, Patel V. Achieving the Millennium Development Goals: does mental health play a role? PLoS Med 2005;2:2291.

16. Wan JJ, Morabito DJ, Khaw J, et al. Mental illness as an independent risk factor for unintentional injury and injury recidivism. J Trauma 2006;61:1299–304.

17. Hiroeh U, Appleby L, Mortensen PB, et al. Death by homicide, suicide and other unnatural causes in people with mental illness: a population-based study. Lancet 2001;358:2110–2.

18. American Psychiatric Association (APA). Diagnostic and statistical manual for mental disorders. 4th edition. Washington, DC: American Psychiatric Association; 2000.

19. World Health Organization (WHO). The ICD-10 classification of mental and behavioural disorders. Clinical descriptions and diagnostic guidelines. Geneva (Switzerland): World Health Organization; 1992.

20. CDC. Adverse childhood experiences reported by adults--Five States, 2009. MMWR Morb Mortal Wkly Rep 2010;59:1609–13.

21. Lasser K, Boyd JW, Woolhandler S, et al. Smoking and mental illness: a population-based prevalence study. JAMA 2000;284:2606–10.

22. Kroenke K, Spitzer RL, Williams JBW, et al. Anxiety disorders in primary care: prevalence, impairment, comorbidity, and detection. Ann Intern Med 2007;146: 317–25.

23. Spitzer RL, Kroenke K, Williams JB, et al. A brief measure for assessing generalized anxiety disorder: the GAD-7. Arch Intern Med 2006;166:1092–7.

24. United Nations. United Nations Millennium Declaration: resolution adopted by the general assembly. No. A/RES/55/2 (8th plenary meeting). New York: United Nations General Assembly; 2000.

25. Patel V, Kleinman A. Poverty and common mental disorders in developing countries. Bull World Health Organ 2003;81:609–15.

26. Patel V, De Souza N. School drop-out. A public health approach for India. Natl Med J India 2000;13:316–8.

27. Patel V, Rahman A, Jacob KS, et al. Effect of maternal mental health on infant growth in low income countries. New Evidence from South Asia. BMJ 2004; 328:820–3.

28. Rahman A, Iqbal Z, Bunn J, et al. Impact of maternal depression on infant nutritional status and illness: a cohort study. Arch Gen Psychiatry 2004;61:946–52.

29. Patel V, Prince M. Maternal psychological morbidity and low birth weight in developing countries. Br J Psychiatry 2006;188:284–5.

30. Chandran M, Tharyan P, Muliyil J, et al. Post-partum depression in a cohort of women from a rural area of Tamil Nadu, India. Incidence and risk factors. Br J Psychiatry 2002;181:499–504.

31. Cooper PJ, Tomlinson M, Swartz L, et al. Post- partum depression and the mother-infant relationship in a South African peri-urban settlement. Br J Psychiatry 1999;175:554–8.

32. Fisher JR, Morrow MM, Ngoc NT, et al. Prevalence, nature, severity and correlates of postpartum depressive symptoms in Vietnam. BJOG 2004;111:1353–60.

33. Oates M. Suicide: The leading cause of maternal death. Br J Psychiatry 2003; 183:279–81.

34. Murray C, Lopez A, editors. Global Burden of Disease and Injury Series. The global burden of disease: a comprehensive assessment of mortality and disability from diseases, injuries and risk factors in 1990 and projected to 2020. Cambridge (MA): Harvard School of Public Health on behalf of the World Health Organization and the World Bank; 1996.

35. Murthy R, Bertolote J, Epping-Jordan JA, et al. The World Health Report Mental Health: new understanding new hope. Geneva (Switzerland): World Health Organization; 2001.

36. Kleintjes S, Flisher A, Fick M, et al. The prevalence of mental disorders among children, adolescents and adults in the Western Cape, South Africa. S Afr Psychiatr Rev 2006;9:157–60.
37. Al-Jawadi AA, Abdul-Rhman S. Prevalence of childhood and early adolescence mental disorders among children attending primary health care centers in Mosul, Iraq: a cross-sectional study. BMC Public Health 2007;7:274.
38. World Health Organization (WHO). Atlas of child and adolescent mental health resources, global concerns, implications for the future. Geneva (Switzerland): World Health Organization; 2005.
39. Das J, Do QT, Friedman J, et al. Mental health and poverty in developing countries: revisiting the relationship. Soc Sci Med 2007;65:467–80.
40. Murali V, Oyebode F. Poverty, social inequality and mental health. Adv Psychiatr Treat 2004;10:216–22.
41. Eaton J. A new movement for global mental health and its possible impact in Nigeria. Nigerian Journal of Psychiatry 2009;7:14–5.
42. Onyut LP, Neuner F, Ertl V, et al. Trauma, poverty and mental health among Somali and Rwandese refugees living in an African refugee settlement: an epidemiological study. Confl Health 2009;3(6). http://dx.doi.org/10.1186/1752-1505-1183–1186.
43. Ssebunnya J, Kigozi F, Lund C, et al. Stakeholder perceptions of mental health stigma and poverty in Uganda. BMC Int Health Hum Rights 2009;9:5.
44. Ndetei D, Khasakhala L, Kingori J, et al. Baseline study: the mental health situation in Kangemi informal settlement Nairobi. Kenya: 2007. Available at: http://www.basicneeds.org.uk. Accessed September 1, 2015.
45. Pailhez G, Bulbena A, López C, et al. Views of psychiatry: a comparison between medical students from Barcelona and Medellín. Acad Psychiatry 2010;34:61–6.
46. El-Gilany A, Amr M, Iqbal R. Students' attitudes toward psychiatry at Al-Hassa Medical College, Saudi Arabia. Acad Psychiatry 2010;34:71–4.
47. Voinescu B, Szentagotai A, Coogan A. Attitudes towards psychiatry – a survey of Romanian medical residents. Acad Psychiatry 2010;34:75–8.
48. Sorsdahl K, Stein DJ, Grimsrud A, et al. Traditional healers in the treatment of common mental disorders in South Africa. J Nerv Ment Dis 2009;197:434–41.
49. Ngoma MC, Prince M, Mann A. Common mental disorders among those attending primary health clinics and traditional healers in urban Tanzania. Br J Psychiatry 2003;183:349–55.
50. Ndetei D, Mutiso V, Khasakhala L, et al. The challenges of human resources in mental health in Kenya. S Afr Psychiatr Rev 2007;10:33–6.
51. Connell J, Zurn P, Stilwell B, et al. Sub-Saharan Africa: beyond the health worker migration crisis. Soc Sci Med 2007;64:1876–91.
52. Kirigia J, Gbary A, Muthuri L, et al. The cost of health professionals' brain drain in Kenya. BMC Health Serv Res 2006;6:89.
53. Stilwell B, Diallo K, Zurn P, et al. Migration of health-care workers from developing countries: strategic approaches to its management. Bull World Health Organ 2004;82(8):595–600.
54. Rohde J, Cousens S, Chopra M, et al. 30 years after Alma-Ata: Has primary health care worked in countries? Lancet 2008;372(9642):950–61.
55. Walley J, Lawn JE, Tinker A, et al. Primary health care: making Alma-Ata a reality. Lancet 2008;372:1001–7.

Childhood Vaccination
Implications for Global and Domestic Public Health

David S. Younger, MD, MPH, MS[a,b,]*, Adam P.J. Younger, MPH[c],
Sally Guttmacher, PhD[b]

KEYWORDS

- Vaccination • Neuroepidemiology • Public health

KEY POINTS

- Vaccination is of indisputable importance in the control and prevention of endemic and emerging domestic and global disease.
- The immunologic basis of vaccination is related to the ability to passively activate the host immune system inducing a salutary host response leading to microbial-specific protective antibodies.
- There are different types of vaccines depending on the methodology used.
- The control of vaccine-preventable diseases is associated with measurable decline in preventable hospitalizations, increased morbidity and mortality, and increased health care costs.
- Improvement in state and local public health infrastructure along with innovative and targeted prevention efforts continues to yield significant progress in controlling infectious illnesses.

INTRODUCTION

This is an era of intense change in exploration and understanding of the complexity of the human microbiome and the surrounding ecosystems. Although humans are hosts to a myriad of microorganisms that have assembled into complex communities outnumbering the human body by a factor of 10-fold providing many of the building blocks for shared immunity, there still exist certain pathogenic microorganisms that cause human and economic devastation, which if prevented by effective vaccination campaigns, could easily be eradicated. This article examines selected aspects of domestic and global vaccination. Vaccination was the topic of a recent book.[1]

[a] Division of Neuroepidemiology, Department of Neurology, New York University School of Medicine, New York, NY, USA; [b] College of Global Public Health, New York University, New York, NY, USA; [c] Public and Nonprofit Management and Policy, The Wagner Graduate School of Public Service, New York University, New York, NY, USA
* Corresponding author. 333 East 34th Street, 1J, New York, NY 10016.
E-mail address: david.younger@nyumc.org

Neurol Clin 34 (2016) 1035–1047
http://dx.doi.org/10.1016/j.ncl.2016.05.004
0733-8619/16/$ – see front matter © 2016 Elsevier Inc. All rights reserved.

HISTORICAL ASPECTS

During the twentieth century, the health and life expectancy of persons residing in the United States improved dramatically. Since the beginning of that century the average lifespan of persons in the United States increased by more than 30 years, with 25 years of the gain attributable to advances in public health. Vaccination of the US public is one of the 10 great public health achievements of the twentieth century.[2] At the beginning of that century, infectious diseases were widely prevalent in the United States and exacted an enormous toll on the population. With few effective antimicrobial treatments and preventative measures available, the first vaccine against smallpox, developed in 1796, was not widely used enough to fully control the disease exacting 894 fatalities of 12,064 reported cases. Four other vaccines against rabies, typhoid, cholera, and plague also developed a century earlier were not widely used by 1900. Since that time, vaccines have been developed or licensed against at least 21 other diseases in the United States, approximately one-half of which are recommended in selected populations at high risk because of areas of environmental factors, age, medical condition, or risk behaviors, whereas 13 are recommended by the Centers for Disease Control and Prevention (CDC) for use in all US children (**Table 1**).

Historically, national efforts to promote vaccines among eligible children began with the appropriation of federal funds for polio vaccination after introduction of the vaccine in 1955, and since then federal, state, and local governments and public and private health care providers have collaborated to develop and maintain the vaccine-delivery system in the United States. By the end of the twentieth century, vaccination coverage was at record levels, exceeding 90% for three or more doses of diphtheria-tetanus-toxoids-pertussis vaccine (DPT), three or more doses of poliovirus vaccine, three or more doses of *Haemophilus influenzae* type b (Hib) vaccine, and one or more doses of measles-containing vaccine. Coverage with four or more doses of DPT was 81% and 84% for three doses of hepatitis B vaccine. There was, however, lower coverage for the then recently introduced varicella vaccine (26%), for the combined series of four DPT/three polio/one measles-containing vaccine/three Hib.[3] By the end of the twentieth century, coverage for children age 5 to 6 years exceeded 95% each school year since 1980 for DPT, polio, and measles-mumps-rubella (MMR) vaccines.

Dramatic declines in morbidity were reported for nine vaccine-preventable diseases for which vaccinations were recommended in US children before 1990: smallpox, diphtheria, paralytic poliomyelitis, and measles caused by wild-type viruses declined 100%; and nearly 100% for pertussis, tetanus, mumps, rubella, congenital rubella, and Hib. The past decade additionally witnessed substantial declines in cases, hospitalizations, mortality, and health care costs associated with vaccine-preventable diseases.[4] In addition, new vaccines were introduced covering rotavirus, meningococcal disease, herpes zoster, pneumococcal bacteremia, and human papillomavirus infection, and tetanus, diphtheria, and acellular pertussis for adults and adolescents, bringing to 17 the number of disease targeted by US immunization policy. One economic analysis[5] showed that vaccination of each US birth cohort with the current childhood immunization schedule feasibly prevented approximately 42,000 deaths and 20 million disease cases, with net saving of nearly $14 billion in direct costs and $69 billion in total societal costs. Pneumococcal conjugate and rotavirus are the two vaccines implemented in the past decade that are particularly striking, preventing an estimated 13,000 deaths and up to 60,000 hospitalizations, respectively, each year, and advances made in the older hepatitis A and B, and varicella vaccines bringing reported cases to record low levels, and reducing age-adjusted mortality in

Table 1
CDC schedule of infant and childhood vaccinations

Vaccine Name	Age at First Dose	Age at Second Dose	Age at Third Dose	Age at Fourth Dose
Hepatitis B (HepB)	Birth	1–2 mo	6–18 mo	—
Rotavirus (RV) RV1 (2-dose series); RV5 (3-dose series)	2 mo	4 mo	6 mo	—
Diphtheria, tetanus, and acellular pertussis (DTaP: <7 y)	2 mo	4 mo	6 mo	15–18 mo
Tetanus, diphtheria, and acellular pertussis (Tdap: >7 y)	11–12 y	—	—	—
Haemophilus influenzae type b5 (Hib)	2 mo	4 mo	6 mo	12–15 mo
Pneumococcal conjugate (PCV13)	2 mo	4 mo	6 mo	12–15 mo
Inactivated poliovirus (IPV: <18 y)	2 mo	4 mo	6–18 mo	4–6 y
Influenza (IIV; LAIV) 2 doses for some	6–18 mo annual vaccination (IIV only) 1 or 2 doses	2–8 y annual vaccination (LAIV or IIV) 1 or 2 doses	8–18 y annual vaccination (LAIV or IIV) 1 dose only	—
Measles, mumps, rubella (MMR)	12–15 mo	4–6 y	—	—
Varicella (VAR)	12–15 mo	4–6 y	—	—
Hepatitis A (HepA)	12–18 mo (2 dose series)	—	—	—
Human papillomavirus (HPV2, females only; HPV4, males and females)	11–12 y (3 dose series)	—	—	—
Meningococcal (Hib-MenCY >6 wk, MenACWY-D >9 mo; MenACWY-CRM >2 mo)	11–12 y	—	—	—

Data from Centers for Disease Control, Atlanta, GA. Available at http://www.cdc.gov/vaccines/schedules.

deaths per million population from hepatitis A from 0.38 by the end of the previous century to 0.26 by the end of the recent decade.[6]

Expanded vaccination coverage has also been historically the most cost-effective means to advance global welfare and one of the 10 great public health achievements worldwide in the past decade,[7] with an estimated prevention of 2.5 million deaths each year among children less than 5 years through use of measles, polio, and DPT vaccines. Polio eradication efforts through mandatory vaccination decreased the number of countries from 20 to 4, with fewer than 1500 cases reported in 2010. With the number of countries using hepatitis B vaccine increasing from 107 in 2000 to 178 in 2009, and global vaccination coverage of 70%, at least 700,000 deaths from cirrhosis and liver cases are expected to be averted in annual birth cohort in the 178 countries. Moreover, during 2000 to 2009, the number of countries using the Hib vaccine worldwide increased from 62 to 161, with a resulting global coverage of 38%, averting an estimated 130,000 pneumonia and meningitis deaths annually among children less than 5 years of age.

The combined achievements in vaccine-preventable diseases mirrored changes in the public health system. These included the greater quantitative capacity of epidemiology in study designs and period health surveys, methods of data collection that evolved from simple measures of disease prevalence to complex studies of precise analysis available in cohort, case-control, and randomized clinical trials to establish the efficacy of vaccination and demonstrate its low risk. The CDC in the United States, which assumed responsibility for collecting and publishing nationally notifiable disease data in 1998, now tracks more than 52 infectious illnesses. Today, public health represents the combined collaboration of governmental federal, state, county, and local governmental health departments, and nongovernmental organization to track infectious illness in the United States and rates of vaccination.

IMMUNE BASIS OF VACCINATION

The human immune system and immunization are inextricably related. In practice, vaccines are most often comprised of an attenuated or weakened version of the pathogenic organism for which immunity is sought. This attenuation is accomplished in such a way that the foreign pathogen is rendered sufficient for invoking an immune response yet incapable of inducing infection. In essence, the immune system processes the immunization as if an infection were present.

Immunity was originally separated into two types, humoral and cell-mediated, based on the purported effects of immunization or vaccine against a given pathogen. Humoral immunity was deemed as the effect of immunization that resulted in definable changes in the cell-free body fluid or serum, whereas the cell-mediated type was ascribed to the observed protective effect associated with multiplication of specific cells. Two primordial types of immune cells are now recognized and contribute to vaccination-induced immunity. One lineage, termed B cells, which mature in the bone marrow, further differentiate into plasma cells and memory cells. Mature plasma cells are capable of producing antimicrobial antibodies capable of latching onto their target in a lock-and-key-specific fashion when their surface antibody receptors recognize other cells displaying foreign infectious antigens, whereas other B-cell types mature into memory B cells that circulate in the bloodstream. T cells, also derived in the bone marrow, pass instead though the thymus gland where they achieve their final immunoreactivity, and are thought to be most protective in recognizing virus-infected cells. These cells participate in the defense against intracellular bacterial, fungal, and protozoan infections; cancers; and transplant rejection. Other aspects of enhanced cellular immunity include the secretion of cell-signaling molecules termed cytokines, which promote cell-to-cell communication in immune responses and stimulate the movement of cells toward sites of inflammation and infection. An important aspect of vaccination-induced immunity is the booster shot, which amplified the immune response by representing the foreign antigen to a nonnaive host immune system.

CATEGORIES OF VACCINES

Vaccines are divided into different categories depending on the way they are prepared and therefore how they confer immunity, including live-attenuated, inactivated, subunit, conjugate, and toxoids. This has been reviewed elsewhere.[8]

Live-Attenuated Vaccine

Most frequently used for viruses rather than bacterial illnesses, the method for preparing live-attenuated vaccines involves passing the viral agent through a succession of cell cultures to weaken it producing a form that is no longer able to replicate in human cells. Still recognized by the body's immune system, it protects against future infection. Examples includes MMR, varicella, and Hib vaccines. Although uncommon it is plausible that the introduced virus can cause illness if it has transformed into a more virulent form through mutation.

Inactivated Vaccine

The microbe is inactivated by heat, irradiation, or certain chemicals to no longer cause illness on vaccination without altering its immune activation properties. Examples are poliovirus and hepatitis A vaccines. However, a disadvantage is the need for multiple boosters to augment efficacy.

Subunit Vaccine

When only a portion of the microbe that acts as an antigen for immune surveillance is needed by the body to confer immunity, subunit vaccination is an appropriate methodology, such as influenza and hepatitis B subunit vaccines.

Conjugate Vaccine

These types of vaccines are prepared from parts of the bacterium combined with a carrier protein, which when chemically linked together to the bacteria coat derivatives and generate a more potent host immune response, such as the pneumococcal vaccine.

DOMESTIC AND GLOBAL VACCINATION PROGRAMS

Vaccination programs in the United States have generally been tied to school entry. The first national push to ensure that every state in the country had vaccination requirements for children entering schools occurred in the 1970s predicated on measles outbreaks during the preceding two decades.[9] Some states acted on their own accord and enacted vaccination laws. However, public opinion has at times been the most useful catalyst, especially outbreaks that remind one of the devastating potential of certain diseases that may have disappeared from public view because of infrequent occurrence. Indeed, a major advance in global public health was the launch of the World Health Organization Expanded Program on Immunization that promoted a schedule of basic vaccines for immunization against polio, measles, tuberculosis, and DPT according to the standard schedule similar to childhood programs in the United States (**Table 2**).

Table 2
World Health Organization schedules of infant and childhood vaccinations

Vaccine Name	Age at First Dose	Age at Second Dose	Age at Third Dose	Age at Fourth Dose
BCG	Birth	—	—	—
Hepatitis B (Option 1)	Birth	4 wk	8 wk	—
Hepatitis B (Option 2)	Birth	4 wk	8 wk	12 wk
Polio (OPV + IPV)	6 wk	10 wk	14 wk	—
Polio (IPV/OPV Sequential)	8 wk	12–16 wk	4–8 wk after second dose	4–8 wk after third dose
Polio (IPV)	8 wk	12–16 wk	4–8 wk after second dose	—
DTP	6 wk	10–18 wk	4–8 wk after second dose	—
Hib (Option 1)	6 wk–59 mo	4 wk after first dose	4 wk after second dose	—
Hib (Option 2)	6 wk–59 mo	8 wk after first dose if 2 doses, 4 wk after first dose if 3 doses	4 wk after second dose	—
Pneumococcal (conjugate) (Option 1)	6 wk	10 wk	14 wk	—
Pneumococcal (conjugate) (Option 2)	6 wk	14 wk	—	—
Rotavirus (Rotarix)	6 wk	10 wk	—	—
Rotavirus (Rota Teq)	6 wk	10–16 wk	4 wk after second dose	—
Measles	9 or 12 mo	4 wk after first dose	—	—
Rubella	9 or 12 mo	—	—	—
Human papillomavirus	As soon as possible from 9 y	6 mo after first dose	—	—

Data from World Health Organization, Geneva, Switzerland. Available at: http://www.who.int/immunization/policy/immunization_tables/en/.

Vaccination as a method of disease prevention has been widely accepted globally. Goal Four of the United Nations Millennium Development Goals to reduce childhood mortality focuses on the delivery of effective vaccinations for children younger than age 5 years. Measles vaccination helped prevent nearly 15.6 million deaths worldwide between 2000 and 2013. The number of globally reported measles cases declined by 67% during the same period; about 84% of children worldwide received at least one dose of measles-containing vaccine in 2013, up 73% from 2000.[10] Chasing a disease down to the last few cases in lesser developed countries to the levels achieved in the more developed world remains a challenge. For example, the goal of malaria eradication faltered in the 1960s in part because of the resistance of *Plasmodium falciparum* to antimicrobial therapy and the development of mosquito vector resistance to insecticides resulting in a worldwide increase in cases. Virtually all vaccines against *P falciparum* (RTS, S/AAS01) have been designed using genetic sequences derived from the single well-characterized reference strain of West African origin (3D7).[11] A multivalent version of RTS, S with carefully chosen sporozoite protein variants, possibly combined with additional antigens, may offer broader protection.[12]

Even though most of the record decline of childhood infectious disease is attributed to increase in the use of vaccines, a small but significant minority of parents in the United States oppose the use of vaccines on children. Thus, the less than perfect effectiveness of certain US vaccination programs, such as childhood pertussis and measles that depend on widespread acceptance, resulted in a record number of cases in the United States in 2015.[13]

Valuable lessons have been learned from the worldwide campaigns to eradicate polio. In 1988, the World Health Assembly endorsed the goal of eradication of polio at a time when the number of new cases of paralysis approximated 350,000 and the disease was endemic in 125 countries.[14] The March of Dimes, established by President Franklin Roosevelt, was set up in the United States to end the epidemic that plagued the nation. Jonas Salk and Albert Sabin were two US scientists who took on the challenge of developing an effective vaccine against polio. To ensure efficacy against wild poliovirus infection, Salk methodically classified circulating polio strains before choosing the three in the final inactivated vaccine.[11] This methodology was implemented in the polio vaccine that achieved strain-specific protective immunity based on the inherent genetic diversity of the poliovirus. Wild-type poliovirus type 2 has since been eradicated in the United States with the last naturally occurring case detected in 1999, and type 3 seems to be close to eradication with virtually no new cases detected. Type 1 poliovirus, however, later emerged during the 2011 outbreak in China suggesting that eradication was incomplete. More recently cases of polio have been diagnosed in Syria, Nigeria, and Bangladesh caused by the disruption of populations by war and antivaccine sentiment expressed by some ultrareligious Muslims. As long as the polio virus circulates anywhere in the world, there is the potential for poliomyelitis to be exported to countries that are disease-free causing serious outbreaks.

LEGAL CHALLENGES TO VACCINATION
The Lessons of Measles Vaccination

The hesitation or refusal of parents to vaccinate children was until recently on the rise in the United States with increasing exceptions granted from school-entry immunization mandates based on personal beliefs and nonmedical reasons. Buttenheim and colleagues[15] noted that while still below levels to maintain herd immunity against measles, there was a 2- to 10-fold underestimate of the true rate of vaccine refusal based on personal beliefs on school entry. This suggests a level of inadequate understanding by parents as to the public imperative of measles immunization or a fear that the vaccine may itself be pathogenic in one form or another.

When an outbreak of measles cases was reported by the CDC in December 2014 at Disneyland in Orange County, California,[16] it was subsequently shown that 7% of children had received two or more MMR vaccinations, 45% were unvaccinated, and 43% had an unknown vaccination status.[17] These findings compelled two California State Senators, both with personal ties to health policy (one a pediatrician and the other the son of a polio survivor), to cosponsor and pass Bill SB 277 eliminating all nonmedical vaccine exemptions, and many other States began to follow California's lead.

There was no greater challenge for public health educators than trying to amend the misunderstanding of the risk of autism following MMR vaccination among concerned lay parent groups at the turn of the twentieth century in the United Kingdom. The basis for this misconception in causality was grounded in a publication in a major medical journal by a UK investigator that was subsequently retracted, which drew attention to cohorts of children with autism presumed to be a result of immune conditioning by early live-attenuated measles vaccination.[18–20] More than a decade later, a retracted US publication cited heightened risk for autism among only African American boys[21] citing a reanalysis of CDC data reported earlier showing no relation of autism in a population of school-matched subjects.[22] Further population-based studies[19] and a recent meta-analysis[23] of case-control and cohort studies have since found no strong evidence for a causal effect of autism by MMR vaccination.

Cawkwell and Oshinsky[24] studied the lessons learned from Mississippi, a state that consistently leads the United States in childhood vaccination with a greater than 99% MMR rate for children entering kindergarten. The fight against compulsory vaccination and the enduring success of Mississippi in repelling challenges to their vaccination requirements were traced to a State Supreme Court decision predicated on a 1972 State code that required vaccination before attending school. In 1979, Charles Brown sued the State of Mississippi claiming a strong religious belief against it, in order for his 6-year-old son to be admitted to Houston Elementary School despite not having been vaccinated. The Court upheld the validity of the State code but went a step further ruling that religious exemptions discriminated against children whose parents did not have those strong religious convictions thus violating the 14th Amendment, which called for equal protection of the law. This line of reasoning, which applied to philosophic and personal belief exemptions, removed any legal pathway to exemptions, with the exception of medical exemptions. The latter were so notoriously strict and required submission to the Department of Public Health by a licensed primary care physician that only 121 were approved in 2013 to 2014. There is no unanimous agreement among scientists and policy experts that removal of all nonmedical exemptions is the most logical path forward in ensuring acceptable rates of vaccination. Tea Party member Senator Chris McDaniel submitted in 2015 SB 2800, a bill that sought to amend the Mississippi code to allow for exemptions to vaccination on a contrary to belief stance that died in Committee. Subsequently, House Bill 130 surfaced supporting a parent's freedom to choose if their child is vaccinated, which although framed differently did not pass.

Strengthening childhood immunization laws is an important public health goal. There is legal precedent for the right of states to mandate vaccination for school entry to protect the public at large, as a social obligation to provide herd immunity, and to protect those who cannot be vaccinated recognizing that it is probably safer to be unvaccinated living in a highly vaccinated community than to be vaccinated but living in an unvaccinated one.[9]

ASSESSING THE IMPACT OF VACCINES FOR ENDEMIC INFECTION

Assessing the impact of vaccination on an individual and population level requires an analysis of the direct and indirect effects of immunization. The theoretic concept of vaccine efficacy describes the individual level benefit or how much less likely an individual is to acquire infection following a given exposure. Most clinical trials, however, assess vaccine effectiveness at the population level. Both may fail to capture the indirect effect of vaccination accounting for the reduction in transmission to unvaccinated subjects in the wider population. Impossible to fully assess from clinical trial data alone, it is this combination of direct and indirect effects that should interest public health experts in fully evaluating the vaccination impact, especially because little may be known about the apparent or real vaccine impacts, and the risk of reinfection or mechanism of protection.

When performing statistical analysis of vaccine efficacy trials with heterogeneous exposure or susceptibility risk, care should be taken to account for the putative mechanism of the vaccine. Halloran and colleagues[25] used the term "leaky vaccine" inspired by the literature on malaria to describe a vaccine that exhibited failure in degree, and all-or-nothing vaccine for one that demonstrates failure in take. A vaccine that displayed only a failure in duration was called a waning vaccine. Farrington[26] cited the vaccine for pertussis as a possibly leaky vaccine, whereas vaccines for measles and rubella were termed all-or-nothing vaccines, and that for cholera as a waning vaccine.

Magpantay and colleagues[27] used mathematical modelling to extrapolate the epidemiologic efficacy and ramifications of such imperfect vaccines considering that an imperfect vaccine might exhibit failures in degree or leakiness and take or all-or-nothingness. These two extremes were reflective of their respective mechanisms of action from all-or-none complete protection of some fraction of subjects, with the remaining fraction remaining unaffected by it, and incomplete or leaky vaccines that reduced the per-exposure transmission rate for all recipients equally. Leaky vaccines again were those for which vaccine-induced protection reduced infection rates on a per-exposure basis, as opposed to all-or-none vaccines, which reduced infection rates to zero for some fraction of subjects, independent of the number of exposures. Leaky vaccines protected subjects with fewer exposures at a higher effective rate than subjects with more exposures. Edlefsen[28] noted that this simple dichotomy had serious implications for analysis of methodologies because leaky vaccines, which in effect protect highly exposed recipients at a lower rate, induce a violation of the proportional hazards condition that is often assumed in survival analysis.

Ragonnet and colleagues[29] applied a dynamic compartmental model to simulate vaccination for endemic infections studying several measures of effectiveness. They used mathematical derivations to calculate and compare the real and apparent impact of vaccination, and to assess the effect of a range of infection and vaccine characteristics on these measures. Their findings showed that vaccine impact was markedly underestimated in the following circumstances: when primary infection provided partial natural immunity, coverage was high, and postvaccination infectiousness was reduced. Leaky vaccines provided the same partial reduction of susceptibility to every vaccinated individual, whereas an all-or-nothing vaccine provided complete protection to a proportion of vaccinated individuals. All-or-nothing vaccines were more effective than leaky ones particularly in settings with high risk of reinfection and transmissibility. Accrued longer latent periods resulted in greater real impacts when risk of reinfection was high, but this effect diminished if partial natural immunity was assumed.

MICROECONOMIC IMPACT OF VACCINATION

Jit and coworkers[30] analyzed the economic impact of vaccination. The authors noted that investment in immunization programs dramatically increased in developed and developing countries over the past two decades as a result of the development of new vaccines against major diseases,[31] and the emergence of new financing mechanisms. Organizations, such as Gavi, the vaccine alliance that subsidizes the cost of vaccines for some lesser developed countries, and the Pan American Health Organization, contributed to this economic feasibility and success of vaccination programs.[32] Spending growth heightened the importance of investing in immunization.[33]

Microeconomic evaluations can be used to facilitate decision-making by national and multinational stakeholders through comparisons of the economic cost of implementing vaccine program infrastructure, purchase, and delivery, against the health and economic benefits of vaccination. Economists have argued that improvements in health can lead to economic growth through longer term mechanisms, such as decreasing birth rates, strengthening macroeconomic stability, and improving educational outcomes.[34,35] Microeconomic theory has been applied to investments in immunization suggesting the separation of benefits into narrow and broad gains. Interest in particular in the former have included health gains; health care cost savings; reductions in the time costs of caring for the sick; and improved economic productivity because of prevention of mental and physical disabilities, improved child survival, the development of herd immunity, and prevention of antibiotic resistance. Bishai and coworkers[36] noted a significant reduction in the poverty-related gradient in younger than age 5 mortality by measles vaccination improving health equity directly. Using a cost-benefit analysis approach to assess the impact of Hib vaccination, Bärnighausen and colleagues[37] demonstrated that past economic evaluations had mostly adopted narrow evaluation perspectives, focusing primarily on health gains, health care cost savings, and reductions in the time costs of caring, while usually ignoring other important benefits including outcome-related productivity gains (improved economic productivity caused by prevention of mental and physical disabilities), behavior-related productivity gains (economic growth caused by declining birth rates because vaccination improves child survival), and community externalities (herd immunity and prevention of antibiotic resistance).

Although vaccination is most cost-effective in low-income groups and regions, the accrual of benefits of vaccination in the poorest countries may be difficult to ascertain, leading to exacerbation or narrowing of the indicators of equity. Using country-level rotavirus vaccination data from demographic and health surveys on within-country patterns of vaccine coverage and diarrhea mortality risk factors, Rheingans and colleagues[38] estimated distributional effects of rotavirus vaccination in 25 Gavi countries. The authors noted the greatest potential benefit of rotavirus vaccination in Gavi countries of the poorest quintiles, although existing rates of vaccination coverage were highly skewed toward the richest quintiles. Therefore, programs that added new vaccines to existing systems without mechanisms to ensure equity in uptake may actually exacerbate rather than reduce existing inequity. Simply adding new vaccines to existing systems could target investments to higher income children because of disparities in vaccination coverage. Maximizing health benefits for the poorest children, while ensuring the best value for money, may require increased attention to these distributional effects.

With an estimated 4% of global child deaths or approximately 300,000 deaths, attributed to rotavirus in 2010, and one-third occurring in India and Ethiopia, Verguet and colleagues[39] hypothesized that public financing of rotavirus vaccination in these two countries could substantially decrease child mortality and rotavirus-related hospitalizations, prevent health-related impoverishment, and bring significant cost savings to households. Using extended cost-effectiveness analysis to evaluate a hypothetical publicly financed program for rotavirus vaccination in India and Ethiopia, the authors measured program impact along the averted dimensions of rotavirus deaths and household expenditures, financial risk protection afforded, and distributional consequences across the wealth strata of the country populations. Their analyses showed direct benefits of rotavirus vaccination in substantially decreasing rotavirus deaths mainly among the poorer, with reduced household expenditures across all income groups, and effective provision of financial risk protection that was concentrated among the poorest. The potential indirect benefits of vaccination of herd immunity would lead to increased program benefits among all income groups.

SUMMARY

Vaccination is a domestic and global imperative not just to prevent certain microbial diseases but to eradicate them. Mass-vaccination campaigns have lowered the incidence of MMR in lesser developed countries to low levels but that may not be good enough because these diseases, like others, can bounce back. At least three big improvements underscore the argument for wider eradication and prevention campaigns, in a list of communicable diseases. The first is better techniques for locating and monitoring cases of disease globally. The second is improved medical technology that has produced superior drugs and vaccines. The third is a change in political attitudes that first sought to effectively deal with AIDS, and then Ebola, and by creating better medical infrastructures.

REFERENCES

1. Largent MA. Vaccine. The debate in modern America. Baltimore (MD): Johns Hopkins University Press; 2012.
2. Centers for Disease Control and Prevention (CDC). Ten great public health achievements—United States, 1990-1999. MMWR Morb Mortal Wkly Rep 1999; 48:241–64.
3. Centers for Disease Control and Prevention (CDC). National, state, and urban area vaccination coverage levels among children aged 19-35 months—United States, 1997. MMWR Morb Mortal Wkly Rep 1998;47:547–54.
4. Centers for Disease Control and Prevention (CDC). Ten great public health achievements—United States, 2001-2010. MMWR Morb Mortal Wkly Rep 2011; 60:619–23.
5. Zhou F. Updated economic evaluation of the routine childhood immunization schedule in the United States. Presented at the 45th National Immunization Conference. Washington, DC, March 28–31, 2011.
6. Vogt TM, Wise ME, Bell BP, et al. Declining hepatitis A mortality in the United States during the era of hepatitis A vaccination. J Infect Dis 2008;197:1282–8.
7. Centers for Disease Control and Prevention (CDC). Ten great public health achievements–Worldwide, 2001-2010. MMWR Morb Mortal Wkly Rep 2011;60: 814–8.
8. Hussein IH, Chams N, Chams S, et al. Vaccines through centuries: major cornerstones of global health. Front Public Health 2015;3:269.
9. Lantos JD, Jackson MA, Harrison CJ. Why we should eliminate personal belief exemptions to vaccine mandates. J Health Polit Policy Law 2012;37:131–40.
10. Available at: www.un.org/millenniumgoals/2015_MDG_Report/pdf/MDG 2015.

11. Plowe CV. Vaccine-resistant malaria. N Engl J Med 2015;373:2082–3.
12. Heppner DG Jr, Kester KE, Ockenhouse CF, et al. Towards an RTS, S-based, multi-stage, multi-antigen vaccine against falciparum malaria: progress at the Walter Reed Army Institute of Research. Vaccine 2005;23:2243–50.
13. Jakinovich A, Sood SK. Pertussis: still a cause of death, seven decades into vaccination. Curr Opin Pediatr 2014;26:597–604.
14. Mundel T, Orenstein WA. No country is safe without global eradication of poliomyelitis. Editorial. N Engl J Med 2013;369:2045–6.
15. Buttenheim AM, Sethuraman K, Omer SB, et al. MMR vaccination status of children exempted from school-entry immunization mandates. Vaccine 2015;33: 6250–6.
16. Clemmons NS, Gastanaduy PA, Fiebelkorn AP, et al. Measles—United States, January 4-April 2, 2015. MMWR Morb Mortal Wkly Rep 2015;64:373–6.
17. Zipprich J, Winter K, Hacker J, et al. Measles outbreak—California, December 2014-February 2015. MMWR Morb Mortal Wkly Rep 2015;64:153–4.
18. Wakefield AJ, Murch SH, Anthony A, et al. Ileal-lymphoid-nodular hyperplasia, non-specific colitis, and pervasive developmental disorder in children. Lancet 1998;351:637–41.
19. Wakefield AJ, Anthony A, Schepelmann S, et al. Persistent measles virus infection and immunodeficiency in children with autism, ileo-colonic lymphoid nodular hyperplasia and non-specific colitis. Gut 1998;42(Suppl 1):A86.
20. Wakefield AJ, Montgomery SM. Autism, viral infection and measles-mumps-rubella vaccination. Isr Med Assoc J 1999;1:183–7.
21. Hooker BS. Measles-mumps-rubella vaccination timing and autism among young African-American boys: a reanalysis of CDC data. Transl Neurodegener 2014;3: 16.
22. DeStefano F, Bhasin TK, Thompson WW, et al. Age at first measles-mumps-rubella vaccination in children with autism and school-matched control subjects: a population-based study in metropolitan Atlanta. Pediatrics 2004;113:259–66.
23. Taylor LE, Swerdfeger AL, Eslick GD, et al. Vaccines are not associated with autism: an evidence-based meta-analyses of case-control and cohort studies. Vaccine 2014;32:3623–9.
24. Cawkwell PB, Oshinsky D. Childhood vaccination requirements: lessons from history, Mississippi, and a path forward. Vaccine 2015;33(43):5884–7.
25. Halloran ME, Haber M, Longini IM. Interpretation and estimation of vaccine efficacy under heterogeneity. Am J Epidemiol 1992;136:328–43.
26. Farrington CP. On vaccine efficacy and reproduction numbers. Math Biosci 2003; 185:89–109.
27. Magpantay FM, Riolo MA, de Cellès MD, et al. Epidemiological consequences of imperfect vaccines for immunizing infections. SIAM J Appl Math 2014;74: 1810–30.
28. Edlefsen PT. Leaky vaccines protect highly exposed recipients at a lower rate: implications for vaccine efficacy estimation and sieve analysis. Comput Math Methods Med 2014;2014:813789.
29. Ragonnet R, Trauer JM, Denholm JT, et al. Vaccination programs for endemic infections: modelling real versus apparent impacts of vaccine and infection characteristics. Sci Rep 2015;5:15468.
30. Jit M, Hutubessy R, Png ME, et al. The broader economic impact of vaccination: reviewing and appraising the strength of evidence. BMC Med 2015;13:209.
31. Plotkin SA. Vaccines: past, present and future. Nat Med 2005;11:S5–11.

32. Leach-Kemon K, Graves CM, Johnson EK, et al. Vaccine resource tracking systems. BMC Health Serv Res 2014;14:421.
33. Kim S-Y, Goldie SJ. Cost-effectiveness analyses of vaccination programmes: a focused review of modelling approaches. Pharmacoeconomics 2008;26: 191–221.
34. Bloom DE, Canning D, Jamison DT. Health, wealth, and welfare. Finance Dev 2004;41:10–5.
35. Belli PC, Bustreo F, Preker A. Investing in children's health: what are the economic benefits? Bull World Health Organ 2005;83:777–84.
36. Bishai D, Koenig M, Khan M. Measles vaccination improves the equity of health outcomes: evidence from Bangladesh. Health Econ 2003;12:415–9.
37. Bärnighausen T, Bloom D, Canning D. Rethinking the benefits and costs of childhood vaccination: the example of the *Haemophilus influenzae* type B vaccine. Vaccine 2011;29:2371–80.
38. Rheingans R, Atherly D, Anderson J. Distributional impact of rotavirus vaccination in 25 GAVI countries: estimating disparities in benefits and cost-effectiveness. Vaccine 2012;30:A15–23.
39. Verguet S, Murphy S, Anderson B, et al. Public finance of rotavirus vaccination in India and Ethiopia: an extended cost-effectiveness analysis. Vaccine 2013;31: 4902–10.

Epidemiology of Zika Virus

David S. Younger, MD, MPH, MS[a,b,*]

KEYWORDS

• Zika virus • Public health • Neuroepidemiology

KEY POINTS

• Zika virus is an arbovirus belonging to the *Flaviviridae* family, originally isolated in Uganda in 1947, known to cause mild clinical symptoms similar to those of dengue and chikungunya and transmitted by different species of *Aedes* mosquitoes. Direct interhuman transmission occurs perinatally, through blood transfusion, and sexually.

• Recent outbreaks in several regions of the world including Egypt, Easter Island, the insular pacific region, and more recently Brazil, highlight the need for the scientific community and public health community to consider it as an emerging global threat.

• Its clinical profile is that of a dengue-like febrile illness, but recently associated Guillain-Barre syndrome and microcephaly have appeared. There is neither a vaccine nor prophylactic medications available to prevent Zika virus infection.

• Public health recommendation advises pregnant women to postpone travel to areas where Zika viral infection is epidemic, and if not, to follow steps to avoid mosquito bites to avert fetal brain injury associated with early and late intrauterine infection.

HISTORICAL ASPECTS

Zika virus was first identified in a rhesus monkey in the Zika Forest of Uganda in 1947.[1] It was later found in people with febrile illnesses in West Africa in 1954.[2] It then spread to Indonesia,[3] Micronesia,[4] the Philippines,[5] French Polynesia,[6] and Easter Island–South Pacific[7] in 2014. Zika virus infections were not documented on mainland South America until the first report of autochthonous transmission in Brazil in May 2015. The conclusion at that time was that Zika virus was introduced into Brazil during the 2014 World Cup Football.[8] This was not supported due to the fact that no Pacific countries with documented Zika virus infection had competed in the World Cup competition. However, Pacific countries had participated in the August 2014 Va'a World Sprints canoe championship, which was held in Rio de Janeiro, suggesting that introduction of Zika virus into Brazil could have occurred then.[9] Another possibility was the introduction of Zika virus to Brazil by travelers from Chile.[10] Since its introduction into Brazil

The authors have nothing to disclose.
[a] Division of Neuroepidemiology, Department of Neurology, New York University School of Medicine, New York, NY, USA; [b] College of Global Public Health, New York University, New York, NY, USA
* 333 East 34th Street, 1J, New York, NY 10016.
E-mail address: david.younger@nyumc.org

in May 2015, Zika virus infection has subsequently spread rapidly across Brazil and the Americas. As of January 28, 2016, autochthonous cases of Zika virus infection have been reported from 26 countries in the Americas: Barbados, Bolivia, Brazil, Colombia, Curacao, Dominican Republic, Ecuador, El Salvador, French Guiana, Guadeloupe, Guatemala, Guyana, Haití, Honduras, Martinique, México, Nicaragua, Panama, Paraguay, Puerto Rico, Saint Maarten, Suriname, Venezuela, Virgin Islands. No autochthonous Zika virus transmission has been reported from European Union countries, and a heightened state of global alert is in place in Europe and the United States to screen for Zika virus in travelers with fever returning from endemic countries. The first travel-associated Zika illness among US travelers was reported in 2007. From 2007 to 2014, a total of 14 returning US travelers had positive Zika testing performed at the US Centers for Diseases Control and Prevention (CDC). In 2015 and 2016, at least 8 US travelers have had positive Zika testing performed at CDC.[11]

INFECTIOUS TRANSMISSION
Mosquito Vectors

Aedes species mosquitoes are present throughout the tropics and are recognized vectors of Zika, chikungunya, dengue, and yellow fever virus.[12–15] Although the main vector associated with transmission of Zika is Aedes aegypti, transmission can also occur with A albopictus, A africanus, A luteocephalus, A vittatus, A furcifer, A hensilii, and A apicoargenteus. A Aegypti mosquitoes live and breed near people and their homes, where they lay eggs in stagnant water and collect in puddles, buckets, flower pots, empty cans and other containers. They bite humans mainly during daytime, outside or inside their houses. A aegypti mosquitoes are widely distributed in the Americas, where the climate is suitable breeding condition. Recognizing that A albopictus has been found in the United States as far north as New York and Chicago, and in parts of southern Europe, Zika transmission will no doubt increase throughout the Americas, with possibility of local transmission within the United States Moreover, as Aedes mosquito species that spread Zika are found in many other locations globally, it is highly likely that outbreaks will spread to new countries.

Sexual Transmission

Whereas Zika virus isolated from semen in returning travelers typically developed up to 6 days after brief travel to Indonesia where Zika was endemic,[16] symptoms in the patient with presumed sexually transmitted infection were noted 10 days after sexual intercourse with the index case.[17,18] Studies are needed to assess how frequently and for how long the Zika virus persists in semen and what precautions should be mandated to prevent sexual transmission of Zika virus short of abstinence during a period of self-imposed quarantine.

Blood Transfusion

Given that many infected individuals with Zika virus infection will be asymptomatic and among them blood donors, transmission of Zika virus via blood transfusion is of concern.[19] This has a parallel in the introduction of West Nile Virus in the United States and Canada, which led to careful screening of donated blood.[20] The outbreak of chikungunya virus, which started in Reunion[21] and spread throughout Asia, similarly prompted screening of blood products. After the introduction of chikungunya virus in Italy, systematic screening by blood banks was considered, but a laboratory test for routine testing was not available.[22] Blood donations from people living in the affected municipalities were discontinued, and a 21-day deferral policy was introduced nationwide for blood donors who visited affected areas even for a few hours. All such stocked blood components collected from donors living in the affected area after the identification of the first case were eliminated. It is likely that blood transfusion-related infection will occur in Zika-endemic areas such that to prevent blood transfusion-related infection, blood donations should also be carefully screened.

ANIMAL AND HUMAN MODELS

Animal and human infectivity have been studied for more than 50 years, revealing the propensity for central nervous system (CNS) involvement. According to Dick and colleagues,[1] Zika virus was first isolated in 1947 from a captive sentinel rhesus monkey caged in the canopy of the Zika forest near Entebbe, Uganda, during the course of research into the epidemiology of yellow fever. The second isolation was made from a lot of *Aedes africanus* taken in 1948 from the same forest. Dick and colleagues[1] carried out cross-neutralization tests indicating that Zika virus was not related to yellow fever, Hawaii dengue, or to Theiler mouse encephalomyelitis virus.

In further experiments of the pathogenicity and physical properties of the virus in experimental animals,[23] Zika virus was found to be highly neurotropic in mice without traces of infection in any tissues other than the CNS at the onset of illness after inoculation. Moreover, the maximum virus titer was present on the first day of signs of illness, with a gradual fall thereafter. After intracerebral inoculation with infected mouse brain homogenates, 1 of 5 experimental monkeys showed mild pyrexia; however, the others showed no signs of infection. Viremia during the first week pi was found in all monkeys tested and antibody was demonstrated by the fourteenth day after inoculation. Among 99 human sera collected for yellow fever studies in Uganda, 6 (6.1%) were considered positive for Zika virus. Antibody was also found in the serum of 1 of 15 wild monkeys tested. The size of Zika virus was estimated to be in the region of 30 to 45 mμ in diameter. The virus was preserved up to 6 months in 50% glycerol and up to 30 months after drying, and susceptible to anesthetic ether; the thermal death point is 58°C for 30 minutes. Neuronal degeneration, cellular infiltration, and areas of softening were present in infected mouse brains sacrificed on the first day of signs of infection and confined to the CNS that was in various stages of infiltration and degeneration including widespread softening, neuronal degeneration, and cellular infiltration in the spinal cord. Minimal inflammatory changes were found in the ependymal membrane. Inclusion bodies of the Cowdry type A were observed in damaged neurons of acutely ill animals, especially in young animals compared with adults. Inclusions were absent from the brains of mice sick for several days or those chronically ill, even though the latter showed extensive round cell infiltration of the brain, and in some, degenerative changes in viscera, although not virus-specific. This histologic picture appeared to differentiate Zika from other neuronotropic viruses.

Two years later, during the investigations of an outbreak of jaundice suspected of being yellow fever in Eastern Nigeria, Zika was isolated from one patient while 2 others showed a rise in Zika virus titers.[2] Patient 1 was a 30-year-old African man with recent cough, diffuse arthralgia, and fever. Patient 2 was a 24-year-old African man who had new onset of fever, headache, and arthralgia. Patient 3 was a 10-year-old girl with recent onset of fever and headache without jaundice. All 3 patients recovered. Acute and convalescent sera from each case were tested by intracerebral protection tests via inoculation into experimental mice, resulting in a mortality rate of 100%. Viral-confirmed neutralization tests using immune monkey serum only in Patient 1, compatible with successful viral isolation. In support of the evidence of viral identification in that case, it was shown that the serum of a monkey immunized by inoculation of the isolated virus had a log neutralization index of 2.24 against the homologous virus, and 2.94 against Zika virus. That patient had no signs of jaundice, unlike the 2 others, in whom viral isolation was unsuccessful.

Following early epidemiologic studies in Uganda indicating that A africanus was probably the Zika vector, Boorman and Porterfield[24] successfully devised a technique employing a mouse skin membrane and heparin-treated blood for infecting mosquitoes. Using this technique, A aegypti mosquitoes were infected with Zika virus and their pathogenicity studied. Little or no virus was detected in mosquitoes on days 5 to 10, but thereafter the viral level rose and remained steady from days 20 to 60. Back-feeding experiments through a mouse skin membrane into uninfected mouse blood resulted in transmission in 12 of 20 cases. Successful infection of a rhesus monkey by the bites of 3 infected mosquitoes was demonstrated 72 days after an infected blood meal.

In the same year, Bearcroft[25] inoculated a 34-year old Nigerian male volunteer with an Eastern Nigerian strain of Zika virus that was comprised of 0.25 mL of 10-3 brain suspension representing 265 mouse lethal dose (LD50) given subcutaneously into the arm and specimens of blood drawn on day 4, 6, and 8 after inoculation. Following an incubation period of 82 hours, a mild, short-lived febrile condition occurred without evidence of involvement of any particular tissue or organ. Zika virus was isolated from the blood during the febrile period, accompanied by a rise in serum antibody to Zika virus by mouse protection and hemagglutination inhibition tests. Both adult and infant mice receiving undiluted serum from the patient between days 4 and 6 died. Histologic examination of portions of the brain showed encephalitis suggestive of viral infection.

CLINICAL ASPECTS

The classic clinical picture of Zika virus infection resembles that of dengue fever and chikungunya and is manifested by fever, headache, arthralgia, myalgia, and maculopapular rash, a complex of symptoms that hampers differential diagnosis. Although the disease is self-limiting, cases of neurologic manifestations including Guillain–Barré syndrome (GBS) have been described in French Polynesia and in Brazil during epidemics. One prototypical 40-year-old Polynesian woman[26] suffered from an influenza-like syndrome with myalgia, febricula, cutaneous rash, and conjunctivitis suspicious for Zika virus infection before development of flaccid paraparesis accompanied by dysautonomia and acquired demyelinating neuropathy. There was no evidence of systemic inflammation. Cerebrospinal fluid showed albuminocytologic dissociation with 1.66 g/L proteins (norm: 0.28–0.52) and 7 white cells/mL (normal <10). Reverse transcriptase polymerase chain reaction (RT-PCR) was negative on blood samples 8 days after the beginning of influenza-like symptoms (corresponding to Day 1) prior to the administration of intravenous immunoglobulin. Blood samples taken at 8 and 28 days after the beginning of the influenza-like syndrome were both positive for Zika-specific immunoglobulin M (IgM) and immunoglobulin G (IgG), assessed by enzyme-linked immunosorbent assay (ELISA). Antibody specificity was determined by plaque reduction neutralization test (PRNT). She slowly improved concomitant with the administration of 2 g/kg body weight of intravenous polyvalent immunoglobulin over 1 month.

A major concern associated with Zika virus infection has been the increased incidence of microcephaly in fetuses born to mothers with Zika virus infection. Ultrasonography in suspected fetuses shows the first signs of fetal anomalies and growth retardation, including a head circumference that is below that expected for fetal age and development. There may be blurred brain structures and calcifications in spite of normal fetal, umbilical, and uterine blood flow on Doppler ultrasonography. A well-studied fetus aborted at 32 weeks from a Brazilian woman[27] had a head circumference in the first percentile as the only external anomaly. However, neuropathologic examination showed agyria, internal hydrocephalus, calcifications, and otherwise normal subcortical development. The most prominent histopathological features included

- Filamentous, granular, neuron-shaped calcifications
- Diffuse astrogliosis; activated microglial cells expressing human leukocyte antigen (HLA)DR
- Scattered perivascular infiltrates of T cells and B cells in subcortical white matter
- Wallerian degeneration of long descending tracts, especially the corticospinal tract
- Granular intracytoplasmic reaction indicative of possible location of the virus in neurons

Electron microscopy showed enveloped structures with morphologic characteristics of *Flaviviridae* virus, and microbiologic investigation was positive for Zika on RT-PCR assay in the fetal brain sample alone. Analysis of the genome showed the highest identity with Zika strain isolated from a French Polynesian patient in 2013 (KJ776791), consistent with an emergence from the Asian lineage. The presence of 2 major amino acid substitutions in nonstructural proteins NS1 and NS4B represented, in all likelihood, an accidental event or adaptation of the virus to a new environment.

MICROBIOLOGIC AND SEROLOGIC CONSIDERATIONS

According to Petersen and colleagues,[28] the CDC recommends specific diagnostic algorithms for Zika virus diagnosis in adults and children.[29,30] The diagnosis of Zika virus can be confirmed by RT-PCR amplification of the viral genome, but it is expensive and prone to contamination. Commercial diagnostic tests for Zika detection are under development but not yet available. The Zika outbreak in the Americas generated renewed interest in development of new rapid diagnostic methods, drugs, and potential vaccines. Ongoing efforts in diagnostics include the standardization of real-time RT-PCR (rRT-PCR) methods for comparative purposes to detect viral RNA; development of rapid specific serologic tests for clinical and epidemiologic studies; determining the role of viral load in pathogenesis; and in utero transmission and validating the use of non-blood specimens. Due of the kinetics of Zika viremia, the clinical utility of rRT-PCR is limited to testing blood samples collected less than 1 week after onset of symptoms. Because Zika virus is excreted for a longer time in urine, such samples are useful for up to 3 weeks after onset of viremia. rRT-PCR can also be performed on amniotic fluid, although the positive and negative predictive values for fetal infection and development of fetal pathology are not well understood. Serum total antibody testing is not reliable because of extensive cross-reactivity against dengue fever and yellow fever, 2 diseases that collocate geographically. This diagnostic limitation to demonstrating seroconversion to Zika in pregnancy hampers the retrospective investigations into the temporal relationship between the Brazilian epidemic and increase in congenital malformations.

The CDC has developed an ELISA technique to detect specific anti-Zika IgM, but the frequency of cross-reactions with other flaviviruses such as dengue and yellow fever make the diagnosis difficult. In the early phase of infection, the rate of IgM and IgG can be low, making confirmation of the diagnosis challenging. The detection of specific antibodies should be confirmed by a complementary seroneutralization assay employing PRNT to demonstrate a fourfold increase of the antibody titer initially found. No commercial kit is currently available for the detection of antibodies specifically related to Zika virus. rRT-PCR is an appealing option as a rapid, sensitive, and specific method for detection of Zika in the early stage of infection. So far, only 1 rRT-PCR assay has been described in the context of the outbreak in Micronesia in 2007. Faye and colleagues[31,32] described a 1-step rRT-PCR test for Zika to detect a wider genetic diversity of Zika isolates from Asia and Africa, including Zika RNA (NS5) and the envelope protein coding region (360 bp) in tissue samples. Next-generation sequencing, complete-genome Zika sequences, multiple-sequence alignments and neighbor-joining phylogenetic trees can be constructed to show phylogenetic relationships for epidemiologic research purposes.

THE HIDDEN TOLL OF ZIKA

The potential hidden toll of Zika virus infection is unknown. Illnesses that occur early in utero can cause fetal wastage, developmental defects, and serious malformations with brain calcification. However later in utero infection can act as a trigger for other CNS sequelae. There has been no research into the long-term sequelae of in utero Zika virus infections. If the rubella epidemic of the United States in the mid-1960s that infected an estimated 12 million Americans and affected 20,000 newborns with significant early and late CNS sequelae including autism and learning and behavioral disabilities is a good analogy, then with an estimated 500 million people residing in countries of Latin America and the Caribbean, Zika spread, there could be devastating consequences on already frail health care systems.

TREATMENT

There is no specific treatment or vaccine. Treatment is symptomatic, combining acetaminophen and antihistaminic drugs. Prevention against the infection relies upon antisectorial protection combining the avoidance of mosquito bites and the eradication of mosquitoes. Prevention at the community level consists in decreasing the number of mosquitoes by decreasing the number of egg-laying sites in potted plant saucers, moats, and water reservoirs by drying them, isolating them, and treating them with insecticides. Individual protection includes wearing long and light-colored clothes and using skin repellents and mosquito bed nets, especially for the protection of babies and bedridden patients, to avoid mosquito bites. There is a role for intravenous immunoglobulin in neurologically affected patients.

PUBLIC HEALTH RECOMMENDATIONS

Adequate public health preventive measures, including public education and mosquito bite prevention, should be implemented quickly after the diagnosis of an imported case. Other control measures include the isolation of the patient during the viremic phase and vector control activities centered on the case's residence, including spraying adult mosquitoes and destruction of larval breeding sites. The roles of clinicians are crucial including the early diagnosis of imported arboviruses such as Zika infection and the timely notification of public health authorities. Clinicians should be aware of current outbreaks in parts of the world that are popular tourist destinations. This is especially important for newly emerging and possibly devastating diseases with specific public health implications. Imported cases should be suspected in travelers who develop compatible symptoms within 1 to 2 weeks after returning from endemic areas. Cross-reactive dengue viral serology (IgG or IgM) during Zika infection may be used as a screening test to identify subjects, since commercial serologic tests for dengue are widely available. Taking into account possible cross-reactions among different viruses belonging to the *Flavivirus* family when using current serologic tests, an approach combining direct and indirect detection techniques, as well as neutralization assay for confirmation, should be utilized. Public health experts highlight the need of improving pretravel advice and consultation for travelers planning to visit countries in which various arboviruses are endemic. Such advice should include effective preventive measures of mosquito bites and avoidance of the use of acetylsalicylic acid, which is contraindicated in suspected or confirmed dengue fever due to the increased risk of bleeding. The explosive spread of Zika in Brazil poses challenges for public health preparedness and surveillance for mass gathering that will occur during the 2016 Brazil Olympic Games and Paralympics in Rio De Janeiro this year. Termed a public health emergency of international concern, the Olympic games constitute an extraordinary event and a public health risk to other countries through the potential for international spread of disease, and as such, will require a coordinated international response.

REFERENCES

1. Dick GW, Kitchen SF, Haddow AJ. Zika virus. I. Isolations and serological specificity. Trans R Soc Trop Med Hyg 1952;46:509–20.
2. Macnamara FN. Zika virus: a report on three cases of human infection during an epidemic of jaundice in Nigeria. Trans R Soc Trop Med Hyg 1954;48:139–45.
3. Olson JG, Ksiazek TG, Suhandiman, et al. Zika virus, a cause of fever in Central Java, Indonesia. Trans R Soc Trop Med Hyg 1981;75:389–93.
4. Duffy MR, Chen TH, Hancock WT, et al. Zika virus outbreak on Yap Island, Federated States of Micronesia. N Engl J Med 2009;360:2536–43.
5. Alera MT, Hermann L, Tac-An IA. Zika virus infection, Philippines, 2012. Emerg Infect Dis 2015;21:722–4.
6. Baronti C, Piorkowski G, Charrel RN, et al. Complete coding sequence of Zika virus from a French polynesia outbreak in 2013. Genome Announc 2014;2: e00500–14.
7. Tognarelli J, Ulloa S, Villagra E, et al. A report on the outbreak of Zika virus on Easter Island, South Pacific, 2014. Arch Virol 2016;161(3):665–8.
8. Zanluca C, de Melo VC, Mosimann AL, et al. First report of autochthonous transmission of Zika virus in Brazil. Mem Inst Oswaldo Cruz 2015;110:569–72.
9. Musso D, Nilles EJ, Cao-Lormeau VM, et al. Rapid spread of emerging Zika virus in the Pacific area. Clin Microbiol Infect 2014;20:O595–6.
10. Salvador FS, Fujita DM. Entry routes for Zika virus in Brazil after 2014 World Cup: new possibilities. Travel Med Infect Dis 2016;14(1):49–51.
11. Smallwood CA, Arbuthnott KG, Banczak-Mysiak B, et al. Euro 2012 European Football Championship Finals: planning for a health legacy. Lancet 2014;383: 2090–7.
12. Terzian AC, Auguste AJ, Vedovello D, et al. Isolation and characterization of Mayaro virus from a human in Acre, Brazil. Am J Trop Med Hyg 2015;92:401–4.
13. Musso D, Cao-Lormeau VM, Gubler DJ. Zika virus: following the path of dengue and chikungunya? Lancet 2015;386:243–4.
14. Marcondes CB, Ximenes MF. Zika virus in Brazil and the danger of infestation by *Aedes (Stegomyia)* mosquitoes. Rev Soc Bras Med Trop 2016;49(1):4–10.
15. Hayes EB. Zika virus outside Africa. Emerg Infect Dis 2009;15:1347–50.

16. Kwong JC, Druce JD, Leder K. Zika virus infection acquired during brief travel to Indonesia. Am J Trop Med Hyg 2013;89:516–7.

17. Foy BD, Kobylinski KC, Foy JLC, et al. Probable non-vector-borne transmission of Zika virus, Colorado, USA. Emerg Infect Dis 2011;17:880–2.

18. Musso D, Roche C, Robin E. Potential sexual transmission of Zika virus. Emerg Infect Dis 2015;21:359–61.

19. Marano G, Pupella S, Vaglio S, et al. Zika virus and the never-ending story of emerging pathogens and transfusion medicine. Blood Transfus 2016;14(2): 95–100.

20. Centers for Disease Control and Prevention (CDC). Investigations of West Nile virus infections in recipients of blood transfusions. MMWR Morb Mortal Wkly Rep 2002;51:973–4.

21. Brouard C, Bernillon P, Quatresous I, et al. Estimated risk of chikungunya viremic blood donation during an epidemic on Reunion Island in the Indian Ocean, 2005 to 2007. Transfusion 2008;48:1333–41.

22. Liumbruno GM, Calteri D, Petropulacos K, et al. The chikungunya epidemic in Italy and its repercussion on the blood system. Blood Transfus 2008;6:199–210.

23. Dick GW. Zika virus. II. Pathogenicity and physical properties. Trans R Soc Trop Med Hyg 1952;46:521–34.

24. Boorman JP, Porterfield JS. A simple technique for infection of mosquitoes with viruses. Transmission of Zika virus. Trans R Soc Trop Med Hyg 1956;50:238–42.

25. Bearcroft WG. Zika virus infection experimentally induced in a human volunteer. Trans R Soc Trop Med Hyg 1956;50:442–8.

26. Oehler E, Watrin L, Larre P, et al. Zika virus infection complicated by Guillain-Barré syndrome—case report, French Polynesia, December 2013. Euro Surveill 2014;19(9):1–3.

27. Mlakar J, Korva M, Tul M, et al. Zika virus associated with microcephaly. N Engl J Med 2016;374(10):951–8.

28. Petersen E, Wilson ME, Touch S, et al. Rapid spread of Zika virus in the Americas—implications for public health preparedness for mass gatherings at the 2016 Brazil Olympic games. Int J Infect Dis 2016;44:11–5.

29. Available at: http://www.cdc.gov/zika/hc-providers/diagnostic.html. Accessed September 1, 2015.

30. Staples JE, Dziuban EJ, Fischer M, et al. Interim guidelines for the evaluation and testing of infants with possible congenital Zika virus infection—United States, 2016. MMWR Morb Mortal Wkly Rep 2016;65:63–7.

31. Faye O, Faye O, Diallo D, et al. Quantitative real-time PCR detection of Zika virus and evaluation with field-caught mosquitoes. Virol J 2013;10:311.

32. Faye O, Faye O, Dupressoir A, et al. One-step RT-PCR for detection of Zika virus. J Clin Virol 2008;43:96–101.

Section II - Health Systems

Assessing the Public's Health

David S. Younger, MD, MPH, MS[a,b,*], Joyce Moon-Howard, DrPH[b]

KEYWORDS

- Public health • Health care • Health systems

KEY POINTS

- The metrics of public health have evolved to accommodate the changing landscape of health care.
- Single measures imperfectly summarize the health of a population with each seeming to describing only a single aspect.
- Summary measures used by the Global Burden of Disease Study allow comparisons along many other lines for communicable and noncommunicable diseases and their burden.
- Community health has been assessed nationally and around the world in rural and urban communities with differing results and policy implications.
- One area of agreement is the importance of addressing population health needs at the community and neighborhood level, a finding that transcends the world megacities.

INTRODUCTION

The health reform debate continues to focus on finding a way to expand health insurance coverage for all Americans,[1] an access issue that is estimated to account for a minority of mortalities,[2] suggesting the contribution of other factors to adequate health. With up to 95% of health spending directed toward medical care and biomedical research,[2] and an increasing body of evidence that health behavior and environment are responsible for up to 70% of avoidable mortalities, there has been increasing awareness of the contribution of other nonmedical factors related to health promotion and mortality. The tide is turning toward a discourse among public health officials, researchers, and health care providers to address the varied social factors and the impact of economic inequality on health.[3] This article describes approaches to the assessment of domestic and global public health. It is strategically placed in this issue

The authors have nothing to disclose.

[a] Division of Neuroepidemiology, Department of Neurology, New York University School of Medicine, New York, NY, USA; [b] College of Global Public Health, New York University, New York, NY, USA
* Corresponding author. 333 East 34th Street, 1J, New York, NY 10016.
E-mail address: david.younger@nyumc.org

Neurol Clin 34 (2016) 1057–1070
http://dx.doi.org/10.1016/j.ncl.2016.06.007
0733-8619/16/$ – see front matter © 2016 Elsevier Inc. All rights reserved.

to follow articles that describe individual diseases and precede descriptions of other national health care systems.

ASSESSING POPULATION HEALTH STATUS

The metrics of public health have evolved to accommodate the changing landscape of health care with no measure perfectly summing the health of a population and each way of estimating seeming to violate some tenet of epidemiology. Measures of risk are generally expressed using mortality rates (MRs) for estimating the frequency of the occurrence of death in a defined population over a specified interval, whether expressed as crude mortality for all causes in a population or a single cause. MRs can be studied in reference to infant and maternal deaths; adjusted for sex, age, race, and ethnicity; or by particular conditions or the proportion thereof to provide insight into public health responses to the leading causes of mortality and health disparities. The global focus on noncommunicable diseases has been driven by the faster rate of decline of communicable, maternal, neonatal, and nutritional causes in an aging world population. It comes as no surprise that global age-standardized MRs significantly increased between 1990 and 2013 for Alzheimer disease and other dementias by 3.2%, and Parkinson disease by 28.2%.[4] According to the National Center for Health Statistics in 2013, the 10 leading causes of death, which accounted for 73.6% of all deaths in the United States (US), included heart disease, cancer, chronic lower respiratory diseases, unintentional injuries, stroke, Alzheimer disease, diabetes, influenza and pneumonia, kidney disease, and suicide. Stroke, the fourth leading cause in 2012, became the fifth leading cause in 2013.[5]

Premature mortality, originally proposed to address the inadequacy of MRs in measuring the burden of disease due to tuberculosis,[6] proved to be a particularly useful way to describe other diseases. In choosing an arbitrary limit to life, the calculation of the difference between the age at death and an arbitrary designated limit measured in years of life lost (YLLs) due to premature mortality became a useful assessment of the impact of premature mortality in a given population. The YLLs rate, which represents years of potential life lost per 1000 populations below an arbitrary endpoint age such as 65 years, was found to be more desirable in comparing premature mortality in different populations because YLLs did not take into account differences in population sizes.[7] Another measure of the burden of disease in a population, disability-adjusted life years (DALYs), captures in a single figure health losses associated with mortality and different nonfatal outcomes of diseases and injuries.[8] DALYs were first described by Murray and Acharya,[8] Murray and Lopez,[9] and Murray and colleagues[10] in the 1990s, with the World Health Organization (WHO) and the Harvard School of Public Health, for the first global burden of disease (GBD) study in 1990 and used in subsequent revisions to the present GBD 2013.

FROM MORTALITY TO DISABILITY MEASURES

Summary measures used by the GBD studies[11,12] of DALYs, such as healthy adjusted life expectancy, are derived from YLL and years lived with disability (YLDs) to compare assessments of broad epidemiologic patterns across countries and time, and to quantify the component of variation in epidemiology related to sociodemographic development. Calculated by adding YLLs and YLDs, DALYs add disability to the measure of mortality and, based on the universal measure of time in life years, have provided a common currency for health care resource allocation and the effectiveness of interventions assessed relative to each other across a wide range of health problems. YLDs, equal to the sum of prevalence multiplied by the general public's assessment of the severity of health loss, has been used as a primary metric to explore disease patterns over time, age, sex, and geography.[13] It recognizes that aging of the world's population has led to substantial increases in the number of individuals with sequelae of diseases. Because YLDs have been declining much more slowly than MRs, the nonfatal dimensions of disease require more and more attention from health systems. Neurologic disorders accounted for 7.7% of all-cause YLDs in 2013, a 5% increase in age-standardized YLDs from 1990 to 2013 (2.4%–7.9%), with the leading causes being Alzheimer disease, Parkinson disease, epilepsy, multiple sclerosis, migraine, tension and medication overuse headaches, and other neurologic disorders.[12]

To appreciate the importance of summary measures compared with traditional epidemiologic metrics, one need only consider the example of the global burden of stroke among developed and developing world nations. Using world mapping, GBD 2013[14] detailed the geographic patterns of incidence, prevalence, MR, DALYs, YLDs, and their trends for ischemic stroke (IS) and hemorrhagic stroke (HS) for 1990 to 2013. Stroke incidence, prevalence, mortality, DALYs, and YLDs were estimated following the general approach of GBD 2010.[13] Age-standardized incidence, MR, prevalence, and DALYs or YLDs declined between 1990 and 2013. However, the absolute number of people affected by stroke substantially increased across all countries in the world during the same period, suggesting that the global stroke burden continues to increase. There were significant country and regional differences in stroke burden in the world, with most of the burden borne by low-income and middle-income countries. Hence, the global burden of stroke has continued to increase despite dramatic declines in age-standardized incidence, prevalence, MR, and disability. Population growth and age played an important role in the observed increase in stroke burden.

Between 1990 and 2013, the outcome of stroke in adults aged 20 to 64 years, for which it carries a particular significance for working individuals, was revealed in the GBD 2013 report[15] using traditional mortality metrics and DALYs important for planning stroke prevention and management in younger adults. Prevalence, age-adjusted MR, DALYs, and their trends for total IS and HS for 1990 to 2013 in adults 20 to 64 years of age were estimated from available data using statistical models with country-level covariates to estimate country-specific stroke burden. Means and 95% uncertainty intervals were calculated for prevalence, mortality, and DALYs. The median of the percent change and 95% uncertainty intervals were determined for the period from 1990 to 2013. Between 1990 and 2013, there were significant increases in prevalent cases, total deaths, and DALYs due to HS and IS in younger adults aged 20 to 64 years. Death and DALY rates declined in both developed and developing countries but a significant increase in absolute numbers of stroke deaths among younger adults was detected in developing countries. Most of the burden of stroke was in developing countries. In 2013, the greatest burden of stroke among younger adults was due to HS. Although the trends in declining death and DALY rates in developing countries are encouraging, these regions still fall far behind those of developed regions of the world. A more aggressive approach toward primary prevention and increased access to adequate health care services for stroke seems to be needed in developing nations.

Such is the example of all types of stroke in African countries undergoing an epidemiologic transition driven by sociodemographic and lifestyle changes that has led to the increased burden of noncommunicable diseases to include cardiovascular risk factors that lead to increased risk of stroke. Accurate and up-to-date information on stroke burden is necessary for the development and evaluation of effective and efficient preventative acute care and rehabilitation programs for stroke patients. A meta-analysis[16] focused solely on the prevalence and incidence of stroke in Africa with pooled data, albeit of uneven quality, of new cases of stroke and number of stroke survivors in populations across 5-year age groups. A total of 1.89 million stroke survivors among people aged 15 years or more were estimated in Africa in 2009, with a prevalence of 317.3 (314.0–748.2) per 100,000 population. Comparable figures for the year 2013 based on the same rates amounted to 535,000 (87.0–625.3) new stroke cases and 2.09 million (2.06–4.93) stroke survivors, suggesting an increase of 10.8% and 9.6% of incident stroke cases and stroke survivors, respectively, attributable to population growth and aging between 2009 and 2013. The prevention of stroke and many noncommunicable diseases in Africa has been affected mainly by weak health systems and poor government response. Hypertension is the main risk factor of all stroke subtypes with odds of about 2.64, and this is more prominent among young Africans who present with stroke unaware of their high blood pressure status. There is an urgent need for more research on stroke, and related vascular disease risk factors, to appropriately quantify this burden. An investment in research capacity, basically to conduct and fund higher quality research, may help raise awareness of stroke burden in Africa. An awareness and fair understanding of stroke burden and disease pattern in Africa may further prompt appropriate policy response and scale up current intervention programs.

HEALTH SYSTEMS MANAGEMENT AND QUALITY OF CARE

It can be said that a national health system reflects the values of the nation in which it exists, although it is hard to find a system embraced by all of its stakeholders, including consumers or patients, health care providers, insurers, and hospital mangers, in public or private institutional, or combination, settings. Health policy and management has been on the frontline of the controversy, confronting the gap between theory, policy, and practice,[17] because of perennial efforts to reform health care systems. Chinitz and Rodwin[17] cite 4 dimensions highlighting this gap in the US. First, the dominance of microeconomic thinking in health policy analysis and design that leads to the cyclical return to financial incentives and market mechanisms as solutions to health systems that cost too much and provide too little. Second, the lack of learning from management theory and comparative case studies, including the high performance health maintenance organizations (HMOs), such as Kaiser Permanente in California and Geisinger in Pennsylvania, or the Mayo Clinics and Cleveland Clinics that have all been touted as being high performers in health care but with little success in generalizing their model across the US. Third, the separation of health policy and management from the rank and file of medical professionals, finding it removed from an understanding of what clinicians and health care managers face in the real world of practice. Fourth, the inability to think about individual health systems in a way that more accurately captures the complexity and conflicts embedded within management and health care practices.

Two separate approaches, each with overlapping metrics for understanding the barriers to adequate health care are described, although their application to neurology has only recently been appreciated. The first approach uses 2 metrics[18,19]: preventable readmissions and hospitalizations for ambulatory care sensitive conditions (ACSCs) developed by the US Agency for Healthcare Research and Quality (AHRQ) in response to the Affordable Care Act mandate to monitor the performance of hospitals and to determine payments to them by the Centers for Medicare and Medicaid Services (CMS) for the care of Medicare and Medicaid beneficiaries. However, these metrics have only recently been investigated for applicability to neurologic disorders.

A second approach has used metrics developed by the World Cities Project (WCP), including discharges for avoidable hospital conditions (AHCs),[20] avoidable hospitalizations,[21] avoidable mortality (AM),[22] and the relation of infant mortality and income.[23,24] The goal of the WCP has been to compare the health, social services, and quality of life in neighborhoods of the urban cores of the world megacities of Paris, Manhattan, and London to better understand the performance of health systems serving population cohorts and potential barriers to adequate health care.

United States Agency for Healthcare Research and Quality Indicators

There are an estimated 6.8 million survivors and approximately 795,000 new and recurrent strokes identified annually.[25] It is among the 10 largest contributors to Medicare costs and, in the elderly, is a leading cause of hospitalization. Reducing readmission rates is a goal of national health care reform. Risk-standardized readmission rates (RSRRs) after hospital discharge are publically reported by the CMS and are used as an indicator of the quality and efficiency of hospital-level care for cardiovascular conditions. The CMS uses risk-adjusted hospital readmission rates as a marker of health care quality.[26,27] The current program uses financial penalties as incentives for hospitals to reduce 30-day readmission rates. Readmissions for myocardial infarction, pneumonia, and congestive heart failure have been the focus of initial CMS tracking; however, neurologic disorders are likely future targets.[28] Readmissions may have little to do with the actual index hospitalization and depend instead more on the quality of follow-up care after discharge. Socioeconomically disadvantaged patients often do not have easy access to outpatient health care and, therefore, are more prone to return to inpatient care. Although it can be argued that this CMS initiative will encourage hospitals to work to improve outpatient care in their communities, this assumes a type of closed network of a host of cooperative payers and patients that most academic hospitals simply do not have in place.[29] Understanding readmissions may eventually help stakeholders involved in the care of neurologic patients anticipate and enact change to maximize the quality of inpatient neurologic care. Although high readmission rates may, in part, reflect unresolved problems at discharge or the quality of immediate after hospital care, they may also reflect a more chronically ill population, social or economic issues, or a combination of these factors.

Lichtman and colleagues[30] analyzed 30-day readmissions for Medicare fee-for-service (FFS) beneficiaries aged 65 years and older who were discharged alive with a primary diagnosis of IS between December 2005 and November 2006. Random-effects logistic regression was used to determine patient-level factors associated with preventable readmissions. Among 307,887 IS discharges, 44,379 (14.4%) were readmitted within 30 days, 5322 (1.7% of all discharges) were the result of a preventable cause, and 39,057 (12.7%) were for other reasons. In multivariate analysis, older age and cardiovascular-related comorbid conditions were strong predictors of preventable readmissions. Preventable readmission rates were highest in the Southeast, mid-Atlantic, and US territories and lowest in the Mountain and Pacific regions. Patient-level proportional hazards analyses confirmed that older age, female sex, and having comorbid conditions often associated with stroke or cardiovascular disease were associated with an increased likelihood of being readmitted for a preventable reason. Those readmitted for a preventable cause were more likely to have congestive heart failure, myocardial infarction, diabetes, and renal failure. Patients with a preventable readmission had a longer length of stay for the index stroke and were more likely to be discharged to a skilled nursing or intermediate care facility. Only a small proportion of readmissions after IS were classified as preventable. The investigators concluded that hospital-level programs intended to reduce all-cause readmissions and costs should target high-risk patients.

Lichtman and colleagues[31] studied FFS Medicare rural and urban beneficiaries aged 65 years and older designated to have access to emergency and inpatient care at a critical access hospital (CAH) or non-CAH, respectively, and discharged with a primary diagnosis of IS in 2006. The investigators performed hierarchical generalized linear models to calculate hospital-level risk-standardized MRs (RSMRs) and RSRRs. Among 10,267 IS discharges from 1165 CAHs and 300,114 discharges from 3381 non-CAHs, the RSMRs of CAHs were higher than non-CAHs (11.9% ± 1.4% vs 10.9% ± 1.7%; $P<.001$) but the RSRRs were comparable (13.7% ± 0.6% vs 13.7% ± 1.4%; $P = .3$). The RSMRs for the 2 higher volume quartiles of non-CAHs were lower than CAHs (posterior probability of RSMRs higher than CAHs = 0.007 for quartile 3; $P<.001$ for quartile 4), without differences for lower volume hospitals; RSRRs did not vary by annual hospital volume. Rural residents tended to be older, uninsured, and have more limited access to primary care services; and rural hospitals had limited availability of specialty caregivers, diagnostic technologies, and acute stroke care teams. Rural and urban gaps were also more likely to adhere to evidence-based guidelines for stroke treatment, although compliance with secondary stroke preventive therapies is similar. There was no difference in stroke mortality between CAHs and similarly sized non-CAHs, suggesting that lower volume, instead of than CAH status per se, explains much of the difference in RSMR and RSRR.

Guterman and colleagues[32] examined national 30-day readmission rates for 554,399 index neurologic admissions from October 2011 to January 2015, noting an unplanned readmission rate of 11% in those aged 65 years and older. Of patients hospitalized with neurologic disorders, rates of unplanned readmission were highest for patients with peripheral nerve disorders (21.9%), central nervous system (CNS) neoplasms (21.0%), nonhypertensive encephalopathy (15.5%), arterial stenosis (15.4%), and bacterial CNS infections (14.5%). With all patients grouped together, median readmission rates increased from minor (6.5%, interquartile range 5.7%–8.9%) to extreme severity of illness (17.3%, interquartile range 14.6%–19.5%, $P<.001$). With patients split by diagnostic category, this same stepwise escalation in readmission rate with higher severity of illness was observed for most diagnoses, although there were some exceptions. For example, some patients with CNS neoplasms and minor severity of illness had higher readmission rates (25.8%) than those with CNS neoplasms and extreme severity of illness (18.8%). Multivariable regression examined predictors of readmission rates by age, race, insurance type, and severity of illness. The severity of illness remained significantly associated with readmission rate in the regression model. Cases with an extreme severity of illness were 2-fold times more likely to be readmitted (odds ratio [OR] 2.4, 95% confidence interval [CI] 2.3–2.5) compared with those with minor severity of illness. Using severity of illness as an ordinal variable in the regression model confirmed this finding, demonstrating increasing readmission with increasing severity of illness (OR 1.9, 95% CI 1.9–2.0). Readmission rates also varied significantly among patients based on primary insurance provider. Patients who were covered by Medicare (OR 1.4, 95% CI 1.3–1.4) and Medicaid (OR 1.2, 95% CI 1.1–1.2) had significantly higher rates of readmission compared with those who carried other insurance types. Although age was not found to be a significant predictor of 30-day readmission, a subset analysis revealed that older age was associated with a lower risk of readmission in both the Medicare (OR 0.5, 95% CI 0.5–0.5) and Medicaid (OR 0.6, 95% CI 0.5–0.7) group. This was not the case for those carrying commercial health insurance (OR 1.0, 95% CI 0.9–1.0). The higher readmission rates among patients with public insurance, and those older in age in particular, might reflect less frequent use of primary and preventative care, unrecognized comorbid illness, and less robust transitions of care, as well as fewer outpatient safety nets. There were demonstrated differences in health care utilization for young adults across race and insurance type and these data suggested that the differences likely extended to inpatient hospitalization as well. The investigators commented that these data should provide insight into management of neurologic disease nationally, offering policymakers realistic goals for standards of care and challenging health care providers to develop systems-based solutions that will improve transitions of care for those at highest risk of readmission with neurologic disease.

Hospitalization admission for ACSCs was studied by Basu and colleagues,[33] who conducted a multivariate cross-sectional design, using compositional factors describing the hospitalized populations and the contextual factors, all aggregated at the primary care service area level in small geographic areas in 2 cross-sections spanning 11 years (1995–2005) using hospital discharge data from the Healthcare Cost and Utilization Project of the AHRQ for Arizona, California, Massachusetts, Maryland, New Jersey, and New York. The investigators noted that ACSC admission rates were inversely related to the availability of local primary care physicians (PCPs), and managed care was associated with declines in ACSC admissions for the elderly. Minorities, aged elderly, and patients under the federal poverty level were found to be associated with higher ACSC rates. The conceptual models for ACSC hospitalizations addresses aspects of supply and demand for outpatient services to explain the variations of admission rates. Consumers, including patients and families, seek, use, and pay for services, whereas PCPs, managed care plans, and hospitals supply services and sometimes make decisions on behalf of patients. ACSC hospitalization occurred when the demand for primary care exceeded its supply or when it was rational not to use primary care because hospital care would be available and better paid for by the insurance. There may be economic, cultural, and social barriers to prevent utilization of primary care. Some of the factors affecting the demand for outpatient care and, inversely, hospitalization for ACSC conditions include poverty, education level, and public and private insurance.[34]

Riley and colleagues[35] noted that, compared with FFS, HMO enrollees were diagnosed at earlier stages for cancer sites for which effective screening services are available. The earlier detection of certain cancers among HMO enrollees resulted from coverage of screening services and promotion by HMOs of such services. Medicare-managed care enrollment was associated with less use of hospitals for ACSC conditions.[36] The supply factors associated with ACSC admissions were inpatient bed supply, PCPs, and physician practice patterns, such that, if all else is equal, a greater supply of PCPs would tend to make primary care more accessible and reduce average prices for primary care for potential patients who could be treated in an ambulatory setting, relative to hospital inpatient stays. Characteristics such as being elderly in poverty or in rural locations would be expected to exert important influences on increased rates of ACSC or preventable admissions. The degree of remoteness and rural or urban residence is expected to be positively associated with ACSC admissions,[37] whereas population density is negatively associated with ACSC admissions.[38]

It is clear from the previously described studies that the indicators of preventable readmissions and hospitalization for ASCS address the fundamental aspects of the barriers to adequate primary care. They also show the difficulties posed by differing severities of hospitalized patients with IS returning to potentially challenged community care settings, which reflects the urgency for adequate community assessment and neighborhood support.

Metrics of the World Cities Project

According to Rodwin and Gusmano,[24] comparing world mega-cities of wealthier nations of the Organization for Economic Cooperation and Development (OECD) is important for 3 reasons. First, it reveals a deeper understanding of emerging global trends in urbanization, health risks, and population aging. Second, each of the cities exert a dominant influence on developing nations globally. Third, it is important to create a foundation to understand their comparative health systems. The framework for the WCP is based on comparisons of urban cores from which inequalities in health care use and health status can be ascertained at neighborhood levels, representing the diversity of socioeconomic strata of the larger urban core and community. Manhattan, London, and Paris are the largest cities of the higher income nations of the OECD and represent enormous and diverse city regions. Paris was originally selected as a prototypical urban core against which those of Manhattan and Inner London would be matched. The definition of the respective urban cores of each world city conformed to 5 criteria.[24] First, each represented historic centers of their respective metropolitan regions. Second, their populations were similar in size, ranging from 1.5 million in Manhattan to 2.1 million in Paris. Third, the urban cores of these cities combined a mix of high-income and low-income populations marked by wide variation in average household income. Fourth, each functioned as a central hub for employment with large numbers of commuters. Fifth, each served as a center for medical resources within their respective regions and nations, having large numbers of teaching hospitals and medical schools, and high rates of acute hospital beds and physicians per capita.

Despite similarities, the WCP investigators[24] found that these cities exist within very different health systems. Manhattan has a high proportion of uninsured patients, whereas those with insurance are covered by a patchwork system of public and private indemnity insurers and managed care organizations. Those residing in Paris are typically covered by National Health Insurance (NHI), whereas Londoners are generally eligible to receive care through the National Health Service. There are differences between the cities in the specialty mix of physicians and the relative size of the public hospital sector that, among other factors, affect use of health services. A similar measure of pretax average household income by neighborhood subunit was available for Manhattan and Paris but absent in London, leading WCP investigators to use a deprivation index. In each city, income strata or deprivation indices were referred to quartiles for comparisons.

Gusmano and colleagues[20] analyzed AHCs as an indicator of access to primary health care in Manhattan and Paris. The selection of AHCs was a dimension of health system performance and a recognized valid indicator of access to primary care.[35] Citing their similarities, Gusmano and colleagues[20] noted that, with populations of 8.0 million and 6.2 million, Manhattan and Paris were, respectively, 2 of the largest cities among the higher income countries of the OECD. Their respective urban cores were centers of medical excellence with a disproportionate share of hospitals, physicians, and indigent patients in comparison with their surroundings. Their per capita rates of physicians and acute hospital beds were virtually the same. Both cities were destinations for large immigrant communities from around the world. Despite their similar characteristics, the investigators[20] noted that the primary care system in France was much stronger than in Manhattan, with approximately 50% of physicians in primary care compared with 30% for Manhattan. NHI, which covers the entire population legally residing in France who met residency requirements, is complemented by a system that resembles Medigap for US Medicare beneficiaries but differs in that French

NHI coverage increases when a patient's costs increase without deductibles, and drug benefits are extensive. French patients with debilitating or chronic illnesses are exempted from coinsurance if they consult physicians who accept NHI reimbursement as payment in full. Patients who choose to consult with physicians who require coinsurance are typically eligible for some coverage under complementary insurance. If this constitutes a financial barrier, they can choose physicians who accept NHI rates as payment in full or can consult physicians at any of 50 health centers located in every arrondissement of the city. In 2000, NHI was extended to the 3% to 4% of Parisians who were previously not covered. In addition to greater income inequality in Manhattan than in Paris, 24% of the population is uninsured, and gaps in access to primary care exist, despite the presence of a strong safety net, including the largest US public hospital system. The calculation of comparative hospital discharge rates for AHCs for the Manhattan and Paris health systems used the definition of AHCs developed by Weissman and colleagues.[39]

Gusmano and colleagues[20] tabulated discharge rates for the marker conditions of appendicitis, gastrointestinal obstruction, and hip fractures; and for referral-sensitive procedures, including lower-extremity joint replacements and organ transplants. The investigators noted that, for people age 18 years and older, the age-adjusted discharge rate for AHCs in Manhattan was more than 2 and a half times that of Paris, a much greater difference than among large US cities. Discharge rates for marker conditions were 20% higher in Manhattan than in Paris, whereas those for referral-sensitive procedures were identical in the 2 cities. Gusmano and colleagues[20] noted that discharge rates for AHCs were higher in lower-income neighborhoods of Manhattan and Paris but the differences among residents of below-median-income neighborhoods compared with residents of above-median-income neighborhoods were 56% greater in Manhattan and 20% greater in Paris. There was no difference in Manhattan and very little difference in Paris between higher and lower income neighborhoods for discharges related to marker conditions. There were 20% fewer discharges for referral-sensitive procedures among residents of lower-income areas in Manhattan. In Paris, however, there was virtually no difference between residents of higher and lower income areas for these procedures. Multiple logistic regression analysis showed a statistically significant influence for age, indices of severity of illness, and number of physicians per 1000 population. Female patients had decreased odds of admission for an AHC by about 30%. The neighborhood income and education variables were not significant in Paris. The odds of AHC discharges were 29% higher among blacks and 47% higher among Hispanics than whites. The odds of AHC discharges for uninsured people were 82% greater than for people with private insurance; and the odds of AHCs were 39% among Medicaid recipients and 21% higher among Medicare beneficiaries than among people with private coverage. Although AHCs were related to neighborhood-level income in both cities, the magnitude of the disparity among high-income and low-income neighborhoods was higher by a factor of 2 in Manhattan compared with Paris. The higher rates of AHCs in Manhattan were explained by multiple barriers to care, including race and ethnicity, income of residence, sex, and insurance status. Medicare beneficiaries, Medicaid recipients, and the uninsured are all more likely than the privately insured to be hospitalized for AHCs. Inadequate insurance coverage and lack of timely effective primary care can thus result in unnecessary illness, loss of productivity, and costly hospitalizations.

Weisz and colleagues[22] studied the association between AM and an income-related variable in the urban cores of Paris, London, and Manhattan. The investigators[22] obtained mortality data from vital statistics sources for each geographic area for the periods from 1988 to 1990 and 1998 to 2000 to assess the correlation between area of residence and age-adjusted and gender-adjusted totals and AM rates. They used regression models to analyze the association of a neighborhood income-related variable expressed as the exponential of the estimate, the estimated incident rate ratio (IRR), that is, the ratio of the value of the AM rate in the low-income (or high-deprivation) areas to that of the ratio of the value of the AM rate in the low-income or high-deprivation areas to that of the rest of the city. Weisz and colleagues[22] noted that, compared with the US and the United Kingdom, France had the lowest age-adjusted and gender-adjusted MRs. Over the 2 periods (1988–90 and 1998–2000), the rates of AM declined in all 3 urban cores but Manhattan experienced the greatest decline (20%) in comparison with Paris (16%) and London (13%). Negative binomial regression results revealed that residence in a low-income neighborhood, compared with the remainder of the city, was significantly associated with increased AM rates per 1000 population in all 3 urban cores, and that the IRR was greatest in Manhattan, followed by London, and least in Paris. The observed differences between France and the US and their world cities were greater with respect to AM than to total mortality, supporting a hypothesis that part of the difference between these countries could be attributed to differences in their health systems. The health of residents of Inner London, measured in terms of total and AM, was worse than that of Manhattan residents, which was not surprising given the concentration of poverty in London, and its reputation for poor primary care. Inequality of access to timely and effective medical care seemed to be a much greater problem in Manhattan than either London or Paris. Weisz and colleagues[22] observed that, in contrast to Inner London and Paris where there was universal access to health care, those living in the lowest income neighborhood of Manhattan exhibited a significantly higher percentage of avoidable deaths than people living in the rest of the borough. This might be related to barriers in access to health care services, poor knowledge of the system's operation, or poorer ability to communicate with providers. Despite the recognition of the steep inverse association between social and economic status,[40,41] and mortality from a wide range of diseases, Weisz and colleagues[22] make compelling arguments for the disparities in AM based on access to disease prevention services and health care to improve population health in these 3 world cities.

EXAMINING COMMUNITY-LEVEL HEALTH INDICATORS

Although epidemiologic studies have traditionally identified risk factors for major disease, only recently have the individually based risk factors been contextualized to devise effective interventions and improve health outcomes by focusing on what puts people at risk of risk. In their theory of fundamental causes, Link and Phelan[42] (1995) argued that the association between socioeconomic status (SES) and mortality has persisted despite improvements in disease outcome and modification of individual risk factors because higher SES protects health no matter what mechanisms are relevant at any given time. Marmot[43] noted that the social determinants of health may be relevant to communicable and noncommunicable disease alike, therefore health status should be of concern to policy makers in every sector, not solely those involved in health policy. The report of the WHO Commission on Social Determinants of Health, contextualized by Marmot and colleagues,[44] concluded that social inequality underlies much of the health inequalities in and among nations. That SES and other similar determinants so prominently affect health inequality and are potent predictors of adverse health outcomes, and even individual diseases, probably stems from their embodiment of multiple mechanisms. Phelan and colleagues[45] advocated policies to promote medical health-promoting advances while weakening the link between these advances and socioeconomic resources by reducing disparities in socioeconomic resources. Heavily influenced by the foregoing observations, public health researchers have been charged with developing interventions to examine health status and health needs of populations by identifying those contextual factors that contribute to health risks and health status of subpopulation groups, particularly those experiencing the greatest disparity in health. Doing so may require drilling down from community levels to examine living conditions and social circumstances that put communities at risk for poor health outcomes, as well as identifying community level needs and assets that provide opportunities for community level interventions to ameliorate or reduce those risks.

Northern Manhattan Stroke Study

Important health indicators to consider in population health are socioeconomics, insurance coverage, and access to adequate primary care in individual neighborhoods. This information can only be gathered by conducting large-scale detailed community assessments and epidemiologic investigations that are rarely available in most neighborhoods. An exception is a study of urban Northern Manhattan, which has been a source of epidemiologic interest to investigators of the Northern Manhattan Stroke Study (NOMASS)[46] that was designed to address IS risk factor and prognosis in that multiethnic population. Using the 1990 census,[47] the initial population of about 260,000 people were racially and socioeconomically heterogeneous and served by the consortium of hospitals and clinics of New York Presbyterian/Columbia Presbyterian Medical Center, the only hospital in the region. They have been exhaustively studied epidemiologically for nearly 2 decades by NOMASS collaborators from the Departments of Neurology and Public Health from Columbia University, the Miller School of Medicine, and the College of Global Public Health of New York University to assess risk factors and prognosis related to IS. Detailed US census survey and descriptive health appraisal data derived from updated versions of Take Care New York community health appraisal of Northern Manhattan, gathered by the New York City Department of Health and Mental Hygiene,[48] made Northern Manhattan a unique setting for the study of IS and emblematic of the potential for community and epidemiologic activism in understanding the dynamics of a community to appropriately target public health and socioeconomic needs. In an exemplary study of the interaction of SES and physiologic predictors of adverse health outcomes in the multiethnic community of Northern Manhattan, Rodriguez and colleagues[49] investigated increased left ventricular mass (LVM) and lower SES as predictors of cardiovascular morbidity and mortality. Socioeconomic data of 1,916 black, Hispanic, and white subjects in a NOMAS population-based sample were characterized based on educational attainment, whereas echocardiography-defined LVM was indexed and analyzed as a continuous variable. LVM varied by race and educational level (P trend $= 0.0004$) with a significant inverse and graded association between mean LVM and SES. Lower SES was an independent predictor of increased LVM among hypertensive and normotensive blacks. Hispanics carried a higher burden of increased LVM than whites at a level similar to that of blacks. The investigators noted that, although their findings did not establish a causative role for SES in the pathogenesis of increased LVM there was a link between SES and LVM. The opportunities for research into socioeconomic and ethnically based risk factors, as well as more aggressive monitoring of cardiovascular risk factors and earlier intervention for those at greatest cardiovascular risk, was suggested.[49]

REFERENCES

1. Schroeder SA. The medically uninsured: will they always be with us? N Engl J Med 1996;334:1130–3.
2. McGinnis JM, Williams-Russo P, Knickman JR. The case for more active policy attention to health promotion. Health Aff 2002;21:78–93.
3. Special Report: World Economy. For richer, for poorer. The Economist 2012;3–24.
4. Wang H, Dwyer-Lindgren L, Lofgren KT, et al. Age-specific and sex-specific mortality in 187 countries, 1970-2010: a systematic analysis for the Global Burden of Disease Study 2010. Lancet 2012;380:2071–94.
5. National Center for Health Statistics. Mortality in the United States, 2013. Atlanta (GA): Department of Health and Human Services; National Center for Health Statistics; 2014. Data Brief No. 178.
6. Dempsey M. Decline in tuberculosis. The death rate fails to tell the entire story. Am Rev Tuberc 1947;56:157–64.
7. National Center for Health Statistics. Health, United States. Hyattsville (MD): Department of Health and Human Services; National Center for Health Statistics; 2004. Available at: http://www.cdc.gov/nchs/hus.htm.
8. Murray CJ, Acharya AK. Understanding DALYs (disability-adjusted life years). J Health Econ 1997;16:703–30.
9. Murray CJL, Lopez AD. The global burden of diseases: a comprehensive assessment of mortality and disability from diseases, injuries and risk factors in 1990 and projected to 2020, vol. II. Cambridge (MA): Harvard School of Public Health on behalf of the World Health Organization; World Bank (Global Burden of Disease and Injury Series; 1996.
10. Murray CJL, Lopez AD, Jamison DT. The global burden of disease in 1990: summary results, sensitivity analysis and future directions. Bull World Health Organ 1994;72(3):495–509.
11. GBD 2013 DALYs and HALE Collaborators, Murray CJ, Barber RM, Foreman KJ, et al. Global, regional, and national disability-adjusted life years (DALYs) for 306 diseases and injuries and healthy life expectancy (HALE) for 188 countries, 1990-2013: quantifying the epidemiological transition. Lancet 2015;386:2145–91.
12. Global Burden of Disease Study 2013 Collaborators. Global, regional, and national incidence, prevalence, and years lived with disability for 301 acute and chronic diseases and injuries in 188 countries, 1990-2013: a systematic analysis for the Global Burden of Disease Study 2013. Lancet 2015;386:743–800.
13. Vos T, Flaxman AD, Naghavi M, et al. Years lived with disability (YLDs) for 1160 sequelae of 289 diseases and injuries 1990–2010: a systematic analysis for the Global Burden of Disease Study 2010. Lancet 2012;380:2163–96.
14. Feigin VL, Mensah GA, Norrving B, et al, GBD 2013 Stroke Panel Experts Group. Atlas of the global burden of (1990-2013): the GBD 2013 study. Neuroepidemiology 2015;45:230236.
15. Krishnamurthi RV, Moran AE, Feigin VL, et al, GBD 2013 Burden of Disease 2013 Study. Stroke prevalence, mortality and disability-adjusted life years in adults aged 20-64 years in 1990-2013: Data from the Global Burden of Disease 2013 Study. Neuroepidemiology 2015;45:190–202.
16. Adeloye D. An estimate of the incidence and prevalence of stroke in Africa: a systematic review and meta-analysis. PLoS One 2014;9(6):e100724.
17. Chinitz DP, Rodwin VG. On health policy and management (HPAM): mind the theory-policy-practice gap. Int J Health Policy Manag 2014;3:361–3.

18. Centers for Medicare and Medicaid Services. Readmissions reduction program. Available at: http://www.cms.gov/Medicare/Medicare-Fee-for-Service-Payment/AcuteInpatientPPS/Readmissions-Reduction-Program.html. Accessed August 1, 2013.

19. Leung KS, Parks J, Topolski J. Preventable hospitalizations among adult Medicaid beneficiaries with concurrent substance use disorders. Prev Med Rep 2015;2:379–84.

20. Gusmano MK, Rodwin VG, Weisz D. A new way to compare health systems: avoidance hospital conditions in Manhattan and Paris. Health Aff (Millwood) 2006;25:510–20.

21. Rosano A, Loha CA, Falvo R, et al. The relationship between avoidable hospitalization and accessibility to primary care: a systematic review. Eur J Public Health 2013;23:356–60.

22. Weisz D, Gusmano MK, Rodwin VG, et al. Population health and the health system: a comparative analysis of avoidable mortality in three nations and their world cities. Eur J Public Health 2008;18:166–72.

23. Rodwin VG, Neuberg LG. Infant mortality and income in 4 world cities: New York, London, Paris and Tokyo. Am J Public Health 2005;95:86–90.

24. Rodwin VR, Gusmano MK. The World Cities Project: rationale and design for comparison of megacity health systems. J Urban Health 2002;79:445–63.

25. Go AS, Mozaffarian D, Roger VL, et al. Heart disease and stroke statistics—2013 update: a report from the American Heart Association. Circulation 2013;127: e6–245.

26. Kocher RP, Adashi EY. Hospital readmissions and the Affordable Care Act: paying for coordinated quality care. JAMA 2011;306:1794–5.

27. Williams MV. A requirement to reduce readmissions: take care of the patient, not just the disease. JAMA 2013;309:394–6.

28. Centers for Medicare and Medicaid Services. Readmissions Reduction Program, Medicare Program; hospital inpatient prospective payment systems for acute care hospitals and the long term care hospital prospective payment system and proposed fiscal year 2014 rates; quality reporting requirements for specific providers; hospital conditions of participation; Medicare program; FY 2014 hospice wage index and payment rate update; hospice quality reporting requirements; and updates on payment reform; proposed rules. Fed Regist 2013;78: 27485–823.

29. Josephson SA, Johnston SC, Hauser SL. The neurologic revolving door: time to pay attention to readmissions. Ann Neurol 2013;73:A5–6.

30. Lichtman JH, Leifheit-Limson EC, Jones SB, et al. Preventable readmissions within 30 days of ischemic stroke among Medicare beneficiaries. Stroke 2013; 44:3429–35.

31. Lichtman JH, Leifheit-Limson EC, Jones SB, et al. 30-day risk-standardized mortality and readmission rates after ischemic stroke in critical access hospitals. Stroke 2012;43:2741–7.

32. Guterman EL, Douglas VC, Shah MP, et al. National characteristics and predictors of neurologic 30-day readmissions. Neurology 2016;86:1–7.

33. Basu J, Mobley LR, Thumula V. The small area predictors of ambulatory care sensitive hospitalizations: a comparison of changes over time. Soc Work Public Health 2014;29:176–88.

34. Billings J, Zeitel L, Lukomnik J, et al. Impact of socioeconomic status on hospital use in New York City. Health Aff 1993;12:162–73.

35. Riley GF, Potosky AL, Lubitz JD, et al. Stage of cancer at diagnosis for Medicare HMO and fee-for-service enrollees. Am J Public Health 1994;84:1598–604.
36. Basu J, Mobley L. Do HMOs reduce preventable hospitalizations for Medicare beneficiaries? Med Care Res Rev 2007;64:544–67.
37. Ansari Z, Laditka JN, Laditka SB. Access to health care and hospitalization for ambulatory care sensitive conditions. Med Care Res Rev 2006;63:719–41.
38. Schreiber S, Zielinsky T. The meaning of ambulatory care sensitive admissions: Urban and rural perspectives. J Rural Health 1997;13:276–84.
39. Weissman JS, Gatsonis C, Epstein AM. Rates of Avoidable Hospitalization by Insurance Status in Massachusetts and Maryland. JAMA 1992;268:2388–94.
40. Marmot MG, Smith GD, Stansfield S. Health inequalities among British civil servants: the Whitehall II study. Lancet 1991;337:1387–93.
41. Pappas G, Queen S, Hadden W. The increasing disparity in mortality between socioeconomic groups in the United States, 1960 and 1986. N Engl J Med 1993; 329:1032–109.
42. Link BG, Phelan J. Social conditions as fundamental causes of disease. J Health Soc Behav 1995;Spec No:80–94.
43. Marmot M. Social determinants of health inequalities. Lancet 2005;365:1099–104.
44. Marmot M, Bell R, Goldblatt P. Action on the social determinants of health. Rev Epidemiol Sante Publique 2013;61(Suppl 3):S127–32.
45. Phelan JC, Link BG, Tehranifar P. Social conditions as fundamental causes of health inequalities: theory, evidence, and policy implications. J Health Soc Behav 2010;51(Suppl):S28–40.
46. Sacco RL, Boden-Albala Bernadette B, Gan R, et al. Stroke incidence among white, black and Hispanic residents of an urban community. Am J Epidemiol 1998;147:259–68.
47. Bureau of the Census. 1990 census of population and housing. Washington, DC: Bureau of the Census; US Department of Commerce; 1990.
48. Community Health Profiles. Take care New York. Inwood and Washington heights. 2nd edition. Manhattan (NY): Department of Health and Mental Hygiene; 2006.
49. Rodriguez CJ, Sciacca RR, Diez-Roux AV, et al. Relation between socioeconomic status, race-ethnicity, and left ventricular mass: the Northern Manhattan study. Hypertension 2004;43:775–9.

Health Care in Brazil
Implications for Public Health and Epidemiology

David S. Younger, MD, MPH, MS[a,b,]*

KEYWORDS

- Brazil • Health care • Public health • Global health • Epidemiology

KEY POINTS

- Health care in Brazil is a constitutionally mandated right.
- The Brazilian health system comprises of a network of complementary and competitive service providers and purchasers, forming a public-private mix.
- A network of family-based community-oriented primary health programs, or Programa Agentes Communitários de Saúde, and family health programs, or Programa Saúde da Família, introduced almost 2 decades ago were the government's health care model to restructure primary care under the Unified Health System, or Sistema Único de Saúde.
- Despite achievements in the last quarter century, access to health services and gradients of health status continue to persist along income, educational background, racial, and religious lines.
- In 2011, approximately 145,000 people died of injuries, and 1 million were hospitalized in Brazil, making it a serious neurologic problem.

INTRODUCTION

The BRICS nations of Brazil, Russia, India, China, and South Africa represent 5 major emerging national economies. Collectively, the BRICS countries are useful comparisons because of their size; racial, ethnic, and geographic diversity; and inherent problems of social inequality, making them more similar to the United States than its European contemporaries. Despite achievement in the last quarter century, access to health services and gradients of health status continue to persist along income, educational background, racial, and religious lines. These findings have relevance for domestic public health in Brazil, and as a global BRICS nation, for the global public health. A series of *Lancet* articles,[1,2] commentary,[3–6] and correspondence[7] emphasize the timely importance of considering the Brazilian health care system.

The author has nothing to disclose.

[a] Division of Neuroepidemiology, Department of Neurology, New York University School of Medicine, New York, NY, USA; [b] College of Global Public Health, New York University, New York, NY, USA
* Corresponding author. 333 East 34th Street, 1J, New York, NY 10016.
E-mail address: david.younger@nyumc.org

Neurol Clin 34 (2016) 1071–1083
http://dx.doi.org/10.1016/j.ncl.2016.06.002
0733-8619/16/$ – see front matter © 2016 Elsevier Inc. All rights reserved.

neurologic.theclinics.com

BACKGROUND

The Brazilian health care sector has historically been driven by civil society rather than by government, political parties, or international organizations. Public health has a long tradition in Brazil dating to the creation of a General Directorate of Public Health at the end of the 19th century. Two of Brazil's revered scientific leaders, Oswaldo Cruz and Carlos Chagas, acted decisively against public health threats such as bubonic plague, yellow fever, and smallpox. The Eloi Chaves Law created a social security system for urban workers employed in the private sector; however, access to health services was not the main objective of the health care system. Instead, there was a system of regulated citizenship whereby social rights including retirement pensions and medical coverage were restricted to private sector workers who earned regular wages. A social security system based on compulsory contributions by employers and employees was tied to the job market, leaving agricultural and informal sector workers uninsured. The Brazilian social security administration provided medical services to its beneficiaries through the private health sector. Brazil was among 61 nations that signed the World Health Organization Constitution in 1946. The Brazilian health system was divided into 2 models of health care delivery, liberal or private practice medicine operating through the market and government-run medicine delivered in public hospitals and clinics. There was an underfunded Ministry of Health (MoH) and social security system that provided medical care through retirement and pension institutes delivered based on occupational categories. Since the 1960s, the social security system has purchased for-profit health services from third parties, allowing doctors and medicine to function as businesses and guaranteeing professional salaries. In the 1970s, the first step of health care reform was to extend coverage for particular health services beginning with urgent and emergency care independent of the system of social security contributions.

The movement for true Brazilian health care reform involved various segments of society from intellectuals and health service researchers to worker's organizations and political parties, as part of the struggle for democratization of the country during periods of military regimes based on the concept of universality and equality of access to health care. Article 198 of the Constitution of 1988 stated the right and responsibility of the state to provide a Unified Health System, or Sistema Único de Saúde (SUS), that regionalized and decentralized the network of health services and coordinated its management at each level of government, with community participation, and an integrated approach to health service delivery. Article 199 of the Constitution defined the role of the private sector.

The Constitution established new revenue sources for social security through mandatory contributions tied to gross revenues and net profits of companies. The MoH became the beneficiary of the new source of revenue created in 1996, that of a tax on all financial transactions. In 2001, a constitutional amendment reverted the system of financing of the health sector to general revenues, and the federal government was required to allocate and spend an amount equivalent to the previous year's budget adjusted for gross national product, the average growth of which has been 2.4% over the last several years, using the 1999 budget as a basis. State and municipal governments mandated to increase their spending on health to 12% and 15% of their respective budgets by 2004 have had to increase their contribution to the health system by approximately 12% per capita, commensurate with a decline in the federal share of spending that decreased from 77% during the 1980s to 53% in 1996.

GEOGRAPHY

The country is divided into 5 geographic regions: north, northeast, center-west, southeast, and south with differing demographic, economic, social, cultural, and health conditions (**Fig. 1**). The north region contains the Amazon rainforest and the lowest population density, whereas the southeast region, which covers only 11% of the total territory, accounts for 43% of the population and 56% of the gross domestic product (GDP).

SOCIAL DEMOGRAPHY AND VITAL STATISTICS

Brazil's vital statistics are shown in **Table 1**. Brazil is a federative republic with an estimated population in 2010 of 190,732,694 persons, making it the fifth most populous country. Its political system comprises several political parties with 3 levels of autonomous vertical governance, a single federal government, 26 states, and 5563 municipalities. It is governed by an independent judiciary with an executive branch led by the president and a bicameral legislature. Brazil was a colony of Portugal from the year 1500, gaining independence in 1822 and forming a republic in 1889. The population is multiethnic with one-half of citizens self-classifying as brown (43%) or black (7%) in race or skin color. It has a demographic advantage of a large working-age population that has steadily increased in age from 2005 to 2010 to between 20 and 59 years.

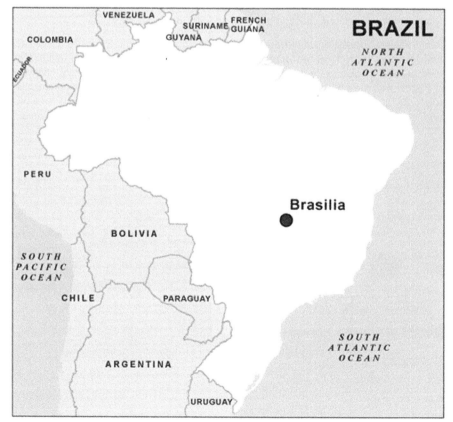

Fig. 1. Geography of Brazil. (*From* MapOpenSource. Available at: http://www.mapsopen source.com/brazil-capital-map-black-and-white.html. Accessed September 1, 2015.)

Table 1
Vital statistics: Brazil

Population	202.7 million (July 2014 est.)
Life expectancy at birth	Total population: 73.3 y Male: 69.3 y Female: 77 y
Maternal mortality ratio	56 deaths/100,000 live births (2010)
Infant mortality ratio	19.21 deaths/1000 live births
Literacy rate	Total population: 90.4% Male: 90.1% Female: 90.7%
GDP	$2.19 trillion (2013)
GDP per capita	$12,100 (2013)
Population below poverty line	21.4% (2010 est.)
Health expenditures	8.9% of GDP (2011)
Physician density	1.76 physicians/1000 population (2008)
Hospital bed density	2.3 beds/1000 population (2011)
HDI	0.744 (2010)
Gini Coefficient	52.7 (2012)

From The world factbook 2016–17. Washington, DC: Central Intelligence Agency; 2016. Available at: https://www.cia.gov/library/publications/the-world-factbook/index.html.

The increasing population of individuals 60 years and older, who are expected to account for more than 13% of the population by 2020 (**Fig. 2**), present an associated health burden of disease anticipating significant health care expenditures. Over the last 2 decades, the poverty rate in Brazil has halved, resulting in a declining inequality

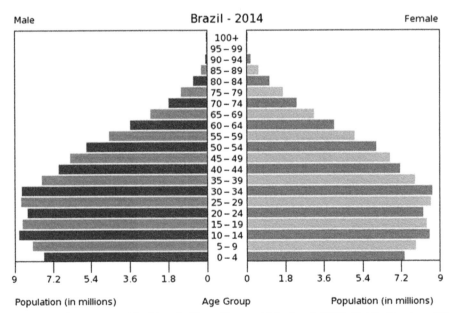

Fig. 2. Population pyramid of Brazil. (*From* The world factbook 2016–17. Washington, DC: Central Intelligence Agency; 2016. Available at: https://www.cia.gov/library/publications/the-world-factbook/index.html.)

as measured by the Gini coefficient, which has decreased by 1.2% per year. With a per-person GDP of about $11,000, Brazil has grown by an average annual rate of 1.7% since 1990, and despite 8.5% of the Brazilian population living on less than 70 reais (R), or $1.50 per day, the estimated growth rate among the poorest citizens places Brazil in a position to reach its 2015 millennium development goal of poverty reduction.

INFRASTRUCTURE

The Brazilian health system (**Fig. 3**) comprises a network of complementary and competitive service providers and purchasers, forming a public-private mix. There are 3 main sectors including public, private for-profit and nonprofit, and the private health insurance sectors. The public sector or SUS operates throughout the country with health professionals and provides for the health needs of 174.6 million people in 5714 hospitals with a demand for services that remains higher than the supply of health facilities and personnel. The private for-profit and nonprofit sector provides services that are financed in various ways with public or private funds. The private health insurance sector provides different forms of health plans, with varying insurance premiums and tax subsidies. People can access each of the sectors depending on ease and ability to pay. Health plans in Brazil are typically small or medium sized, operating by contractual arrangements and providing care in doctor's offices and hospitals.

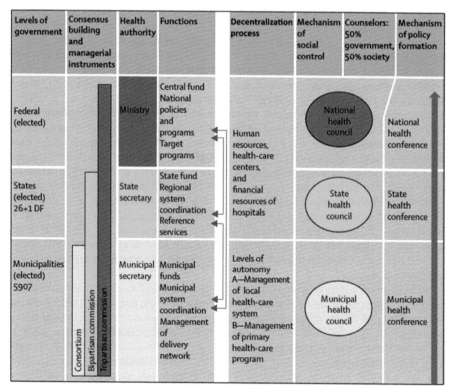

Fig. 3. Sistema único de Saúde: process and decision-making structure for formation of policy in Brazil. DF, fedal district. (*From* Fleury S. Brazil's health-care reform: social movements and civil society. Lancet 2011;377:1724–5; with permission.)

Managed care, a recent development in Brazil, has not been accompanied by health maintenance organizations or preferred provider organizations. In 1998, 24% of the population had health insurance including 18% private and 6% for civil servants. This proportion grew slightly to 26% in 2008 resulting in revenues of R63 billion. Those with private health plans or insurance policies report having better access to preventative services and higher health care use rates than those without such plans or policies. A National Supplementary Health Agency formed in 2000 to provide legal and administrative oversight of the private health insurance market deemed it illegal to deny coverage to any patient with a pre-existing disorder or to set limits on the use of specific health care services or procedures. Funding for the SUS comes from general tax revenues, out-of-pocket spending, and employers' health care spending and social contributions from federal, state, and municipal budgets. The SUS has been perpetually underfinanced. Federal spending on health care has increased since 2003, although with adjustment for inflation there has been a net decrease.

The family-based community-oriented primary health program, or *Programa Agentes Communitários de Saúde* (PACS), and the Family Health Program, or *Programa Saúde da Família* (PFS), introduced between 1991 and 1994, were the government's health care models to restructure primary care under the SUS. An innovative feature of the PSF model was the reorganization of primary clinics that focus on families and communities and the integration of medical care, with health promotion and public health actions. A family health care team in the SUS is composed of a doctor, nurse, auxiliary nurse, and 4 to 6 community health workers, of which, there were 17,807 in 2009. The teams are located at PSF clinics and assigned to specific geographic areas, serving 600 to 1000 families. They are the first point of contact with the local health system, coordinating care and working toward integration of diagnostic, specialist, and hospital care. Their services have been associated with improved health outcomes. Secondary care by the SUS has been problematic because service supply is restricted and given preferentially to those with private health plans. Tertiary care, including high-cost procedures, is carried out predominantly by contracted private sector providers and public teaching hospitals and is funded by the SUS at above market value. The likelihood of a patient being admitted to a hospital increases with the availability of beds, and the likelihood of primary care lessens both with the distance between the municipality in which the patient resides and the municipality in which care can be provided. In 2010, there were 29,347 specialty clinics and 39,518 primary care clinics with 16,226 diagnostic and therapeutic support services. With 6384 hospitals nationwide, 69% were private, and only 35% of hospital beds were in the public sector available to the SUS through contracts. One-quarter of public hospitals are controlled by municipal governments. With many new hospitals set up by decentralization, most averaging 35 beds each, those in the municipal sector and others for-profit, tend to be less effective and less efficient than larger ones.

The SUS offers comprehensive coverage to all, although it is used by those of lower income, and despite achievement in the last quarter century, access to health services and gradients of health status continue to persist along income, educational background, racial, and religious lines. In 2008, 83% of the population with a monthly per capita family income more than 5 times the minimum salary of 510R, had additional health insurance, and opted out of the public health system wherever possible, whereas only 2% of those with monthly per capita family incomes of less than a quarter of the minimum salary had additional insurance.

There are 3 reports of the impact of primary care on the need for hospitalization in Brazil,[8–10] and 2 reports[11,12] that explored adverse events in the hospitals.

Macinko and colleagues[8] examined aggregated data on 60 million public sector hospitalizations between 1999 and 2007 among Brazil's 558 microregions. The study modeled rates of hospitalization as a function of area-level socioeconomic factors, health service supply, PFS availability, and heath needs, controlling for endogenous explanatory variables. The study found that ambulatory care sensitivity (ACS) hospitalizations declined by more than 5% annually, and PFS availability was associated with lower ACS hospitalizations. Areas with the highest predicted ACS hospitalization rates were those with the highest private or nonprofit hospital bed supply and lowest (<25%) PFS coverage, whereas the lowest predicted rates of ACS hospitalizations were noted in areas with the highest (>75%) PFS coverage and the presence of few private or nonprofit hospital beds. Guanais and Macinko[9] provided evidence of the effectiveness of PACS created in 1991 on avoidable hospitalization related to circulatory diseases, and the effectiveness of the PFS introduced in 1994, on avoidable hospitalizations related to diabetes mellitus and respiratory diseases between 1998 and 2002. During that period, hospitalizations for circulatory conditions decreased in both men and women (6.5% and 8.8%, respectively) commensurate with a 2-fold increase in services of the PACS, whereas ACS hospitalizations for respiratory diseases decreased and those for diabetes mellitus increased for men and women commensurate with a 5-fold increase in coverage of the PFS. It is estimated that between 1999 and 2002, the expanded access to primary care services resulted in nearly 126,000 fewer hospitalizations representing an overall cost savings of R120 million or $63 million. Macinko and colleagues,[10] who used data from a population-based cohort of elderly Brazilians to assess predictors of hospitalization during 10 years of follow-up, noted the risk of hospitalization was positively associated with male sex, increased age, chronic conditions, and visits to the doctor in the previous 12 months; being underweight was a predictor of any hospitalization, whereas obesity was an inconsistent predictor of hospitalization.

Mendes and colleagues[11] studied adverse drug events (ADE) in hospital patients admitted in 2003. These authors found an incidence of adverse events of 7.6% and overall proportion of preventable adverse events of 66.7%, with an incidence density of 0.8 adverse events per 100 patient-days. The most frequent location was the patient's ward, and most were surgical in nature. Cano and Rozenfeld[12] collected studies published from 2000 to 2009 from a Medline search, identifying 29 studies. These authors found a proportion of ADE that ranged from 1.6% to 41.4% of inpatients and rates ranging from 1.7 to 51.8 events per 100 patient admissions, a considerable share of which were avoidable. One retrospective Brazilian cohort analysis of hospitals in Rio de Janeiro noted ADE in 1.8 cases per 1000 hospitalizations.

Macinko and colleagues[13] noted that from 1999 to 2007, hospitalizations in Brazil for ACS chronic diseases including cardiovascular disease, stroke, and asthma decreased at a rate that was statistically significant and almost twice the rate of decline in hospitalizations for all other causes. In municipalities with high PFS enrollment, chronic disease hospitalization rates were 13% lower than in municipalities with low enrollment, when other factors were held constant. These results suggested that the PFS improved health system performance by reducing the number of potentially avoidable hospitalizations.

REFORM

The impact of income inequality on life expectancy in Brazil was studied by Rasella and colleagues[14] using a panel dataset created for 27 Brazilian states from 2000 to 2009. The investigators[14] noted that the Gini index, as did other measures of income inequality, were negatively associated with life expectancy (P<.05) even after adjustment for all of the socioeconomic and health-related covariates. Primary care rendered through the National Health System was positively associated with increased life expectancy (P<.05). Using a fix-effect linear regression model, there was a statistically significant association between the Gini index and life expectancy, even after controlling for income per capita, demographic and socioeconomic variables, and health care–related variables. Thus, reducing income inequality represents an important step in the improvement of health and in increasing life expectancy in Brazil. Among several indicators of income inequality including the Gini coefficient, top 10% to bottom 40% income ratio, illiteracy rate, poverty index, median income, and demographic density indicator, Szwarcwald and colleagues[15] noted correlation between the poverty index and the Gini coefficient in administrative regions of Rio de Janeiro, with higher homicide rates in sectors of the city that had the greatest concentration of slum residents and the highest degree of income inequality. Lima-Costa and colleagues[16] examined socioeconomic inequalities in health among older adults in Brazil and England noting worse health in Brazilians than English respondents with country-specific differences higher among the poorest but also affecting the wealthiest persons. There was a strong inverse gradient of similar magnitude across education and household income levels for most health indicators in each country. Prevalence ratios of lowest versus highest education level of poor self-rated health were 3.24 in Brazil, and 3.50 in England. Macinko and Lima-Costa[17] further studied trends in horizontal equity in the utilization of health care services from 1998 to 2008, during a major period of economic and social change in Brazil, noting that the probability of having at least one doctor visit in the preceding 12 months became substantially more equitable over time, ending with a slightly prorich orientation in 2008. Factors associated with greater equity included health needs, schooling, and enrollment in the PFS. Macinko and colleagues[18] later explored the prevalence of correlates of perceived discrimination in a large multiracial Brazilian metropolitan area noting that nearly 9% of the samples reported some type of discrimination. In multivariate analysis, reports of any discrimination were higher among people who were identified as black versus white (odds ratio [OR], 1.91), higher (OR, 1.21) among women and people in their 30s (OR, 1.33), and lower (OR, 0.63) among older individuals. Those with many health problems (OR, 4.97) were more likely to report discrimination than those with few health problems. There seems to be multiple factors associated with perceived discrimination in this population that may affect health. Policies and programs aimed at reducing discrimination in Brazil will likely need to address this wider set of interrelated risk factors across different populations.

In 2005, the MoH provided $2 million to 27 state capital cities in Brazil that promoted a broad health promotion policy including a series of actions in intersectorial articulation and policy development, health education, disease and risk factor monitoring and health care provision centered on healthier diets, physical activity, reduction of smoking, and harmful use of alcohol. By 2009, this allocation increased to $25 million distributed on a competitive basis to states and municipalities. The SUS, which aims for universal access at all levels of care, is increasingly supported by the PFS to expand access to integral and continuous care while providing a platform for the prevention and management of chronic diseases. In 2001, there was a national reorganization for the care of diabetes and hypertension that included a nationwide screening program with implementation of evidence-based norms to guide primary care and widespread availability of low-cost, generic medications such as aspirin and statins for those with absolute risks for cardiovascular disease. In 2001, the MoH expanded the People's Pharmacy program, which offers basic medications for diabetes and hypertension free of charge and other medications for chronic diseases, such as asthma, osteoporosis, and glaucoma, at discounts up to 90%. A nationwide smoking cessation program has been implemented. With major gaps in primary care provision, important aspects of a chronic care model are beginning to emerge to increase access to specialty clinics.

Neonatal mortality (which is strongly influenced by the availability and quality of care during and after delivery), special care for low birth weight babies, and some aspects of prenatal care are likewise influenced by the implantation of public policies in basic sanitation and nutrition, and the availability of primary care services, especially maternal and child health programs. Childhood mortality is reduced when there is promotion of breastfeeding, prenatal care, immunizations, and prevention and treatment of infectious diseases especially those associated with diarrhea and lower respiratory tract illnesses. The PSF, which has its roots in the community health programs of the state of Ceara from the early 1990s, by 2007 grew to encompass more than 26,000 community-based teams responsible for providing care to almost 85 million people, making it one of the largest systems of community-based primary care. The program's decentralized approach to primary care addresses every health care need, is person focused over the lifetime of the individual, and coordinates the care of different providers and types of health services. The program is financed on a capitation basis with incentives to increase its numbers and municipalities. Several peer-reviewed studies of the impact of the PSF on infant and childhood mortality have been reported.[19–27] Rasella and coworkers[21] reviewed vital information from Brazilian municipalities noting a statistically significant negative association between PFS coverage levels and all analyzed mortality rates (notably 31% and 19% from diarrheal and lower respiratory tract infection, respectively). Aquino and coworkers[20] collected data on PFS coverage and infant mortality rate (IMR) from Brazilian municipalities and noted reduction in the IMR from 13% to 22% for all 3 levels of PFS coverage that were greater in municipalities, leading investigators to conclude that PFS contributed to a reduction in health inequalities. A pooled, cross-sectional ecologic analysis using panel data from Brazilian microregions and controls for confounders showed that IMR was reduced by about 13% between 1999 and 2004, whereas PFS coverage increased from14% to 60%.[19] Victora and colleagues[22] measured how many of 11 essential procedures recommended by the MoH were carried out at least once during antenatal care from among measurement of uterine height and blood pressure, gynecologic and breast examination, screening for cervical cancer by Pap smear, administration of tetanus toxoid, prescription of iron and vitamins, breastfeeding counseling, blood and urine analyses, and number of ultrasound examinations, even though the latter were not considered essential by the MoH. In 2004, the investigators[22] studied antenatal care as measured by utilization of the essential procedures in 98% of 4244 women and found that care was higher among economically better-off patients who were also more likely to start antenatal care in the first trimester. Five procedures were nearly universally performed (uterine height and blood pressure, blood and urinalysis, and ultrasound scan) in the public and private sector, whereas those with private insurance were more likely to have had breast and gynecologic examinations, screening for cervical cancer, counseling about breast feeding, and iron and vitamin prescriptions ($P<.001$).

The economic development of Brazil between 1985 and 2004 had been slow-growing, with a highly unequal middle-income economy influenced by 2 important sources: low growth rates and low growth elasticity of poverty reduction consistent with the country's high level of inequality. With an annual growth in per capita GDP that averaged just less than 0.5% between 1985 and 2004, the elasticity of poverty reduction rate was just more than one-half the normal for developing countries, computed according to Ravillion.[28] Brazil's period of economic stagnation in the 1980s was marked by hyperinflation as a result of accumulated fiscal deficits and an accommodating monetary policy. The 1990s saw an expansion of Brazil's social security and social assistance programs, driven by increases in coverage and benefits, motivated and mandated by the 1988 Constitution, which extended noncontributory pension rights to former agricultural workers or poor urban workers who became elderly or disabled. When Brazil emerged from a military dictatorship in 1988, it was an unequal society with the wealthiest 10% of the population holding almost 50% of the national income and the poorest 10% with only 0.7%. The redemocratization included a new federal constitution that obliged the state to provide universal and equitable access to health services, so an integrated health system was established, coordinating services at all levels of government following the principal of decentralization.

The global crisis made children and women the most vulnerable to inequalities of health care services, focusing greater attention on achieving a reduction of child mortality and improving maternal health (Millennium Development Goal 5) by 2015. Barros and colleagues[24] compiled and reanalyzed data from vital statistics and population-based surveys and explored the roles of broad socioeconomic and demographic changes and the introduction of reform measures in Brazil. The investigators[24] noted a decline in the IMR from 47.1 per 1000 live births in 990 to 20 in 2007, an average yearly decline of 5.1%, although increasing at a somewhat slower rate of 5.5% per year in the 1990s to 4.4% after 2000. Mortality rates among children age 1 to 4 years were considerably lower between 2006 and 2007, declining from 6 per 1000 live births in the early 1990s to 3 per 1000 live births after 2000.

Macinko and colleagues[25] performed a longitudinal ecological analysis using panel data from secondary sources, controlled for state level measures of access to clean water and sanitation, average income, women's literacy and fertility, physician and nurses per 10,000 population, and hospital beds per 1000 population. They found that from 1990 to 2002, the IMR declined from 49.7 to 28.9 per 1000 live births. During the same period, the PFS coverage was associated with a 4.5% decrease in IMR controlling for all other health determinants (P<.01). Access to clean water and hospital beds per 1000 live births was negatively associated with IMR, whereas female literacy, fertility rates, and mean income were positively associated with IMR. These findings suggested that the PFS was an important although not unique contributor to the declining IMR in Brazil. Rasella and colleagues[26] analyzed data on mortality rates and the family health program (FHP) coverage for 5.507 Brazilian municipalities in Brazil between 2000 and 2006 and carried out multivariate regression analysis of panel data using fixed effects models to control for relevant covariates. These investigators found a significant negative association between PFS coverage levels and all analyzed mortality rates with a reduction of 17% (rate ratio [RR], 0.83; 95% confidence interval [CI], 0.79–0.88) to 60% (RR, 0.40; 95% CI, 0.37–0.44), respectively, for those municipalities with none to the highest PFS coverage, supporting the important role of the PFS in reducing unattended deaths and improving quality of vital information in Brazil.

Szwarcwald and colleagues[27] examined temporal trends of the adequacy of indicators to advance the vital information provided by the Mortality Information System and the Live Birth Information System in Brazil between 2003 and 2005, for which live birth data were available in 80.3% of municipalities, representing 87.3% of the population and 63.6% of municipalities. The most important limitation of the 2 systems was deaths from undetermined causes in areas of extreme poverty, so noted in samples of municipalities with very deficient information wherein only 175 (33.7%) were reported to the Mortality Information System. Community and FHP in the North East reports were the best sources of information, in which 52% of infant deaths were reported, followed by national health facilities and hospital. The main flaws found in the issuance of death certificates and reporting infant deaths were the occurrence of deaths without the completion of the standardized forms, absence of strategies for certification in cases of household deaths in rural areas, incorrect classification of fetal and neonatal deaths, completion of certificates by nondoctors, problems with the flow and transfer of local data to the national database, and lack of perception of the importance of death registration by the local community including community health workers.

GLOBAL BURDEN OF DISEASE: IMPLICATIONS FOR NEUROLOGY

In 2011, approximately 145,000 people died of injuries, and 1 million were hospitalized in Brazil, making it a serious neurologic problem. Survivors of injury often experience temporary or permanent disabilities and consequently decreased capacity to work and quality of life. Injuries have a correspondingly high impact on the health care system. In Brazil, injury deaths and hospitalizations are tracked through the Mortality Information System (Sistema de Informação sobre Mortalidade) and the Hospitalization Information System (Sistema de Informações Hospitalares) of the Unified Health System (SUS). Both datasets are maintained by Brazil's Ministry of Health. With no national information system systematically recorded in emergency room visits, the only source for such data is the Surveillance System for Violence and Accidents, a survey conducted by the Ministry of Health of Brazil in 2006, 2007, 2009, and 2011, which collected data on violence and accidents to analyze trends and describe the profile of ER visits. The Disability-Adjusted Life Year (DALY) is an indicator of years of life lost from death or disability. It is used to demonstrate changes in population health, particularly in the context of the demographic and epidemiologic transition, and is considered a better way to measure the impact of injuries than raw incidence, as it takes into account the duration and severity of such events. DALYs are composed of 2 parts: (1) an estimate of years of life lost from premature mortality (Years of Life Lost) and (2) an estimate of years of life lived with disability (Years Lived with Disability [YLD]). DALYs are estimated using clinical and epidemiologic parameters: incidence, prevalence, lethality, remission, duration, and proportion of treated cases. There have been 2 editions of the global burden of study (GBD) study in Brazil (GBD-Br): the first produced estimates for 1998[11] and the second for 2008.[12] Important methodologic adjustments for estimating injury-related YLDs were applied in the 2008 GBD-Br,[28] which incorporated data from the 2009 VIVA Rio survey, allowing for more reliable assessment of the impact of injuries in Brazil. Injuries accounted for 10.0% of the total burden of disease in Brazil in 2008, corresponding to 19 DALYs per 100,000 inhabitants. DALYs for injuries were skewed toward men, with a male/female ratio of 4.8; among women, unintentional injuries predominated. The 15- to 29-year age group experienced the highest burden. YLD accounted for 10% of total DALYs, with most (95%) coming as a result of unintentional injuries; of these, falls accounted for the largest proportion (36.3%) with other unintentional injuries, transport-related injuries, fire/burns, assaults/homicides, intentional self-harm/suicides, and all other groups combined representing less than 1%.

REFERENCES

1. Palm J, Travassos C, Almeida C, et al. The Brazilian health system: history, advances, and challenges. Lancet 2011;377:1778–97.

2. Victora CG, Barreto ML, do Carmo Leal M, et al. Health conditions and health-policy innovations in Brazil: the way forward. Lancet 2011;377:2042–3.
3. Buss P. Brazil: Structuring cooperation for health. Lancet 2011;377:1722–3.
4. Fleury S. Brazil's health-care reform: social movements and civil society. Lancet 2011;377:1724–5.
5. Almeida-Filho N. Higher education and health care in Brazil. Lancet 2011;377:1898–900.
6. Uauy R. The impact of the Brazil experience in Latin America. Lancet 2011;377:1984–6.
7. Gusso G, Fernández MP, Gérvas J. Brazilian health-service organization: problems at a glance. Lancet 2011;378:316–7.
8. Macinko J, de Oliveira VB, Turci MA, et al. The influence of primary care and hospital supply on ambulatory care-sensitive hospitalization among adults in Brazil, 1999-2007. Am J Public Health 2011;101:1963–70.
9. Guanais F, Macinko J. Primary care and avoidable hospitalization: evidence from Brazil. J Ambul Care Manage 2009;32:115–22.
10. Macinko J, Camargos V, Firmo JOA, et al. Predictors of 10-year hospital use in a community-dwelling population of Brazilian elderly: the Bambui Cohort Study of Aging. Cad Saude Publica 2011;27(Suppl 3):S336–44.
11. Mendes W, Martins M, Rozenfeld S, et al. The assessment of adverse events in hospitals in Brazil. Int J Qual Health Care 2009;21:279–84.
12. Cano FG, Rozenfeld S. Adverse drug events in hospitals: a systematic review. Cad Saude Publica 2009;3)(25(Suppl):S360–72.
13. Macinko J, Dourado I, Aquino R, et al. Major expansion of primary care in Brazil linked to decline in unnecessary hospitlalization. Health Aff 2010;29:2149–60.
14. Rasella D, Aquino R, Barreto ML. Impact of income inequality on life expectancy in a highly unequal developing country: the case of Brazil. J Epidemiol Community Health 2013;67:661–6.
15. Szwarcwald CL, Bastos FI, Viacava F, et al. Income inequality and homicide rates in Rio de Janeiro, Brazil. Am J Public Health 1999;89:845–50.
16. Lima-Costa MF, De Oliveira C, Macinko J, et al. Socioeconomic inequalities in health in older adults in Brazil and England. Am J Public Health 2012;102:1535–41.
17. Macinko J, Lima-Costa MF. Horizontal equity in health care utilization in Brazil, 1998-2008. Int J Equity Health 2012;11:33.
18. Macinko J, Mullachery P, Proietti A, et al. Who experiences discrimination in Brazil? Evidence from a large metropolitan region. Int J Equity Health 2012;11:80.
19. Macinko J, de Fatima M, de Souza M, et al. Going to scale with community-based primary care: an analysis of the family health program and infant mortality in Brazil, 1999-2004. Soc Sci Med 2007;65:2070–80.
20. Aquino R, de Oliveira NF, Barreto ML. Impact of the family health program on infant mortality in Brazilian municipalities. Am J Public Health 2009;99:87–93.
21. Rasella D, Aquino R, Barreto ML. Reducing childhood mortality from diarrhea and lower respiratory tract infections in Brazil. Pediatrics 2010;126:e534–40.
22. Victora CG, Matijasevich A, Silveira MF, et al. Socio-economic and ethnic group inequities in antenatal care quality in the public and private sector in Brazil. Health Policy Plan 2010;25:253–61.
23. Matijasevich A, Victora CG, Barros AJ, et al. Widening ethnic disparities in infant mortality in southern Brazil: comparison of 3 birth cohorts. Am J Public Health 2008;98:692–8.

24. Barros FC, Matijasevich A, Requejo JH, et al. Recent trends in maternal, newborn, and child health in Brazil: progress toward Millennium Development Goals 4 and 5. Am J Public Health 2010;100:1877–89.

25. Macinko J, Guanais FC, de Fáima M, et al. Evaluation of the impact of the Family Health Program on infant mortality in Brazil, 1990-2002. J Epidemiol Community Health 2006;60:13–9.

26. Rasella D, Aquino R, Barreto ML. Impact of the Family Health Program on the quality of vital information and reduction of child unattended deaths in Brazil: an ecological longitudinal study. BMC Public Health 2010;10:380.

27. Szwarcwald CL. Strategies for improving the monitoring of vital events in Brazil. Int J Epidemiol 2008;37:738–44.

28. von-Doellinger V, Campos M, Mendes L, et al. The 2008 Global Burden of Disease study in Brazil: a new methodological approach for estimation of injury morbidity. Rev Panam Salud Publica 2014;36:368–75.

Health Care in the Russian Federation

David S. Younger, MD, MPH, MS[a,b,*]

KEYWORDS

- Russia • Health care • Public health • Global health • Epidemiology

KEY POINTS

- The Russian Federation has shown a willingness to work domestically to advance public health reform, and has increasingly asserting its global role in development, financial, environmental, and security matters, recalibrating its relations with international partners.
- Showing a commitment to the equal right of all citizens to health with emphasis on vulnerable groups, the government has prioritized efficient, high-quality health services; promoted a healthy lifestyle; and introduced innovative methods and medical interventions to respond to population needs.
- With ground-breaking legislative platform for improving the health care system by creating federal laws on compulsory medical insurance, there has been an attempt to create a sustainable national policy on the leading risk factors for communicable and noncommunicable diseases.
- With a global estimated prevalence of headache at 11%, the finding of the Global Burden of Disease Study 2010 of 14.7% indicates a major public health problem in Russia, not adequately addressed by the health care system.

INTRODUCTION

Brazil, Russia, India, China, and South Africa are members of the BRICS nations. Collectively, the BRICS are useful comparisons because of their size; racial, ethnic, and geographic diversity; and inherent problems of social inequality. Their lower per capita expenditures on health care and technological investments, incremental reforms, and exclusion of a large proportion of the population from health insurance make the BRICS nations useful comparisons to the United States. Russia's total health expenditures as a share of gross domestic product (GDP) have been low in comparison to other countries of the World Health Organization (WHO) European Region and, in comparison to other countries of the Group of Eight (G8), Russian health

The author has nothing to disclose.
[a] Division of Neuroepidemiology, Department of Neurology, New York University School of Medicine, New York, NY, USA; [b] College of Global Public Health, New York University, New York, NY, USA
* 333 East 34th Street, 1J, New York, NY 10016.
E-mail address: david.younger@nyumc.org

Neurol Clin 34 (2016) 1085–1102
http://dx.doi.org/10.1016/j.ncl.2016.06.001
0733-8619/16/$ – see front matter © 2016 Elsevier Inc. All rights reserved.

neurologic.theclinics.com

expenditures as a proportion of GDP have continued to trend downward. Public health funding is also very low in the Russian Federation in comparison to the WHO European Region in line with the inordinate level of out-of-pocket payments, particularly in outpatient pharmaceuticals that are excluded from guaranteed insurance packages. This article considers the background, social demography, health statistics, health care infrastructure, public health reforms, and global burden of neurologic disease.

BACKGROUND

The present Russian Federation health system has its roots in the country's complex political history and its major leaders. At independence from the United Soviet Socialist Republics (USSR), or Soviet Union, in 1991, the health system of the Russian Federation inherited an extensive and highly centralized Semashko system embodying the legacy of Nikolai Aleksandrovich Semashko,[1] a Russian statesman who served as the first People's Commissar of Public Health from 1918 to 1930, essentially organizing the extensive centralized Soviet health system. The Semashko model was constructed as a multitiered system of care with a strongly differentiated network of service providers, where each of the 5 levels (district, central rayon, municipal, oblast, and federal hospitals) corresponded to the severity of the disease and were connected by a referral system. Central to the model was the element of team work, overseen by a district physician responsible for providing and coordinating the medical care for the population in a given catchment area, making it possible to integrate the activities of other medical services with low-cost universal health care coverage.[2] Outpatient care, traditionally provided by state owned multispecialty polyclinics, district physicians, and specialists in their staff, served the local population with district physicians acting as the first contact provider and gatekeeper, referring patients to specialists and hospitals. The shift to the general practitioner model, common for most Eastern European countries, did not happen in the Russian Federation, wherein the number of general practitioners was only 0.7 per 10,000 residents in 2010[3] compared with the average of 8.2 for the European Union.[4] The hospital sector also inherited the Semashko model, constructed as a multilevel system of inpatient care serving rural, central rayon, city, regional, and federal hospitals as well as numerous specialty care facilities, with a referral system from one level to another. Hospitals varied substantially in their size and internal structure, with some having the polyclinic as a structural unit but without distinction between acute and long-term hospital care, a phenomenon that prevails in the Russian Federation.

The traditional Soviet health system was criticized for its lack of incentives, distorted structure of skewed inpatient care, predominance of administration over management, and a desire to promote integration through central administrative instruments. In 1994, 1 year after the transition, Sheiman[5] summarized the weaknesses of the traditional Soviet system referring to 6 other areas of deficiency. First, government dominance of the management, finance, and provision of health care wherein medical institutions, including primary care providers, were state owned and directly managed by health authorities. Second, lack of consumer choice of medical care providers such that citizens registered with a specific polyclinic were assigned a physician responsible for the community. Polyclinics unable to choose secondary care providers meant a lack of competition for patients such that the interests of providers dominated over those of the consumer. Third, hospital budgeting was based on the number of beds and failed to offer incentives to all actors in the inpatient care sector, with wide variations in performance. Fourth, polyclinics were paid according to the number of visits and staff, and physicians were remunerated by a salary lacking economic incentives.

Fifth, having developed primarily by increasing the number of poorly qualified physicians and expanding the bed capacity, there were nearly twice as many Soviet physicians and hospital beds per 1000 inhabitants per capita as in Organisation for Economic Co-operation and Development (OECD) countries.[6,7] Sixth, the defects in the Soviet health care system were aggravated by gross underfunding, with expenditures amounting to 3% of the GNP compared with 6.5% to 12% in OECD Western countries. Moreover, medical institutions lacked elementary drugs, materials, instruments, and were typically unable to pay staff wages. Finally, it became evident in the late 1980s that poor health outcomes were due to inadequate health care management, not only underfunding.

According to Field,[8] regression of the Soviet system from its undeniable achievements can be traced to the period of Brezhnev during the period of stagnation beginning in 1964, when shortages and corruption became endemic. A series of political and social reforms that called for *perestroika* (restructuring), *glasnost* (transparency), and *demokratizatsiya* (democratization) culminated in health financing reforms and the introduction in 1993 of a mandatory health insurance (MHI) model.[9]

The system of MHI as the Soviet insurance model for the Russian Federation, argued Sheiman,[5] it served three purposes was seen first as a way to strengthen the financial base of Soviet health care by relieving the health sector from competing with other budget priorities earmarked or purpose-oriented insurance contributions added to health insurance contributions of employers adding an additional 30% to the planned health sector budget. Second, MHI was chosen to offer economic incentives and add a third party, making it possible to shift from an integrated to a contractual model of relationship between fundholders and providers of medical care. Insurance carriers, it was argued, would be driven by economic interests to choose the most competent physicians and medical institutions. Third, the system of MHI was chosen with the intention of shifting emphasis to primary medical care and support of the most competent providers, with subsidies for setting up their own practices. A network of insurance organizations would be freer to purchase medical care; moreover, MHI introduced tighter financial controls, inviting providers to become more interested in increasing efficiency and collecting information about performance.

Final MHI legislation was adopted and enacted in February 1993 with the following major points: (1) universal MHI for all citizens of the Russian Federation, specifying a package of basic medical benefits with cost sharing for nonincluded services and supplementary benefits under voluntary health insurance (VHI) plans; (2) the selected health insurance carrier was obliged to take all applicants with a valid contract for 1 year, with the choice of a medical professional and institution; (3) individuation of its own health insurance program by each of the 83 designated regions with a population ranging from 500,000 to several million residents; (4) the creation of Regional Funds for Mandatory Health Insurance (RFMHI) for each region, an autonomous nonprofit entity accountable to the regional government that did not act so much as an insurance carrier but regulated the regional system according to the rules of the MHI authority and the regional government; (5) income-related insurance contributions by employers equaling 3.4% for the RFMHI and 0.2% for the federal fund were coupled with insurance for nonemployed pensioners and children through the local government; (6) the financing of competing insurers according to a weighted capitation formula reflected the risk of medical expenditures by the RFMHI; and (7) the entrance of insurers into contracts with public and private hospitals and polyclinics enabled them to sell their services to different purchasers resembling the National Health Service trust of the United Kingdom.

Regional experiments with the concept of MHI, which started in the autumn of 1993, provided some experience of forming markets for both third-party purchasers of providers of medical care. One such regional experiment, termed regulated competition approach, combined market incentives and regulation. The regulatory regime of the MHI was summarized as follows: (1) 1-year enrollment; (2) insurers and providers complying with a negotiated General Tariff Agreement specifying the method of payment to providers, universal rates of payment, and procedures of setting individual rates; (3) insurer obligation to broaden risk bearing by creating reserves amounting to 2% of their capitation payment; (4) the requirement of insurers to itemize MHI and VHI along the items of insurance contributions, payment to providers, formation and distribution of reserve funds, and income distribution; and (5) capitation payments, controlled by insurers, divided into 4 purpose-oriented funds, including payments to providers, the reserve fund of preventative measures, and administration costs, with the caveat that additional "free money" could not be used for financial operations.

A weighted capitation formula was based on a 2-step calculation using first, a set of coefficients reflecting the value of predicted expenditures for local areas, and second, a set of coefficients for different groups of subscribers to estimate average weighted capitation payments for the area under consideration, multiplied by the coefficient for a particular group. At its creation, it was uncertain what market form MHI would take and whether it would be pluralistic, with competition of a large number of insurers; regional monopsony, associated with fewer incentives for insurers to be innovative and responsive to a subscriber's needs; a general insurer model; or a version of regional monopsony with some elements of a pluralistic model. Abel-Smith[10] likened the evolution of Soviet health care reform to the transition from a Beveridge-like model of highly centralized tax-financed health care system with an emphasis on universal access to comprehensive care, to that of a Bismarck-like model,[11,12] politically and economically decentralized and financed by earmarked payroll tax and general budget revenue and MHI. With the passage of time, these changes led to tension over financing and provision of health care services in the setting of later economic hardship.

GEOGRAPHY

The Russian Federation is the largest country in the world, with a surface area of 17 million km^2 land boundaries of more than 20,000 km bordering Azerbaijan, Belarus, Democratic People's Republic of Korea, Estonia, Finland, Georgia, Kazakhstan, Latvia, Lithuania, Mongolia, Norway, People's Republic of China, Poland, and Ukraine (**Fig. 1**).

SOCIAL DEMOGRAPHY AND VITAL STATISTICS

The vital statistics of the Russian Federation are shown in **Table 1**. The population peaked in the 1990s and has been shrinking ever since[13] due to falling fertility and birth rates coupled with a high death rate. Its population pyramid is shown in **Fig. 2**. The inflated death rate, however, which has been more severe in the Russian Federation than in neighboring states due in part to accidents and alcoholism, affected mainly men of working age. More than 150 minority nationalities and 100 different languages in addition to Russian reflect the country's diverse cultural and ethnic background. According to a 2002 census, the largest populous groups were Russian (79.8%), Ukrainian (2%), Bashkir (1.2%), Chuvash (1.1%), and others (12.1%). Although a majority of Russians are nonpracticing believers, the dominant religion is Russian Orthodox (in up to 20%) followed by Islam (in 15%) and other denominations.

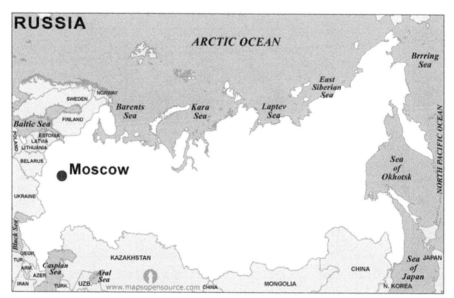

Fig. 1. Geography of the Russian Federation. (*From* MapOpenSource. Available at: http://www.mapsopensource.com/russia-capital-map-black-and-white.html.)

The aftermath of the political transformation of the Soviet Union in 1992 impacted unfavorably on the country's economy with a cumulative GDP decline of 40% from the 1990 level over 7 consecutive years. Macroeconomic indicators, including GDP and GDP per capita from 1990 to the 2000, exemplified the significant decrease in

Table 1 Vital statistics: Russia	
Population	142.5 Million (July 2014 estimated)
Life expectancy at birth	Total population: 70.2 y Male: 64.4 y Female: 76.3 y
Maternal mortality ratio	34 Deaths/100,000 live births (2010)
Infant mortality ratio	7 Deaths/1000 live births
Literacy rate	Total population: 99.7% Male: 99.7% Female: 99.6%)
GDP	$2.11 trillion (2013)
GDP per capita	$18,100 (2013)
Population below poverty line	11% (2013 est.)
Health expenditures	6.2% of GDP (2011)
Physician density	4.31 Physicians/1000 population (2006)
Hospital bed density	9.7 Beds/1000 population (2006)
Human Development Index	0.778 (2012)
Gini doefficient	39.7 (2009)

From The world factbook 2016-17. Washington, DC: Central Intelligence Agency; 2016. Available at: https://www.cia.gov/library/publications/the-world-factbook/index.html.

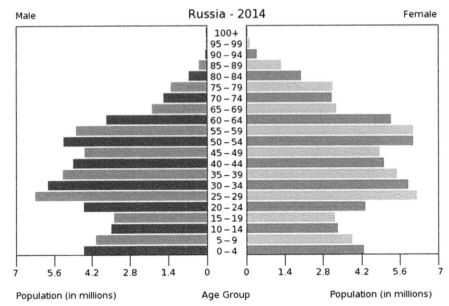

Fig. 2. Population pyramid of the Russian Federation. (*From* The world factbook 2016–17. Washington, DC: Central Intelligence Agency; 2016. Available at: https://www.cia.gov/library/publications/the-world-factbook/index.html.)

employment, labor market problems, wage arrears, budgetary deficits, and failing banking sector facing a transformation of the economy from an administrative command system to a more market-based system that continued for years even after inflation was brought under control in 1995, and until the economy showed signs of recovery in 1997. The impact of these political changes resulted in gross economic inequalities of regions of the Russian Federation, some of which persist to the present.

The Russian Federation is a federalized political system with an executive branch headed by the President who is elected by popular vote to a 4-year term, which was increased to 6 years in 2012, but who cannot serve more than 2 consecutive terms. A bicameral Federal Assembly is the legislative branch, which consists of the upper house (Federation Council) and lower house (State Duma). The judiciary consists of the Constitutional Court of judges appointed by the Federation Council on the recommendation of the President. The Constitution is strongly presidential, with the government responsible not to the Parliament but to the President, with constraints imposed on him by the Parliament in his choice of Prime Minister.

There are 83 regions or subjects in the Russian Federation, including 46 oblasts, 21 republics, 9 krais, 4 autonomous okrugs, 1 autonomous oblast, and others in the cities of Moscow and St. Petersburg, all with equal rights. The regions are subdivided into municipalities, which in 2009 included 23,907 such municipalities, including 1829 municipal regions, 512 urban okrugs, and 21,300 settlements,[14] each with lower levels of governments typically devoid of power yet important in shaping the lives of the local population. A process of political recentralization contemporaneously began with Vladimir Putin in the introduction first of extra tiers of federal administration by grouping the subjects into 7 *federal 'nye okruga* (federal administrative districts) headed by specially appointed presidential representatives, followed by an additional federal administrative district and enactment of the Federal Law on General Principles of

Organization of Legislative and Executive Bodies of State Power of a Subject of the Russian Federation and the Federal Law on Main Guarantees of Electoral and Rights to Participate in Referendum.[15,16] Presidential power was further fortified by an executive directive to send envoys to each federal administrative district ensuring that federal agencies at the regional level functioned in accordance with federal directives and policies rather than looking to local governmental structures. A consequence of recentralization has been that regional leaders have stronger incentives to comply with ministerial programs and policies answerable to the presidential administration rather than the local electorate. In 1997 the Russian Federation became a member of the G8 countries and a permanent member of the Paris Club, with accession status with the World Trade Organization and OECD and a full member of the United Nations with a seat on the Security Council, the Commonwealth of Independent States, the Organization for Security and Co-operation in Europe, and the Council of Europe. Notwithstanding, calls for suspension of the Russian Federation membership to the Council to be revoked followed more than 115 judgments of serious human rights abuses, including extrajudicial executions and torture. The Russian Federation scored 2.2 on the 2009 Corruption Perception Index, where 10 equals the absence of corruption.

INFRASTRUCTURE

The infrastructure of the Russian Federation's health care system is shown in **Fig. 3**. The Ministry of Health and Social Development (MoHSD) and its associated federal services, *Rospotrebnadzor* (Federal Consumer Right Protection and Human Wellbeing Surveillance Services), *Roszdravnadzor*, the Federal Medical and Biological Agency (FMBA), and the Federal MHI Fund, are the principal institutions. Regional and municipal health authorities oversee and monitor regional and respective municipal facilities and health authorities, which in urban municipalities consist of multipurpose, specialized hospitals, specialized clinics, outpatient facilities, diagnostic centers, and specialized emergency care facilities, whereas networks in rural municipalities generally consist of central and general rayon hospitals, small village uchastkovye village hospitals, and primary care facilities are provided by outpatient departments and feldshers. Several ministries operate parallel health systems of ministerial polyclinics, hospitals, sanatoria, and public health facilities. Funding for the health system goes through 2 channels: the general revenue budget managed by federal, regional, and local health authorities, and the MHI system managed by federal and territorial MHI funds.

In accordance with the 1993 Constitution of the Russian Federation, health issues were placed under the joint jurisdiction of article 72 of the Russian Federation and Subjects of the Russian Federation envisioning under the Foundations of the Legislation of the Russian Federation on the Protection of Citizens' Health, that there would be delineation of responsibilities among different levels of government and stakeholders. The principal entities included the federal, regional, and municipal authorities; Parliament; Presidential Executive Office; Ministry of Finance; Ministry of Economic Development; MoHSD; the subordinated bodies of the Rospotrebnadzor, Rospotrebnadzor, FMBA, and the Federal MHI Fund and its Territorial MHI Fund; as well as parallel systems of medical facilities run by ministries other than the MoHSD and the private and voluntary sectors, professional groups, and pharmaceutical commercial players.

The federal authorities were empowered to provide a unified health policy and federal programs and to coordinate the activities by state, regional, and municipal authorities as well as federal subjects and municipal and private health systems, setting

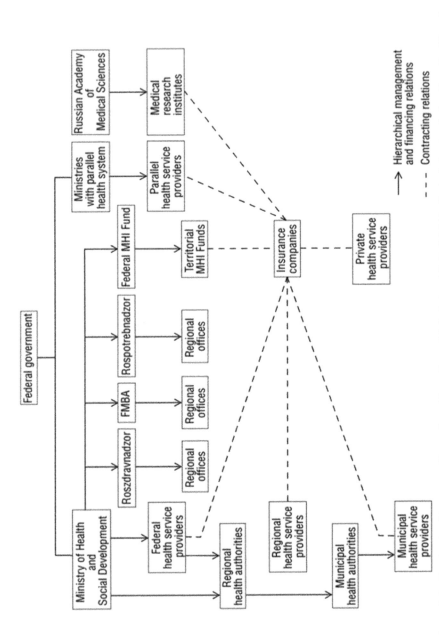

Fig. 3. Overview of the Russian health system. (*Reproduced from* Popovich L, Potapchik E, Shishkin S, et al. Russian federation. Health system review. Health Syst Transit 2011;13:1–90; with permission.)

federal standards in health care, providing unified training programs for medical and pharmaceutical workers, and licensing of health system activities. With the caveat that regional authorities did not have the right to approve laws in the area of health that contradicted federal law, both federal authorities and regional authorities were responsible for the organization of tertiary care, state sanitation and epidemiologic surveillance, pharmaceutical policy, and setting medical standards. Municipal authorities by contrast were responsible for the formation of their health authorities, development of the medical facility network, and provision of primary care, and public health education for their population. The municipal health management bodies in urban municipalities included health care departments whereas in rural ones there was a chief physician of the central district hospitals.

The Parliament, which consisted of the State Duma and the Federation Council, was responsible for the adoption of the federal legislation. In the State Duma, a Health Protection Committee was responsible for subcommittees on health care, medical science, budgetary funding, medical education, rehabilitation policy, maternal and child health protection, MHI and expenditure policy, drug circulation, and the medical industry. In the Federation Council, a Committee on Social Policy and Health Care was responsible for developing and implementing the MHI Fund budget for health, health insurance, drug manufacturing, and public health; preparing preliminary drafts of laws for the State Duma; organizing and conducting parliamentary hearings; and preparing conclusions and suggestions related to draft laws.

The Presidential Executive Office was charged with the preparation of analytical materials and recommendations required for the President to fully implement his authority. In 2005, a presidential executive [advisory] committee was formed to ensure cooperation between federal governmental authorities, government authorities of the subjects of the Russian Federation, local government authorities, and nongovernmental organizations to implement national priority projects. Their decisions were forwarded to the President, Government office, Federation Council, State Duma, and regional government authorities. The Government Office, a government authority supporting the activity of the government and the Prime Minister, monitored the fulfilment of the decisions made by the executive authorities in areas related to health and the Department of Social Development. The Department of Social Development was thus charged with ensuring collaboration between the government, chambers of the Parliament, and federal ministries, services, and agencies; drafting laws; appeals; and decisions of executive authorities.

In 2004, the Ministry of Health merged with the Ministry of Labor to form the MoHSD, the highest administrative level of the state health system, and some functions, previously granted to the Ministry of Health, were subordinated to federal governing bodies under its jurisdiction to separate out regulatory functions from policy making, which stayed in the MoHSD. The Ministry of Finance was given the role of determining funding levels for health and developing the state budget, including that of the MoHSD and its subordinated agencies as relayed by the MoHSD, who in turn submitted the requests for funding to the lower house for approval. The MoHSD was charged with the core functions instead of elaborating health policy and legislative regulation in the areas of health, health prevention, medical care, pharmaceutical activity, drug safety and efficacy, sanitation and epidemiology, social development including living standards and income levels of the population, demographic policy, pensions, labor and working conditions, and consumer rights. Moreover the MoHSD was made responsible for executing federal targeted programs funded through the federal budget and in prevention of socially significant diseases, child health, and traffic safety. Appointed by the President on the recommendation of the Prime Minister, the MoHSD carried out its functions through subordinate organization and other federal institutions of executive power, local government institutions, and public associations. In the health sector, the MoHSD coordinated and regulated the activities of the Rospotrebnadzor, Roszdravnadzor, and FMBA in addition to the Federal MHI Fund. The head of the Rospotrebnadzor, appointed by the government on the recommendation of the MoHSD, was responsible for regulation and monitoring in the areas of population sanitation, epidemiology, and consumer protection and licensing and registration of food, chemical substances, radiation catastrophes, emergency containment of communicable disease, and quarantines. The head of the Roszdravnadzor, also appointed by the government on the recommendation of the MoHSD, with regional offices and 4 research institutes, was responsible for surveillance of pharmaceutical activities and medical equipment compliance, social service monitoring and conformity, drug licensures, and monitoring of medical facilities, and social protection organizations.

The head of the FMBA, also appointed on the recommendation of the MoHSD, was a body responsible for monitoring the sanitary and epidemiologic well-being of employees in certain branches of the economy in potentially dangerous working conditions; signing government contracts for chemical and nuclear power facilities and the space program; and medical, medicosocial, and pharmaceutical care of employees its serves. The director of the Federal MHI Fund, an independent state noncommercial financial and credit organization under the jurisdiction of the MoHSD, was appointed by the government on the recommendation of the MoHSD. The agency, managed by a board and MoHSD, supervised and regulated the Territorial MHI Funds at the regional level. The Territorial MHI Funds, also independent state noncommercial financial and credit organizations, pooled resources for the MHI system of contributions from employers, payments for the insurance of nonworking population, supplements from the Federal MHI Fund, subsidies and subventions from the federal budget resources, and any revenues. A parallel system of medical facilities run by ministries other than the MoHSD traditionally provided health services to the presidential administration and ministries of defense, interior, economy, and others in inpatient and outpatient facilities. There was a private sector that existed from a legal perspective that pertained to owners not part of the state. Existing laws allowed for participation of private providers in publically financed medical care. At the regional level, however, officials could exclude private firms for ideological reasons or to protect state facilities from participation from competition. Official data of the Federal State Service, dated 2010, showed 124 private hospitals of a nationwide total of 6545 hospitals, with a total capacity of 3900 beds in 2008. A majority or 120 were located in cities and 4 in rural areas. The share of private providers was higher for outpatient care, with 2432 private outpatient providers of a nationwide total of 12,278 outpatient facilities. From 2007 to 2008, the number of private providers in inpatient and outpatient sectors fell by 32% and 53%, respectively. The Soviet Union had a wide range of scientific and professional organizations that the state curtailed; however, since 1991, several entities were founded, including the Russian Association. There have been several pubic-professional activities that have been consolidated. The voluntary sector of patient organizations has become prominent, initially concentrating on specific medical problems and geographic locations, with gradual momentum to develop a common strategy for patient rights. The main commercial players are the pharmaceutical industry with prominent commercial lobbying activities to sway ministerial policy and legislation.

Although private in nature, health insurance companies in the Russian Federation possess authorized funds within the MHI to provide VHI and must legally organize their activity in accordance with Russian Federation legislation. In accordance with the 1993 Law on Health Insurance, health management bodies and health facilities do not have the right to found insurance companies; however, they may own shares up to 10% of the insurance companies. Moreover, they generally do not have the right to provide insurance other than VHI, and when they do provide both VHI and MHI insurance, they are obligated to have separate budget managements for each type. Health insurance companies were also obligated to have reserve funds to ensure sustainability without the right to refuse coverage for a given individual. They operate in accordance with contracts signed between them and the Territorial MHI Fund on a nonprofit basis, signing contracts with facilities as well as individuals.

Pharmaceutical regulation falls under the MoHSD, which approves the list of medications to be distributed to citizens covered by the Provision of Supplemental Medicines, which currently includes approximately 375 medications divided into 31 groups. There are limited resources to cover costly medications. Because Russian physicians tend not to practice evidence-based medicine, there have been no incentives to limit overprescribing of medications by practicing physicians. Physicians trained at universities rarely undertake continuing medical education, especially those in rural areas. The MoHSD determines the size of the medical school classes, which depends on the medical workforce needs. There are mismatches between the numbers of staff and the activity required. Although a patient has the right to choose a medical facility and physician within the medical facility, in practice most citizens use local polyclinics and are unaware that they may switch away from an unsatisfactory physicians, and others are unaware of the right to a second opinion or legal representation. Moreover, patients making decisions about health care purchases in the Russian Federation have limited access to the information they need to make informed decisions.

Robbins and colleagues[17] observed that although the Soviet Union was the first country in the world to guarantee free medical care as a constitutional right to all its citizens, the quality and accessibility have been in question. The total health expenditures as a share of GDP in the Russian Federation were 5.2% in 2008, low in comparison to other countries of the WHO European Region. In comparison to other countries of the G8 that averaged more than 7%, in recent years health expenditures as a proportion of GDP have continued to trend downward. Total health expenditures in the Russian Federation are lower than the average level for countries of the European Union and Commonwealth of Independent States countries, based on per capita health expenditures. Public health funding is also low in the Russian Federation in comparison to the WHO European Region, falling from 73.9% in 1995 to 64.4% in 2009 in line with the inordinate level of out-of-pocket payments, particularly in outpatient pharmaceuticals, which are excluded from guaranteed insurance packages.

The system has a relatively even mix of financing from compulsory sources, including general taxation and payroll contributions for MHI and out-of-pocket expenses, with growing private expenditures since the1990s, accounting for 35.5% of the total health expenditure in 2009, of which 28.8% was paid out of pocket. The 2 main types of pool for prepaid funds are the MHI through its federal and territorial funds, and the federal, regional, and territorial budgets. Purchasing through MHI takes place at the regional level through Territorial MHI Funds on a contractual basis. Russian citizens are guaranteed universal access to services irrespective of whether they hold MHI policies; however, up to 1.8% of the population did not have MHI policies in 2010. The scope of coverage as determined by the PGG, the state medical package, which had 2 parts: a basic MHI package that covers everyday needs and the budget package that covers specialized and high-technology medical care and outpatient pharmaceutical costs and emergency care. Although federally mandated, local and regional authorities are responsible for maintaining the network of polyclinics and hospitals.

Danichevski and colleagues[18] summed up the basic aspects of health care financial support in 2006, noting that the Russian health system was financed from 3 major sources: taxation and duties, compulsory health insurance, and transfers from enterprises and other government ministries channeled through several parallel subsystems, further noting that there were widespread informal payments and a small voluntary insurance sector as well as some formal payments for privately delivered care and in public facilities, for extra services. Although the legal framework covering the actors in the health insurance system was set out in the 1993 Health Insurance Law, the procedures for collection and distribution of these 3 main sources of finance are characterized by a mix of formal procedures and informal realities.

Four informal aspects of financing critical to the operation of the Russian health system, without procedural transparency include the following: (1) the municipality budget that receives a small share of taxes; (2) the regional health insurance fund that collects premiums on the basis of 3.6% of payroll costs, 0.2% of which is transferred to the federal fund for redistribution between regions; (3) municipal government payments for nonworking residents; and (4) other parallel systems of financing, including voluntary insurance and unofficial payments, the latter of which was a characteristic feature in Russia. The collection of taxes or government revenues emanates from 3 sources: value added tax equaling 18%, excise tax, corporate income tax, social security contributions, and natural resource extraction tax, all at the federal level; corporate and transport taxes and a share of personal income tax revenue at the regional level; and land tax, individual property tax, and personal income tax at the local level. Payroll contributions to MHI funds were initially collected through a separate earmarked tax set at 3.6% of the wage bill, 3.4% of which was directed to the Territorial MHI Fund and 0.2% to the Federal MHI Fund. Since 2011, a unified social tax became social insurance contributions and the rate was set at 34% of the wage bill, 26% of which goes to the Pension Fund and 2% for social insurance. MHI contributions in 2011 were set at 5.1% of the wage bill, 2.1% for Federal MHI Fund, and 3% for Territorial MHI Fund. The share of the unified social tax and payroll contribution earmarked to the MHI system has been consistently insufficient. The proportion of pooled funds derived from the budget system and MHI funds from over the past 2 decades. Currently the share of MHI funds in total public spending varies greatly from region to region, ranging from 18% to 89%, and fostering inequalities in the Russian Federation. Moreover MHI funds were used to cover nonworking individuals. Out-of-pocket payments, which accounted for 28% of total health expenditures in 2008, include payments for services and medications as well as informal payments. The latter were frequent during the Soviet era, as a form of gratuity or under the table, and have become widespread, especially to assure a favorable outcome in surgical and obstetric procedures.

There is a hierarchy of clinics and hospitals at the municipal, regional, and federal levels to which more complex cases can be referred. Secondary care is rendered in specialized ambulatory care and inpatient care facilities organized on a territorial basis. The basic units of secondary and tertiary care include small rural hospitals, district hospitals, central district hospitals, and city hospitals; regional hospitals, federal hospitals, and specialized clinics; and hospitals and specialized clinics in parallel systems that render care through private payments and VHI schemes. Long-term care for the chronically ill and elderly is provided in acute care settings, rarely in geriatric beds. Palliative or hospice care was not well developed but was growing, with an estimated

33 inpatient palliative care units in 2005, with 74 hospices and 17 consultant teams in hospitals nationwide. Mental health services have been a low priority in the Russian system, funded through general budgetary revenues. People with mental illness or disabilities unable to live at home are referred to institutions for inpatient care but may not receive the psychiatric treatment they need. Andreyev[19] and Wilkinson[20] comment that in the prior USSR, political dissenters were labeled as schizophrenic and detained to prevent them from opening disparaging the state.

PUBLIC HEALTH REFORM

Between 2003 and 2004, overall administrative reform was introduced in the Russian Federation that began the period of recentralization. The first development was the enactment of 3 federal laws: Federal Law on General Principles of Organization of Legislative and Executive Bodies on State Power of a Subject of the Russian Federation, Federal Law on General Principles of Organizing Local Government in the Russian Federation, and Federal Law on Monetization of Benefits. The second was enactment of the National Priority Project-Health (NPPH), leading to a substantial increase in the share of federal expenditures in total public health expenditures. A third development was the Law on Mandatory Health Insurance, which centralized the financial administrative aspects of the MHI system at the federal level, modifying the role of the major players in the MHI system. A fourth development was placement of the Federal MHI Fund under the jurisdiction of the MoHSD.

Gordeev and colleagues[21] appraised 2 decades of reforms in the Russian public health care sector in 2010, noting that available empirical data were not sufficient for an evidence-based evaluation of the reforms and that more studies on the quality, equity, efficiency, and sustainability impact of the reforms were needed. Future reforms should focus on the implementation of cost-efficiency and cost-control mechanisms, providing incentives for better allocation and distribution of resource; tackling of problems in equity in access and financing; and finally the need to implement a system of quality controls and stimulate healthy competition between insurance companies.

Sheiman and Shevski[3] provided a recent review of health care integration in the Russian Federation. In the decade after 1991, there was a 16% reduction of the number of hospitals and outpatient facilities, whereas in the second decade there was a reduction of 40% in the number of inpatient facilities and 28% reduction in the number of outpatient facilities. Despite the contraction in the size of the network of health facilities in all levels of medical care, obsolescence and maintenance were pervasive problems among a significant number of health facilities under control of the MoHSD. The condition of health care facility buildings serving inpatients and outpatients indicates a lack of basic services, such as sewage, hot water, telephones, and information systems, with rural facilities more severely lacking than those in urban settings. Commensurate with a reduction in hospital numbers, there was a reduction in the number of hospital beds by 25% from 1990 to 2006. The average length of stay in acute care hospitals in 2006 of 11.5 days[13] fell from 14.3 days in 1997, whereas bed occupancy remained constant at 85.6% in 2006.[13] According to the MoHSD, 25% of medical equipment was re-equipped under the NPPH from 2002 to 2010; more than 112,000 units of different level medical equipment remain to be replaced especially in areas of cardiology, cardiovascular surgery, oncology, obstetrics, and gynecology, and others. The development of communications technology and a national information technology infrastructure are core elements of the Russian Federation economic policies, with only 42% of the population accessing the Internet in 2009, lower than OECD countries that averaged 74% according to the World Bank in 2011. For this reason, access to the Internet has not had an impact on the health sector. From 1990 to 1995, the total number of physicians initially fell from 45 per 10,000 population to 44.4 per 10,000 population, recovering at 50.1 per 10,000 in 2009.

Training for physicians in the Russian Federation takes 6 years of general medical education followed by 2 years of internship toward specialization. The MoHSD and the Ministry of Education and Science set target admissions level for medical schools and agree on course length and curricula to ensure the quality of the workforce; however, their efforts have been undermined by some faculty members charging for passing grades on tests.[22] The percentage of medical school graduates increased by 39% between 2000 and 2008. Danichevski and colleagues[23] studied maternity care in the Russian Federation in the Tula region of south Moscow in 2002, noting that in the preceding year the infant mortality rate was 19.5 per 1000 compared with 15.3 per 1000 in Russia as a whole, with 19 health facilities of various sizes providing obstetric care with the aim of determining how normal deliveries were managed. Their findings demonstrated a widespread divergence from internationally accepted practices using non–evidenced-based medical practices and, in some instances, heavily influenced by pharmaceutical companies. In many instances, medications were used not known to have any role in pregnancy elsewhere or for indications different from those in other countries. Their findings gave evidence for ineffective and potentially dangerous care. The reasons cited for these departures included inadequate training, corruption, and the effects of informal payments from pharmaceutical companies to physicians rendering maternity care. Stickley and colleagues[24] studied the sharp growth in the use of complementary and alternative medicine noting rates that ranged from 3.5% to 25%, with a greater likelihood of their use in rural than in urban residents as well as in those with greater wealth and a distrust of doctors.

Kutzin and colleagues[25] reviewed lessons from health financing reform in central and eastern Europe and the Russian Federation, identifying several pitfalls and lessons for successful reformers, including logical prioritization, lack of attempt to implement models developed elsewhere, attention to the sequencing of reform steps, treating of the definition of a benefits package as a policy instruments rather than an accounting exercise, and implementation of reform accompanied by analysis, reporting, learning and adaption. Rechel and McKee[26] identified 3 concerns of current health reforms in Eastern Europe, including the universal switch to health insurance systems, a growing reliance on formal and informal out-of-pocket payments, and efforts to strength primary care with a family model delivered by general practitioners. In 2005, outpatient pharmaceutical coverage was launched through a Federal Program for Supplementary Medicine Provision at the same time major reforms to social welfare were taking place for certain beneficiaries. In 2006, approximately 14.5 million people or 10% of the population qualified for these benefits. In 2013, Rechel and colleagues[27] noted that cardiovascular disease were more worrisome factors of mortality in the Russian Commonwealth of Independent States than in Western Europe. Moreover, negative mortality trends were much more pronounced in disadvantaged than in privileged groups. In the early years of the Russian transition, mortality increased by 57% in those with lower levels of education compared with 35% in men with higher education.

In 2005, Putin announced 4 national priority projects targeting housing, agriculture, education, and health, launching the NPPH, with the aim of improving population health by improving material, technological, and human resources in the health sector. Four important results of the NPPH were the increase in primary care physicians and nurses, increased salaries, and reduced waiting time for medical procedures and ambulance wait times. Pilot programs in health system reform were launched in 2008 in 19 regions at past of NPPH. Health worker payrolls have been reformed with the switch to a New Payroll System that rejected a unified salary scale and introduced more flexible payroll systems linking wages with performance and salary differentiation within certain categories.

A new National Health Concept committee was set in 2008 by MoHSD in 2008 and a dedicated Web site to encourage public participation in shaping the health priorities and policy direction was envisioned that included reduction in the risk factors for noncommunicable disease, health education, providing healthier food, and other innovative health concepts. National standards of care provision will be set assuring government guarantees and improved organization of medical care, drug supply and improved human resources.

In 2000, Vlassov[28] noted that even by 2000, Russian medical research used less frequent advance study designs and methods of data analysis and medical students were taught that epidemiology was the science of the spread of infectious diseases. With no department of epidemiology in Russian universities where epidemiology was taught in the modern sense, and no available epidemiologic and biostatistical periodicals, epidemiology in Russia has remained an archaic state. Gotsadze and colleagues[29] studied sanitary surveillance and epidemiologic in the Russian Federation and among 24 former Soviet Union communist countries undergoing reform from 1990 to 2009 as a clue to reforms in the Russian Federation. The investigators noted that progress in reform of public health services varied considerably. Decentralization often took the form of delegation from health ministries to separate agencies with the aim of improving performance and accountability, much like the present-day Russian Federation.

WORLD CUP 2018: IMPLICATIONS FOR PUBLIC HEALTH

There may be unexpected health-related dangers in the pursuit of politics of isolating the Russian Federation, in particular as concerns its preparation for the upcoming World Cup event.[30] This megaevent will be hosted in 11 cities across European Russia and could draw more than a million international spectators. The health risks involved in mass gatherings are well documented, and addressing them requires a collective multidisciplinary approach with regional, national, and international partners. The World Cup poses logistical and planning challenges, especially in terms of managing health risks and antiterrorism. Implementing strategies to minimize these risks is a global priority that requires coordinated international effort and planning. The primary risks in mass gatherings are noncommunicable diseases and injuries, although the potential global spread of communicable diseases also requires active monitoring. A proactive international approach that focuses on prevention and surveillance has provided a high level of public health protection during previous mass gatherings. New technological solutions, such as Web-based health surveillance networks and crowd-modelling software, are important for planning and executing a safe event. Unlike annual mass gatherings, the World Cup is a 1-time ambulatory megaevent held at different locations. When the Russia 2018 Local Organizing Committee published its report on their preparatory activities, it made no mention of health planning. The Russian Ministry of Health has secured funding for the repair and modernization of 13 state-run health facilities in host cities. But a safe megaevent requires more than new infrastructure: the protection of health depends on rigorous surveillance and emergency planning. This advance work is contingent on extensive international collaboration, especially for the deployment of new technologies. Russia needs

Western partners to share best practices for risk assessment, communicable disease surveillance, and capacity building. The current context of sanctions and mistrust, however, hampers this international cooperation. Russia needs immediate international expert support to undertake effective public health measures in the 11 host cities, starting with risk assessments, disaster simulations, crowd behavioral models, and infectious disease surveillance mechanisms. For nearly a century, Russia has largely existed apart from Western technological and economic flows, and even the fall of the Soviet Union did not eliminate the tendency of western policy makers and commentators to view Russia as an antagonist rather than as a partner.

BURDEN OF DISEASE: IMPLICATIONS FOR NEUROLOGY

With a global estimated prevalence of headache at 11%, the finding of the Global Burden of Disease Study 2010 of 14.7%[31] indicates a major public health problem in Russia, not adequately addressed by the health care system. Wolfe[32] reviewed the unmet health care needs of people with headache in Russia focusing on 3 major aspects of headache-attributed burden: (1) functional disability, including lost productive time; (2) impact on quality of life (QOL); and (3) willingness to pay for an adequate headache service if it were available. Using a countrywide population-based random sample, 2725 biologically unrelated adults (ages 18–65 years) in 35 cities and 9 rural areas of Russia were interviewed in a door-to-door survey; the mean lost paid-work days due to headache in the previous 3 months were 1.9 ± 4.2 and mean lost household work days were 3.4 ± 5.7. The estimated annual indirect cost of primary headache disorders was $22.8 billion, accounting for 1.75% of GDP. QOL was reduced by all types of primary headaches. According to WHO QOL-8, it was significantly lower in those with headache on greater than or equal to 15 days per month than in those with episodic headache (24.7 ± 4.6 vs 28.1 ± 5.0; $P<.05$) and lower in those with migraine than in those with tension-type headache (27.1 ± 4.9 vs 28.8 ± 5.0; $P<.05$). Average willingness to pay for adequate headache treatment was RUB $455 \pm$ RUB 494 per month (median RUB 300), a sum sufficient in most cases, and correlated with illness severity (higher for headache on ≥ 15 d/mo than for migraine and higher for migraine than for tension-type headache). Headache was thus burdensome and costly in Russia and, manifestly, poorly mitigated by existing health care. Structured health care services for headache need to be urgently put in place.

REFERENCES

1. Popovich L, Potapchik E, Shishkin S, et al. Russian federation. Health system review. Health Syst Transit 2011;13:1–190.
2. Sheiman I. Rocky road from the Semashko to a new health model. Interview by Fiona Fleck. Bull World Health Organ 2013;91:320–1.
3. Sheiman IK, Shevski V. Evaluation of health care delivery integration: the case of the Russian Federation. Health Policy 2014;115:128–37.
4. World Health Organization/Europe (WHO). European health for all database. Updated: 2012.
5. Sheiman I. Forming the system of health insurance in the Russian Federation. Soc Sci Med 1994;39:1425–32.
6. Sidel VW. Feldshers and "feldsherism". The role and training of the feldsher in the USSR. N Engl J Med 1968;278:987–92.
7. OECD Health Data File. Paris: OECD; 1990.
8. Field MG. Noble purpose, grand design, flawed execution, mixed results: Soviet socialized medicine after seventy years. Am J Public Health 1990;80:144–5.

9. Paton CR. Perestroika in the Soviet Union's health system. BMJ 1989;299:45–6.
10. Abel-Smith B. The beverage report: its origins and outcomes. Int Soc Secur Rev 1992;45:5–16.
11. Or Z, Cases C, Lisac M, et al. Are health problems systemic? Politics of access and choice under Beveridge and Bismarck systems. Health Econ Policy Law 2010;5:269–93.
12. Antoun J, Phillips F, Johnson T. Post-Soviet transition: improving health services delivery and management. Mt Sinai J Med 2011;78:436–48.
13. WHO Regional Office for Europe. 2011.
14. Rutland P. Putin's economic record. In: White S, Gitelman Z, Sakwa R, editors. Developments in Russian politics 6. Basingstoke (United Kingdom): Palgrave Macmillan; 2005. p. 186–203.
15. Federal State Statistics Service. 2010.
16. Hahn G. Reforming the federation. In: White S, Gitelman Z, Sakwa R, editors. Developments in Russian politics 6. Basingstoke (United Kingdom): Palgrave Macmillan; 2005. p. 148–66.
17. Robbins A, Caper P, Rowland D. Financing medical care in the new Soviet economy. JAMA 1990;264:1097–8.
18. Danichevski K, Balabanova D, McKee M, et al. The fragmentary federation: experiences with the decentralized health system in Russia. Health Policy Plan 2006; 21:183–94.
19. Andreyev HJN. Political dissent and "sluggish" schizophrenia in the Soviet Union. BMJ 1986;293:822.
20. Wilkinson G. Political dissent and "sluggish" schizophrenia in the Soviet Union. Br Med J 1986;293:641–2.
21. Gordeev VS, Pavlova M, Groot W. Two decades of reforms: appraisal of the financial reforms in the Russian public healthcare sector. Health Policy 2011;102: 270–7.
22. Geltzer A. When the standards aren't standard: evidence-based medicine in the Russian context. Soc Sci Med 2009;68:526–32.
23. Danichevski K, McKee M, Balabanova D. Prescribing in maternity care in Russia: the legacy of Soviet medicine. Health Policy 2008;85:242–51.
24. Stickley A, Koyanagi A, Richardson E, et al. Prevalence and factors associated with the use of alternative (folk) medicine practitioners in 8 countries of the former Soviet Union. BMC Complement Altern Med 2013;13:83.
25. Kutzin J, Jakab M, Cashin C. Lessons from health financing reform in central and Eastern Europe and the former Soviet Union. Health Econ Policy Law 2010;5: 135–47.
26. Rechel B, McKee M. Health reform in Central and Eastern Europe and the former Soviet Union. Lancet 2009;374:1186–95.
27. Rechel B, Roberts B, Richardson E, et al. Health and health systems in the Commonwealth of Independent states. Lancet 2013;381:1145–55.
28. Vlassov V. Is there epidemiology in Russia? J Epidemiol Community Health 2000; 54:740–4.
29. Gotsadze G, Chikovani I, Goguadze K, et al. Reforming sanitary-epidemiological service in Central and Eastern Europe and the former Soviet Union: an exploratory study. BMC Public Health 2010;10:440.
30. Wolfe SD. 2018 FIFA World Cup: isolating Russian could harm global health. Lancet 2015;385:749–50.

31. Vos T, Flaxman AD, Naghavi M, et al. Years lived with disability (YLDs) for 1160 sequelae of 289 diseases and injuries 1990–2010: a systematic analysis for the Global Burden of Disease Study 2010. Lancet 2012;15:2163–96.
32. Ayzenbrg I, Katsarava Z, Sborowski A, et al. Headache-attributed burden and is impact on productivity and quality of life in Russia: structured healthcare is urgently needed. Eur J Neurol 2014;21:758–65.

Health Care in India

David S. Younger, MD, MPH, MS[a,b,]*

KEYWORDS

- India • Health care • Public health • Global health • Epidemiology

KEY POINTS

- Equal access to health care in India has been impeded by socioeconomic barriers.
- There is a 3-tier public system of public health care centers in villages, district hospitals, and tertiary care hospitals.
- Government expenditure in India is inordinately low with a disproportionate emphasis on private health spending.
- The poorest receive a minority of the available subsidies, whereas only the richest obtain more than a third, fostering a divide in the health care infrastructure across the rich and poor in urban and rural settings.
- The global dimensions of the medical, sociologic, psychological, and financial consequences of epilepsy result in maximal affliction in developing countries. A large proportion of patients with epilepsy in these countries never receive appropriate treatment.

INTRODUCTION

The BRICS nations of Brazil, Russia, India, China, and South Africa are collectively useful comparisons because of their size, racial, ethnic, and geographic diversity and inherent problems of social inequality, making them more similar to the United States than their European contemporaries.

India has experienced a remarkable epidemiologic and demographic transition during the past several decades. This article examines the health care system and the global burden of diseases in India.

BACKGROUND

The right of all Indians to health care[1,2] has been interpreted as the need to eliminate barriers to care in most states in India and the achievement of equitable access irrespective of income or socioeconomic status through universal access. In 2004, Sharma[3] commented that a coalition of health and medical voluntary organizations

The author has nothing to disclose.
[a] Division of Neuroepidemiology, Department of Neurology, New York University School of Medicine, New York, NY, USA; [b] College of Global Public Health, New York University, New York, NY, USA
* Corresponding author. 333 East 34th Street, 1J, New York, NY 10016.
E-mail address: david.younger@nyumc.org

Neurol Clin 34 (2016) 1103–1114
http://dx.doi.org/10.1016/j.ncl.2016.06.005
0733-8619/16/$ – see front matter © 2016 Elsevier Inc. All rights reserved.
neurologic.theclinics.com

in India, led by the People's Health Movement, urged political parties to support the right to health noting that the constitution provided a basis for such a right without the operational framework in place to ensure universal access to public health services. With its 3-tier public system of public health care centers (PHCs) in villages, district hospitals, and tertiary care hospitals, government expenditure in India has been shrinking, composing 0.9% of its gross domestic product (GDP) on health care, lower than the 2.8% of GDP expended by less developed countries. There has instead been an explosion in private health spending approaching 82% of all health spending. The paradox in health equity in India is exemplified by the poorest 20% receiving only 10% of available subsidies, whereas the richest 20% obtain 33% of them.

A call for action by the India Group for Universal Health Care toward achieving universal health care in India by 2020[4] was termed timely and overdue but dangerously unrealistic for 2 reasons. One was an underestimation of the severe degree of persistent and ubiquitous poverty that characterized the era of economic growth with up to 77% of Indians in extreme poverty, and the other was the dependence on the need for integration of the private sector into a universal Indian health system. The Indian private sector, which has been corporate led, is unlikely to be controlled by integration; unless made to compete against a funded well-resourced managed public system throughout India, it will continue to exert more influence over the public system.

The current health care infrastructure fosters a divide across the rich and poor in both rural and urban settings. Two target-based programs intended to remediate growing negative trends of inequity of health care access exemplify the depth of the problem in health care reform. The National Rural Health Mission (NRHM) was launched in 2005 to strengthen the public health systems by addressing key features of financing, shortage of human resources, infrastructure, and quality of care among the poor and marginalized in less well-developed states in cooperation with the private sector.[2,5] Preliminary evidence from existing studies on NRHM suggested that its efficacy varies from state to state with those lagging behind failing to show any remarkable improvement.[6] The other program, Rashtriya Swasthya Bima Yojana, launched in 2008 as an insurance program entitling below-poverty-line families secondary level inpatient care up to an annual sum equal to $500, was challenged as unimpressive, with variable enrollment across states and districts and deemed to be socially noninclusive, achieving limited success in providing financial support to the poor.[7–10]

GEOGRAPHY

The geography of India is shown in **Fig. 1**. India is bordered by the Arabian Sea to the southwest and by the Bay of Bengal to the southeast. The Palk Strait and Gulf of Mannar separate India from Sri Lanka to its immediate southeast. The northern frontiers of India are defined largely by the Himalayan mountain range, where it borders China, Bhutan, and Nepal. Its western border with Pakistan lies in the Punjab Plain and the Thar Desert. Far northeast, the Chin Hills and Kachin Hills separate India from Burma. To the east it borders with Bangladesh where it is largely defined by the Khasi Hills and Mizo Hills. The Ganges, the longest river originating in India, occupies the northern, central, and eastern India, whereas the Deccan Plateau lies to the south.

SOCIAL DEMOGRAPHY AND VITAL STATISTICS

The vital statistics of India are listed in **Table 1**. The population of India reflects the predominance of younger-aged individuals of both sexes in the younger-than-50-years range, with males in all ages (**Fig. 2**). The 2011 census,[11] which spread across 28 states and 7 union territories, covering 640 districts, 5767 tehsils, 7933 towns, and

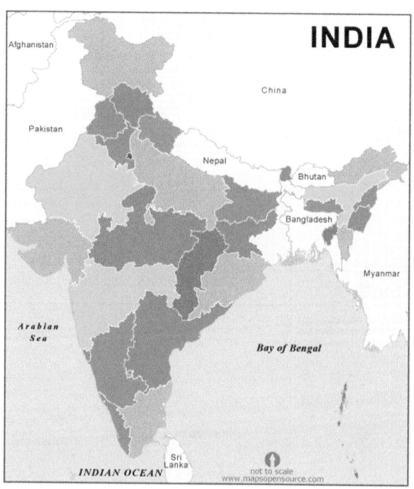

Fig. 1. Geography of India. (*From* MapOpenSource. Available at: http://www.mapsopen source.com/india-states-outline-map-black-and-white.html.)

more than 600,000 villages, sampled households in 7933 towns and 600,000 villages and classified the population according to sex, religion, education, and occupation. Now the second most populated country in the world with more than 1.21 billion people composing more than one-sixth of the world's population, India is projected to be the world's most populous country by 2025, with a population growth rate of 1.41%, ranking 102 in the world in 2010.[12] More than one-half of the population of India is younger than 25 years and more than 65% are younger than 35 years. In 2020, the average age of an Indian is projected to be 29 years compared with 37 years for China and 48 years for Japan. With more than 2000 ethnic groups and every major religion represented, there are 4 major spoken languages, including Indo-European, Dravidian, Austroasiatic, and Tibeto-Burman. Further complexity is evidenced by the great variation that occurs across this population in per capita income and level of education. Occupying about 2.8% of the world's land area, 72.2% of the population[13] resides in about 638,000 villages, with the remaining 27.8% residing in more than 5100 towns and more than 380 urban agglomerations.

Table 1
Vitals statistics: India

Population	1.2 Billion (July 2014 est)
Life expectancy at birth	Total population: 67.8 y Male: 66.7 y Female: 69.1 y
Maternal mortality ratio	200 Deaths per 100,000 live births (2010)
Infant mortality ratio	43.2 Deaths per 1000 live births
Literacy rate	Total population: 62.8% Male: 75.2% Female: 50.8%
GDP	$4.99 Trillion (2013)
GDP per capita	$4000 (2013)
Population below poverty line	29.8% (2010 est)
Health expenditures	3.9% of GDP (2011)
Physician density	0.65 Physicians per 1000 population (2009)
Hospital bed density	0.9 Beds per 1000 population (2005)
HDI	0.554 (2012)
Gini coefficient	33.9 (2010)

Abbreviations: est, estimated; HDI, human development index.
   From The world factbook 2016–17. Washington, DC: Central Intelligence Agency; 2016. Available at: https://www.cia.gov/library/publications/the-world-factbook/index.html.

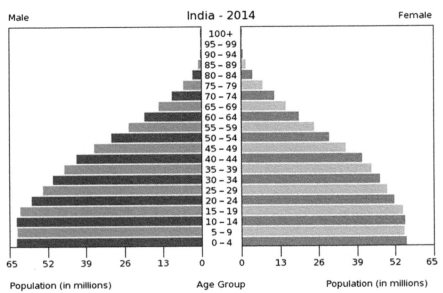

Fig. 2. Population pyramid of India. (*From* The world factbook 2016–17. Washington, DC: Central Intelligence Agency; 2016. Available at: https://www.cia.gov/library/publications/the-world-factbook/index.html.)

INFRASTRUCTURE

India has a 3-tier apex public health system, which at the base includes a vast network of about 22,370 PHCs each serving about 30,000 individuals; in the middle, a community health center serving about 100,000 followed by district level hospitals; and at the apex, tertiary-level centers typically in medical schools. With more than 200 medical schools in major cities countrywide, and an increasing burden in the private health sector, the government has chosen to invest heavily in rural health ultrastructure under the NRHM. The private health care sector is heterogeneous both in demographics with respect to states, rural and urban localities, and in the quality and distribution of health providers. The expansion of the private and public sectors in India has compelled the government to enforce several regulations to promote quality of care and protect consumers.

Insurance has a deep-rooted history in India dating back to 1818, when Oriental Life Insurance Company was forced to cater to the needs of the European community. The preindependence era in India saw discrimination between English foreigners and endemic Indian citizens enforcing higher premiums for the latter. In 1870, Bombay Mutual Life Assurance Society became the first Indian insurer. At the turn of the twentieth century, insurance companies were founded under the 1912 Life Insurance Companies and Provident Fund Acts, which in turn regulated the industry, making premium-rate tables and periodic evaluations certifiable by actuaries. Nonetheless, the disparity between Indian and foreign insurance companies persisted. A 1956 ordinance nationalized the Life Insurance creating the Life Insurance Corporation (LIC) that brought together Indian and foreign insurers. The 1972 General Insurance Business Act, which effectively nationalized 107 other insurers, grouping them into 4 companies, including, the National Insurance Company Ltd, the New India Assurance Company Ltd, the Oriental Insurance Company Ltd, and the United India Insurance Company Ltd. So named, the General Insurance Corporation (GIC) of India was incorporated and commenced business in 1973. With only 2 state insurers, the LIC and GIC and its subsidiaries, insurance was reopened to the private sector in 1990. Effective in 2000, the subsidiaries were separated from the parent company and recreated as independent insurance companies. The LIC of India, a state-owned insurance group and investment company headquartered in Mumbai, is the largest insurance company in India with an estimated asset value of 1,560,481.84 crore. By 2012 Indian insurance was a $72 billion industry; however, only 0.2% of the 1 billion citizens were covered.

Policy makers struggling with private and state health insurance recognized 7 attributes of households in arriving at viable insurance schemes, especially applicable to the poorest households, recently summarized by Dror.[14] They included (1) willingness to pay 1% of the household income on health insurance; (2) recognition that the cost of drug consumption is preferable to hospitalization; (3) inclusion of large households with lesser illness episodes and less risk to insurers; (4) information, resource, and asset sharing within a household and demographic balancing to lower the prevalence of illness; (5) active participation in the health insurance package; (6) recognition and implementation of an insurance package that suits the needs of the poorest households; and (7) significant contribution of the cost of insurance by all of the people.

Nonphysician clinicians are being used to provide cost-effective primary care,[15] especially rural regions where they have become the main providers, and in some instances even specialist services; however, their clinical competence has been questioned. One Delhi-based cross-sectional study stratifying Primary Health Center medical providers[16] that included medical officers, Ayurveda, yoga, unani, siddha, and homeopathy (AYUSH) physicians trained in Indian systems of medicine, rural medical associates (RMAs), and paramedical providers, found that physicians in government or private service were more competent than AYUSH-trained physicians, whereas RMAs were the least competent. Another study found that medical officers and RMAs were equally competent in managing common primary care problems, such as malaria, diarrhea, pneumonia, tuberculosis, preeclampsia, and diabetes, consistent with the experience of other countries.[17] AYUSH medical officers were less competent than medical officers and RMAs, raising concern about the practice of allopathic medicine in primary care settings; paramedics were the least competent of the clinical care providers surveyed.[15] Das and colleagues[18] used a standardized methodology to measure the quality of health care in rural surrounding areas of urban Delhi noting that urban-trained health care providers had better diagnostic skills and rates of treatment rates compared with their rural colleagues. With just more than one-half reporting some education beyond high school, 67.0% of rural providers have no medical qualifications and only 22.5% report some training in traditional medicine. With low levels of history taking, examinations, and emphasis on providers offering medications to their patients, only 14% of rural physicians even questioned their patients about the location of chest pain in those with unstable angina and often performed only brief consultations resulting in poor adherence to checklist formation and treatment.

Emergency medical services (EMS) in India are still in its infancy and very fragmented, without standardized EMS training courses.[19] There are 3 recognized levels of prehospital care, basic, advanced and paramedics. Dial 108 is a free ambulance service provide in public-private partnership with respective state governments for medical, police, and fire emergencies, where dial 1298 is a paid service while 108 is free of charge. With no centralized EMS systems, there is a shortage of properly equipped ambulances and the fee for use of private hospitals is very costly.

With approximately 65% of the Indian population residing in rural areas, many of the Indian medical graduates who derive from rural areas choose to relocate to urban areas where most of the surgeons practice.[20] Clinics located at the village level, in cottage hospitals for a block of villages, and government hospital for the district, are all understaffed with little supplies. One rural surgeon may be the only medical person available in the region treatment all ages of patients and in virtually every body system. Despite being a long way from achieving universal accessible health care, there is interest in recruiting doctors into primary care. In fact, free primary care to achieve universal health care coverage[21] was incorporated in the revised draft of the health chapter for India's 12th Five-Year Plan for 2012 to 2017. With general practice slowly phasing out in India, physicians working in the community tend to operate private practices outside the governmental funded health care system with a large proportion of the population in India relying on government funded hospitals.

The Indian health workforce is composed of a range of health workers who offer health care services in different specialties. Informal medical practitioners are usually the first point of contact for most of the population especially the poor. One study[22] noted that among 25% of self-characterized allopathic providers, 42% practiced in rural areas, and 15% practiced in urban settings without formal medical training. According to self-reported census estimates,[23] other health care workforce members include registered allopathic medical practitioners often with strong professional connections to the private practice, pathology laboratories run by government physicians, and corporate hospitals to which they refer for a commission, as well as, nurses, midwives, pharmacists, and traditional yoga, naturopathic and homeopathic practitioners. With more than 80% of outpatient visits and 60% of hospital admissions in the private sector, 71% of health spending was out of pocket each year, inadvertently forcing 4% of the population into poverty.[24,25] Compared with 1947, when India first gained independence and had few adequately trained workers with a rate of 1.6 doctors per 10,000 population,[26] 70% of whom worked in private urban sectors,[27] often in hospitals that functioned without trained nurses, the rate of allopathic physicians per 10,000 population in 2009 was 11.9 per 10,000 population, a substantial increase over the 1947 figures, yet less than one-half of the World Health Organization's benchmark of 25.4 workers per 10,000 population.[22]

Although mandated to train physicians in clinical skills and public health according to a single system of medical education, public health has been largely restricted to medical schools, with preventative and social medicine departments maintaining low prestige, poor staff quality, and inadequate facilities, thus, rarely attracting competent physicians. Along with the provision of health care and maintenance of the workforce allocated to the states, leaving the central government with a restricted role, well-trained Indian physicians often leave for other countries with a more promising financial future. Therein, Indian physicians composed the largest group of foreign-trained physicians in the United States and the United Kingdom, accounting for 4.9% and 10.9%, respectively; with the second largest group in Australia composing 4% of physicians; and the third largest group of foreign-trained physicians in Canada, accounting for 2.1%. Kaushik and colleagues[28] noted that the migration was substantially higher for graduates of the better medical colleges, with 54% of graduates from India's premier medical colleges emigrating between 1989 and 2000, mostly to the United States, leaving a void in the best-trained physicians at home. With medical education suffering from various shortcomings at conceptual and implementation levels,[29] and the expansion of medical education leading to increases in doctor to patient ratios, Indian medical education continues to suffer from maldistribution of resources, unregulated private sector growth, lack of uniform admission procedures, and traditional curricula lacking innovated approaches.

Preventive health care services, including immunization, antenatal, maternity and postnatal care, contraceptives, family planning measures, and community-based services, such as spraying for malaria and health education, are not high priorities in the India health care budget; moreover, there has been a decline in public health expenditures for antimalaria programs, leprosy, and tuberculosis control, although allocations have increased in AIDS and blindness control programs. With dwindling public health spending and increasing requirements to meet the expansion of primary services in remote areas, many states are exploring new routes of health care financing, including the introduction of user fees, public-private partnerships (PPPs), including the voluntary sector of nongovernmental agencies (NGOs), dual pricing systems, increases in registration fees, effective regulation of the private sector, and achieving cost-effectiveness through better planning at all levels in the health care system. PPPs have assumed the greatest importance, with the justification being improved distribution of the financial burden, improvement in the quality and quantity of health care services, and a strengthening of the capacity of the private sector. There are successful PPP models being practiced in different states of India that include subsidies for infrastructure to open superspecialized hospitals; the handing over of primary health center management to NGOs; involvement of industry to adopt local primary health centers or subcenters allowing industrial corporate houses to adopt villages for health improvement; and encouragement and mobilization of patients to self-organize into health action associations.

REFORM

Inequity in health care financing and delivery of services in India has a global and countrywide impact on levels of morbidity and mortality, especially among households with the most limited financial resources who seek treatment for preventive and immediate care. A report by the State of the World's Mothers from the Save the Children charity[30] found that 29% of babies who died on the day of their birth were born in India, followed by Nigeria, Pakistan, and China. An analysis of life expectancy and healthy life expectancy in India longitudinally over 2007 to 2020 provided projections into the future according to the Indian Healthy Life Expectancy Projection model.[31] From 2000 to 2006, the investigators noted a decrease in mortality rates with increasing rate trends in women, in men aged 35 to 39 years, and in the occurrence of disability given the burden of infectious diseases and malnutrition; the rapid growth of noncommunicable diseases, such as diabetes, cardiovascular disease, and hypertension; as well as disability caused by age-related changes in physical health. India is poorly positioned to meet 16 of the Millennium Development Goals adopted in 2000 for 2015,[32] notably in regard to the proportion of the population below the poverty line; undernourishment in the total population; literacy rates; ratio of girls to boys in primary and secondary education; younger-than-5-years' mortality rate, infant mortality rate per 1000 live births, maternal mortality rate per 100,000 live births; population with sustainable access to improved water source or sanitation; and deaths due to malaria, tuberculosis, human immune deficiency virus, cardiovascular disease, and chronic obstructive pulmonary disease, which account for most out-of-pocket health expenditures.

The National Commission on Macroeconomics and Health, which sought to identify major health conditions in terms of the contribution to India's burden of disease, including causal factors, incidence, prevalence, and the most cost-effective solutions for interventions identified 17 priority health conditions[33] among categories of maternal and childhood communicable diseases, noncommunicable conditions, blindness and oral diseases, accidents, and injuries.

Low levels of public financing, lack of a comprehensive risk-pooling mechanism, and high out-of-pocket expenses in the setting of increasing health costs have been significant factors in health financing and risk protection in the Indian health care system. The utilization of health services among primary, secondary, and tertiary care settings between 2001 and 2002 were, respectively, 48%, 24%, and 15% in the private sector compared with 60%, 21%, and 19% in the public sector,[34] underlying the somewhat greater utilization of primary care in the private sector. Although the utilization of health services in the lower quintiles of both sectors is about 35%, that of the higher quintiles increases in favor of the private sector to almost 70% with a positive relation to increasing income.[35] With health expenditure in the public sector of about 20.0%, and NGO supplying 2.3%, public expenditures in India are among the lowest in the region behind that of Pakistan, Bangladesh, and Sri Lanka. However, with 98% of private health expenditures from households in the form of out-of-pocket payments, a very small portion of private expenditures derives from health premiums, which are otherwise paid by employees and insurance plans. National expenditure surveys[23] suggest that inequities in health care financing has worsened over the last 2 decades, with only about 10% of the Indian population covered by any form of social or voluntary health insurance, which is mainly offered through governmental programs for selective employment groups in the organized sector, such as the Employee State Insurance Scheme or Central Government Health Scheme.[36] After passage of the Insurance Regulatory and Development Authority Bill in 1999, when private insurance entered the Indian market, private insurance companies accounted for only 6.1% of health expenditure on insurance,[37] whereas community-based health insurance schemes and those for the informal public sector, which encouraged risk pooling, accounted for less than 1.0% of the population.[38]

A decade ago, the total health expenditure was 4.63% of the GDP and, respectively, 0.94% and 3.58%, of GDP for the public and private sectors compared with estimates for 2008 to 2009 of 4.13% total health expenditure and 1.10% for public expenditures of the share of GDP.[33] With one of the highest proportions of household out-of-pocket expenditures worldwide estimated at 71.1% in 2008 to 2009, out-of-pocket expenditures on health as a proportion of household expenditure have increased over time in both rural and urban areas.[23,37] Expenditures on both inpatient and outpatient health were consistently higher in private facilities compared with public facilities with the expense of noncommunicable diseases outweighing those of communicable diseases.[38] One impact of out-of-pocket payments in vulnerable poor households has been the exacerbation of poverty due to inadequate financial risk protection in rural areas and poorer states where a greater proportion of the population live near the poverty line, with the burden falling heavily on tribes and castes.

With health insurance placed forward as a measure to protect against catastrophic health expenditures (CHE), and little evidence from low-income countries to support this hypothesis, Devadasan and colleagues[39] studied the circumstances and intensity of CHE among 2 Indian community health insurance schemes, action for community organisation, rehabilitation, and development (ACCORD) and self employed women's association (SEWA), each serving indigenous populations of India's informal sectors and providing low-cost health care through integrated medical insurance packages. The two differed in that admissions for ACCORD were all in a designated not-for-profit institution, whereas those for SEWA were in private for-profit institutions leading to median hospital bills, respectively, of $12 and $46. With 74% of claims covered in the former and 38% of claims reimbursed in the latter, typically at a mean interval of 6 weeks, those subscribing to SEWA had to mobilize financial resources during the time of illness. Of all insured households, 8% of those subscribing to ACCORD compared with 49% of households with SEWA would have been catastrophically affected by hospital costs if not insured. Whether one defines CHE as 10% of annual or disposable income, health expenditures have the capacity to be catastrophic. To that end, it is important to expand the maximum limit of the benefit package to cover common and potentially devastating surgical and medical conditions, especially for poorer households.

GLOBAL BURDEN OF DISEASE: IMPLICATIONS FOR NEUROLOGY

Epilepsy is a major public health concern, affecting an estimated 50 million people worldwide. Of these, nearly 80% live in developing countries. The global dimensions of the medical, sociologic, psychological, and financial consequences of epilepsy result in maximal affliction in developing countries. A large proportion of patients with epilepsy in these countries never receive appropriate treatment. A recent systematic analysis of the magnitude of the treatment gap found a treatment gap of 56% in India.[40] The main causes of this large treatment gap include high cost of treatment, unavailability of antiepileptic drugs, and faith in traditional treatments, superstitions, and cultural beliefs. Many patients, although diagnosed and initiated on treatment, soon discontinue drugs because of their inability to afford the treatment and ignorance of the effects of discontinuation. A study from India reported that 43% discontinued their treatment after 1 year.[41] The social stigma attached to this condition creates further difficulties in its management. The quality of life of patients with epilepsy is affected by the prejudices prevalent in society, such as when epileptic children find it difficult to attend school if they are affected patients because of the stigma.

REFERENCES

1. Bhore J, Amesur R, Banerjee A. Report of the Health Survey and Development Committee. Delhi (India): Government of India; 1946.
2. Government of India. Draft National Health Bill. New Delhi (India): Ministry of Health and Family Welfare; 2009.
3. Sharma DA. Indian health groups demand right to health. Lancet 2004;363:1044.
4. Sengupta A, Prasad V. Towards a truly universal Indian health system. Lancet 2011;377:702–3.
5. Mills A, Ataguba JE, Akazili J, et al. Equity in financing and use of healthcare in South Africa, Ghana, and Tanzania: implications for paths to universal health coverage. Lancet 2012;380:126–33.
6. Gill K. A primary evaluation of service delivery under the National Rural Health Mission (NRHM): findings from a study in Andhra Pradesh, Uttar Pradesh, Bihar and Rajasthan. Working paper 1. New Delhi (India): Planning Commission of India; 2009.
7. Ghosh S, Thakur H. Social exclusion and Rashtriya Swasthya Bima Yojana in Maharashtra: a case study. Mumbai (India): Tata Institute of Social Sciences; 2013.
8. Sun C. An analysis of RSBY enrollment patterns: preliminary evidence and lessons from the early experience. In: Palacious R, Das J, Sun C, editors. India's health insurance scheme for the poor: evidence from the early experience of the Rashtriya Swasthya Bima Yojana. New Delhi (India): Centre for Policy Research; 2011.
9. Narayana D. Review of the Rashtriya Swasthya Bima Yajana: evaluating utilization. Roll-out and perceptions in Amravati District, Maharashtra. Econ Polit Wkly 2012;47:57–74.
10. Salvaraj S, Karan A. Why publicly-financed health insurance schemes are ineffective in providing financial risk protection. Econ Polit Wkly 2012;47:60–8.
11. Census India SRS bulletins. Registrar General of India, Government of India. 2011.
12. World Bank indicators databank. The World Bank. January 2012.
13. Rural-urban distribution Census of India: census data 2001. India at a glance. Rural-urban distribution. Office of the Registrar General and Census Commissioner, India.
14. Dror DM. Health insurance for the poor: myths and realities. Econ Polit Wkly 2006; 14:4541–4.
15. Rao KD, Sundararaman T, Bhatnagar A, et al. Which doctor for primary health care? Quality of care and non-physician clinicians in India. Soc Sci Med 2013; 84:30–4.
16. Das J, Hammer J. Location, location, locations: residence, wealth, and the quality of care in Delhi, India. Health Aff 2007;26:338–51.
17. Wilson A, Lissauer D, Thangaratinam S, et al. A comparison of clinical officers with medical doctors on outcomes of caesarean section in the developing world: meta-analysis of controlled studies. BMJ 2011;342:d2600.
18. Das J, Holla A, Das V, et al. In urban and rural India, a standardized patient study showed low levels of provider training and huge quality gaps. Health Aff 2012;31:2774–84.

19. Sharma M, Brandler ES. Emergency medical services in India: the present and future. Prehosp Disaster Med 2014;29:1–4.
20. Mehendale V. Rural surgery in India. World J Surg 2007;31:1898–9.
21. Kay M. India proposes free primary care to help achieve universal healthcare coverage. BMJ 2012;345:e7347.
22. Rao K, Bhatnagar A, Berman P. India's health workforce: size, composition and distribution. In: La Forgia J, Rao K, editors. India health beat. New Delhi (India): World Bank: New Delhi and Public Health Foundation of India; 2009.
23. Selvaraj S, Karan A. Deepening health insecurity in India: evidence from national sample surveys since 1980s. Econ Polit Wkly 2009;44:55–60.
24. Government of India. National health accounts 2004-2005. New Delhi (India): National Health Accounts. Ministry of Health and Family Welfare. Government of India; 2009.
25. Government of India. Report on the health survey and development committee survey, vol. 1. Delhi (India): Manager of Publications; 1946.
26. Government of India. Compendium of recommendations of various committees on health development 1943-1975. New Delhi (India): Central Bureau of Health Intelligence, Directorate General of Health Services, Ministry of Health and Family Welfare. Government of India; 1985.
27. Kaushik M, Jaiswal A, Shah N, et al. High-end physician migration from India. Bull World Health Organ 2008;86:40–5.
28. Solanki A, Kashyap S. Medical education in India: current challenges and the way forward. Med Teach 2014;36(12):1027–31.
29. Bhaumik S. India tops world table for number of babies who die on day of birth. BMJ 2013;346:13123.
30. Lau RS, Johnson S, Kamalanabhan TJ. Healthy life expectancy in the context of population health and aging in India. Asia Pac J Public Health 2012;24:195–207.
31. Elizabeth KE. India's progress toward achieving the targets set in the Millennium Development Goals [editorial]. J Trop Pediatr 2008;54:287–90.
32. NCMH Background Papers. Burden of disease in India. New Delhi (India): National Commission on Macroeconomics and Health. Ministry of Health & Family Welfare, Government of India; 2005.
33. National Health Accounts INDIA. 2001-2002. National Health Accounts Cell, Ministry of Health and Family Welfare. Government of India (In collaboration with WHO India Country Office).
34. Sundar R, Sharma A. Morbidity and utilisation of healthcare services: a survey of urban poor in Delhi and Chennai. Econ Polit Wkly 2002;37:4729–40.
35. Eleventh five year plan. 2007-12. Social sector. Volume II. Planning Commission, Government of India.
36. Yip W, Mahal A. The health care systems of China and India: performance and future challenges. Health Aff 2008;27:921–32.
37. Devadasan N, Ranson K, Van Damme W, et al. The landscape of community health insurance in India: an overview of based on 10 case studies. Health Policy 2006;78:224–34.
38. Garg CC, Karan AK. Reducing out-of-pocket expenditures to reduced poverty: a disaggregated analysis of rural-urban and state level in India. Health Policy Plan 2009;24:116–28.
39. Devadasan N, Criel B, Damme WV, et al. Indian community health insurance schemes provide partial protection against catastrophic health expenditure. BMC Health Serv Res 2007;7:43.

40. Mbuba CK, Ngugi AK, Newton C, et al. The epilepsy treatment gap in developing countries: a systematic review of the magnitude, causes, and intervention strategies. Epilepsia 2008;49:1491–503.

41. Das K, Banerjee M, Mondal G, et al. Evaluation of socioeconomic factors causing discontinuation of epilepsy treatment resulting in seizure recurrence: a study in an urban epilepsy clinic in India. Seizure 2007;16:601–7.

Health Care in China

David S. Younger, MD, MPH, MS[a,b,*]

KEYWORDS

- China • Health care • Public health • Global health • Epidemiology

KEY POINTS

- China has recently emerged as an important global partner with its immense population and size are such that what happens has a worldwide impact.
- China's major role as health innovator is paralleled by its importance in the control and prevention of epidemic and endemic diseases.
- China has experienced dramatic demographic and epidemiologic changes in the past few decades, including striking decline in fertility and child mortality and increase in life expectancy at birth, prompting major reforms.
- Timely and accurate assessment of the provincial burden of disease is useful for evidence-based priority setting at the local level in China.
- The most common noncommunicable diseases, ischemic heart disease, stroke, chronic obstructive pulmonary disease, and cancers (liver, stomach, and lung), contributed much more to years of life lost in 2013 compared with 1990.

INTRODUCTION

The BRICS nations of Brazil, Russia, India, China, and South Africa, collectively, are useful comparisons because of their size, racial, ethnic, and geographic diversity and inherent problems of social inequality, making them more similar to the United States than its European contemporaries.

China has experienced a remarkable epidemiologic and demographic transition during the past 3 decades. Far less is known about this transition at the subnational level. Timely and accurate assessment of the provincial burden of disease is useful for evidence-based priority setting at the local level in China. This article examines the health care system and the global burden of diseases of China.

BACKGROUND

As one of the world's oldest cultures, China has recently emerged as an important global partner. Several reasons account for this evolutionary trend: first, China's

The author has nothing to disclose.
[a] Division of Neuroepidemiology, Department of Neurology, New York University School of Medicine, New York, NY, USA; [b] College of Global Public Health, New York University, New York, NY, USA
* Corresponding author. 333 East 34th Street, 1J, New York, NY 10016.
E-mail address: david.younger@nyumc.org

Neurol Clin 34 (2016) 1115–1125
http://dx.doi.org/10.1016/j.ncl.2016.06.003
0733-8619/16/$ – see front matter © 2016 Elsevier Inc. All rights reserved.

neurologic.theclinics.com

immense population and size such that what happens has a worldwide impact; second, China's major role as health innovator; third, China's importance in the control and prevention of epidemic and endemic diseases; fourth, China's assumption of greater authority and global responsibility. However, like other developing nations, China has experienced dramatic demographic and epidemiologic changes in the past few decades, including a striking decline in fertility and child mortality and an increase in life expectancy at birth.

Population discontent with the health care system has led to major reforms. The Global Burden of Diseases, Injuries and Risk Factor Study 2010[1] demonstrated that age-standardized years of life lost (YLL) in China were lower in 2010 than all emerging economies in the G20 and only slight higher than those noted in the United States. With the lowest years lived with disability rate in the G20 in 2010, China ranked 10th for healthy life expectancy and 12th for life expectancy.[2] In spite of a mainly urbanized and aging population, and important health threats from infectious outbreaks, reproductive health problems, and health inequality, China has, nonetheless, been on track to reach the Millennium Development Goals 4 and 5 by 2015, respectively, in the reduction of child and maternal mortality rates.[3]

Several other factors characterize the distinctive nature of the Chinese health care system, including its unique history, vast infrastructure, the speed of health reform, and economic capacity to make important advances in health care.[4] With incomplete insurance coverage for urban and rural dwellers, uneven access, mixed quality of health care, increasing costs, and risk of catastrophic health expenditures, China advanced the Healthy China 2020 initiative to encourage disease prevention, health promotion, health care service delivery, expand pharmaceuticals, and promote health care coverage.[4,5] The *Chinese dream* is an extremely popular slogan that refers to the realization of a prosperous and strong country with rejuvenation, sustained well-being, and health care reform.

Dong and Phillips[5] and Blumenthal and Hsiao[6] summarized the evolution of the Chinese health care system as a progression through 5 historical phases, evolving from a socialistic and collectivistic society of the mid-twentieth century emphasizing social equality to a decentralized market-driven system fostering disparities in access to services and the well-being of urban and rural communities.

The first or Post-Liberation phase, from 1949 to 1965, commenced with the establishment of the People's Republic of China. With government ownership of the health care system, bold preventative measures were implemented to treat and prevent infectious diseases and integrate Western and traditional Chinese medicine while health services were provided in urban government-funded hospitals and village and township rural clinics. Communes that owned the land, organized and distributed its harvest, supplied social services, and provided health care by a cooperative medical system. Staffed by practitioners with basic training, so-called barefoot doctors met the basic needs of the rural populations.[7] The second or Cultural Revolution phase, from 1966 to 1976, coincided with university and medical school closers for 5 years sending students and faculty to work in the countryside. The third or Early Reform phase, from 1977 to 1989, heralded a period of rapid economic expansion associated with decentralization of political and economic power and opening China to the global economy. There were many well-coordinated health initiatives, such as the control of vectors[7,8] to diminish infectious diseases, prevention of infant mortality, and increased longevity, whereas chronic cardiac, cancer, cerebrovascular, and mental illness arose as major causes of death and disability. From 1952 to 1982, infant mortality decreased from 200 to 34 per 1000 live births and life expectancy increased from 35 to 68 years, reflecting major investments in public health through a centralized government modeled essentially after the Soviet Union system.[9] Disturbing policies, such as one child per family, along with the accelerated aging of the population and the movement of rural workers to urban areas led to a demographic shift that further exacerbated disparities between the wealthy and impoverished classes. Several decisions leading up the dismantling of its apparently successful health care and public health system in the early 1980s preceded the fourth and final phase of Late Reform, from 1990 to 2002, associated with the reigning in of health care costs.

The first decision was the change in financing of health care reducing the government's investment that amounted to a spending decrease from 32% to 15% at the same time transferring the responsibility for funding of health care services to provincial and local entities through local taxation.[10] A second factor was the imposition of price regulation and tight controls over the amount that publicly run clinics and hospitals could charge for visits, services and pharmaceuticals despite encouragement of profits through markup of 15% or more.[11] Physician salaries were tied to bonuses and revenue generated by their activities, especially in their use of profitable new drugs and high technologic services available in the West. This practice led to a rapid overall increase in health care prices and spending available only to the wealthy through out-of-pocket payments. A third factor was the sudden and complete dismantling of communes that privatized the Chinese agricultural economy separating rural citizen from their cooperative medical systems, removing nearly 900 million Chinese peasants from risk pools and a health safety net. Barefoot doctors, unemployed, switched to more lucrative activities. A final factor was the decentralization of the public health system, which, encumbered by reductions in public funding as a proportion of local public health revenues from 60% to 42%, completed the partial privatization of China's public health system.[10]

GEOGRAPHY

China is the third largest country in the world in terms of land area (**Fig. 1**). It is situated in Eastern Asia sharing borders with Mongolia and Russia to the north; Pakistan, India, Nepal, Bhutan, and Myanmar to the west; Laos and Vietnam to the south; and North Korea to the east. China borders the South China Sea, East China Sea, and Yellow Sea as well as the Gulf of Tonkin. The country is divided into 3 geographic regions, including mountains and plateaus to the west, deserts and basins in the northeast, and the low-lying valleys and plains in the east.

SOCIAL DEMOGRAPHY AND VITAL STATISTICS

The vital statistics for China are shown in **Table 1**. The population pyramid is shown in **Fig. 2**. China has the largest world population with more than 1.36 billion people, with a life expectancy at birth of 75.2 years. Women have a higher life expectancy than men, 77.4 and 73.1 years, respectively. The maternal mortality ratio in 2010 was 37 per 100,000 births, and the infant mortality ratio was 14.8 per 1000 live births. The literacy rate for men was 97.5% and 92.7% for women. With one of the largest and fastest growing work economies with a total gross domestic product (GDP) of $13.4 trillion in 2013 and GDP per capita of $9,800, 6% of the population was below the poverty line with a human development index and Gini coefficient at 0.699 and 42.1, respectively. Health expenditures compose about 5.2% of the GDP.

INFRASTRUCTURE

China's present health care infrastructure can be divided into primary health care and hospital care in primarily rural and urban communities. Although guided by a market

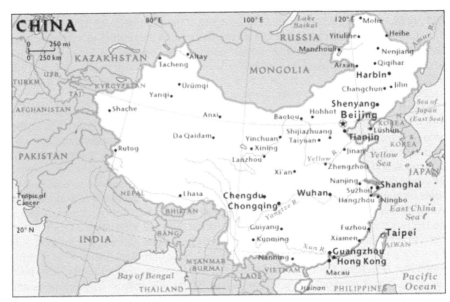

Fig. 1. Geography of China. (*Data from* Available at: https://maps.google.com/maps/ms?msa=0&msid=200187709978753177644.0004cb2a594bbc55b1164&dg=featureFigure 9. Accessed September 1, 2015.)

approach, the central government has responded to growing public criticism for affordable access to health care services with greater financial risk protection from out-of-pocket spending on health services. Funding for health care in China derives from several newly enacted governmental sources.[12] They include subsidies to rural and

Table 1	
Vital statistics	
Population	1.36 Billion (July 2014 est)
Life expectancy at birth	Total population: 75.2 y Male: 73.1 y Female: 77.4 y
Maternal mortality ratio	37 Deaths per 100,000 live births (2010)
Infant mortality ratio	14.8 Deaths per 1000 live births
Literacy rate	Total population: 95.1% Male: 97.5% Female: 92.7%
GDP	$13.39 Trillion (2013 est)
GDP per capita	$9800 (2013 est)
Population below poverty line	6.1%
Health expenditures	5.2% of GDP (2011)
Physician density	1.46 Physicians per 1000 population (2010)
Hospital bed density	3.8 Beds per 1000 population (2009)
HDI	0.699
Gini coefficient	42.1

Abbreviations: est, estimated; GDP, gross domestic product; HDI, human development index.
From The world factbook 2016–17. Washington, DC: Central Intelligence Agency; 2016. Available at: https://www.cia.gov/library/publications/the-world-factbook/index.html.

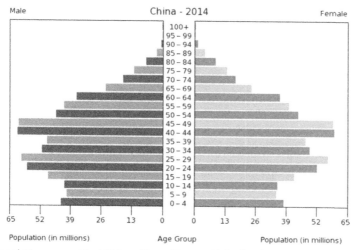

Fig. 2. Population pyramid of China. (*From* The world factbook 2016–17. Washington, DC: Central Intelligence Agency; 2016. Available at: https://www.cia.gov/library/publications/the-world-factbook/index.html.)

urban residents not covered by the Urban Employee Basic Medical Insurance (UEBMI) program through the New Cooperative Medical Scheme (NCMS) or the Urban Resident Basic Medical Insurance Program (URBMI), respectively. With a goal of increasing funding to cover at least 75% and 50% for hospital admissions and outpatient services, more than 96% of the population is covered together by NCMS, URBMI, and UEBMI. There has been a parallel increase in governmental health service coverage for hospital payments. Primary health care providers receive governmental funds to deliver a package of basic health services. Health care providers and government-appointed hospital officials, motivated by profits and behavior similar to other for-profit organizations, have been incentivized to prescribe excessive and high-tech diagnostic tests and to prescribe pharmaceuticals to earn profits for later distribution. In 2011, expenditures on drugs accounted for 43% of total health expenditures,[12] nearly triple the Organization for Economic Cooperation and Development's (OCED) average of 16%. With providers permitted to charge a 15% markup on pharmaceuticals, and public hospital profits tied to utilization of services, there is neither the motivation nor the incentive to find cost-effective approaches to health care service delivery focusing on aspects of disease prevention, health promotion, and disease management or a more functional coordination between primary, secondary, and tertiary health care providers.

Bhattacharyya and colleagues[13] studied primary care in China over the past 2 decades noting that the current performance of community health facilities suffered from inadequacy of providers, increasing funding for community health services, unaffordability, and safety concerns regarding community health service providers. An important part of the Chinese Urban Health Reform System, community health centers (CHCs) were established throughout the country numbering in excess of 2406 CHC and 9700 service stations in autonomous regions and central government-ruled cities, such as Beijing, Shanghai, Chongqing, and Tianjin. Although regarded as basic networks for medical treatment and public health surveillance,[14] CHCs are facing many problems in the deliverance of their 6 main services: disease prevention and control, health care services, health education, family planning, medical treatment service, and community rehabilitation. In competing with local hospitals for acute and chronic care services, CHCs have had difficulty in winning the trust of local residents because of scarcity of medical resources, lack of funds, absence of newest medical technology, and few professional and qualified medical staff, especially in rural areas.

Among several factors that mitigate physician behavior, including, training, education, professional ethics, altruism, practice norms, regulatory oversight, and financial incentives, the incentive system of fee for service of the past 2 decades has slowly eroded primary care and hospital delivery of services in China. This system has led to artificially high price schedules, overpayment for pharmaceuticals, overuse of expensive high technologic testing, increase in health costs, and an erosion of professional ethics and practice norms.[15] Ethical codes for medicine in China have been based on principles of autonomy, beneficence, and justice; however, in recent years the potential for conflicts of interest has undermined ethical relations between medical professionals, researchers, drug companies, and even regulatory agencies.[16]

The Chinese government has piloted new ways of dealing with misdirected provider financial incentives, including the change from fee for service to aggregated and prospective payments for performance and treatment protocols that assure improved quality and emphasize prevention and primary care of chronic disease in place of curative services more appropriate to infectious illness. In 2005, the Ministry of Health (MoH) piloted a new system of primary care funding of providers that separated revenue and charges[17] and another payment reform pilot in 2005 in which CHCs were paid fees for service according to a government price schedule and distinct health bureaus that were given a yearly budget subject to end-year reassessment. Preliminary results showed that such pilots were associated with a reduction in per-visit outpatient expenditures. There are fewer pilot programs for provider payment methods in villages where health care workers are the main source of prevention and primary care for rural residents. However, their situation differs in that the motivation to dispense drug prescriptions, including antibiotics and intravenous injections, for simple health problems, is the return to their net income. Whereas inpatient services have typically been billed based on the utilization of services, so-called case-based systems of payment have been piloted based on payment rates for each disease in its *International Classification of Diseases* code, with expenditure caps or a prospective budget to reduce incentives for providers to increase volume or transfer expenditures to nonintervention cases.[18]

REFORM

With only 29% of Chinese people in possession of health insurance, out-of-pocket expenses accounted for 58% of health care spending in 2002 as compared with 20% in 1978.[18] In a 2001 survey of residents from 3 Chinese provinces, one-half responded that they had given up health care in the previous 12 months because of its cost.[19] With increasing health costs, annual per capita spending on personal health services increased in China by a factor of 40 from roughly $1.35 to $55.00 from 1978 to 2002, whereas national spending on health care increased from 3.0% to nearly 5.5% of the GDP.[6] The decline in efficiency of the Chinese health care system has affected both urban and rural communities, however, more so in severely rural communities where only 3% of China's poorest rural western provinces have health insurance compared with 49% of urban Chinese. Notwithstanding, the quality of care in rural communities is generally inferior to that of its urban counterparts because of inadequately trained professionals, leading to relative underuse of rural services and overuse of urban ones. Such gaps in wealth, financial and physical access to care, and governmental and public health expenditures have had a differential effect on children less than 5 years of age and maternal mortality. In 2002 the former was comparatively worse in rural than urban areas, respectively, at 39 versus 14 per 1000 for children less than 5 years of age, as was the latter, maternal mortality, at 72 versus 54 per 100,000, respectively.

Anand and colleagues[20] studied human resources of doctors and nurses using year-end data in China at the province level during 1990 to 2005 to assess levels of education, health-care-worker density, measures of inequality for density of health workers, and provider quality. The investigators noted that about two-thirds of doctors and nearly all nurses were educated up to junior college only despite a massive expansion of medical education countrywide. There was significant inequality in the distribution of both doctors and nurses within provinces that varied with respect to health outcomes, which in some cases showed that the density of health workers was linked to rates of infant and maternal mortality.

China's performance in health care delivery was studied nationally and regionally using indices of health system coverage and catastrophic medical spending,[21] noting that provision of maternal and child health services was well addressed but poor in addressing noncommunicable diseases, notably hypertensive treatment. Those with low income received lower health system coverage than those with higher incomes but had an increased probability of either not seeking health care when ill or undergoing catastrophic medical spending. With mortality analysis showing a parallel transition in the major causes of death in the past 3 decades in China from communicable diseases and maternal and perinatal infectious conditions to noncommunicable chronic diseases, respectively accounting for 41% in 1973% and 74% of mortality in 2005, there was a staggering pace of increased age-standardized mortality of 10% from noncommunicable disease between 1991 and 2000.[22] Modification and prevention of behavioral risk factors, diet, hypertension, obesity, tobacco use, and the response to chronic disease have, thus, claimed center stage in China. Xiao and Kohrman[23] suggested integrating medical anthropological solutions in conjunction with legislation banning smoking in public places, uniformly high cigarette prices, and tobacco advertising bans[24] in arriving at a solution to tobacco use in China citing that smoking has been encouraged in Chinese society among men as a means of development, both economic and personal.[25]

Since 1978, after China adopted reform policies and opened up to the global community, the medical care system and health of residents have improved. Nevertheless, the main orientation of health care reform in the 1980s and 1990s was to render autonomy to government-owned public hospitals without contribution of public expenditures. With the emergence of for-profit privately owned hospitals, health care expenditures increased along with disparities between urban and rural areas and different provinces increased at the expense of health care coverage and access to services for most of its citizens, most of whom were the poorest. By absorbing and integrating experiences domestically and abroad, the new guidelines for China's health care reform have addressed core issues of equity and accessibility with strong public support.[26] According to Chen,[27] China's 2009 plan for health care reform marked the first phase toward achieving comprehensive health coverage by 2020. There are 5 essential components: first, systematic reform and affirming the government's role in wide medical research coverage for more than 90% of Chinese citizens; second, a national essential-drug system to meet the basic needs for treatment and prevention of diseases and to ensure safety, quality, and supply; third, improved grassroots-level medical care, with emphasis in rural areas on infrastructure and human resources in a 3-tier network at county, town, and village levels, and urban CMCs to alleviate overcrowding in city hospitals and foster a gatekeeper system led by family doctors and nurses; fourth, promotion of basic public health services; fifth, pilot program reforms to direct substantial increases in public investment, restricting of hospital management, and correction of commercialization and skewed financial incentives.

Eggleston and colleagues[28] proposed that improvement in quality of care, responsiveness to patients, efficiency, cost escalation, and equity could be improved not simply by shifting ownership to the private sector or by encouraging providers both public and private to compete with one another for individual patients but by changing the way providers were paid, shifting away from fee for service and amending the distorted price schedule. Other elements of active purchasing might contribute to improved outcomes in health services in China. With most patients continuing to receive treatment in government-owned facilities, the private sector has grown more rapidly than the public sector, especially in rural areas because many village clinics have been sold or taken over by individuals. With at least one government-owned township health center and other private clinics in each village area, the government has called for policies on subsides, taxation, and price setting for hospitals whether for profit or not or government or nongovernmentally owned. Basic medical insurance based on medical saving accounts combined with a social risk-pooling fund have been rolled out in urban communities, whereas the NCMS cooperative medical scheme, combining household contributions with central and local government subsidies, has been available since 2003. In 2013 a new health department, the national health and family planning commission (NHFPC), was established, merging with the MoH to improve medical and health care services and to deepen institutional reform in the medical care and public health sectors.[29]

Tian and colleagues[30] conducted a cross-sectional survey in 2011 of 12 randomly sampled counties and 118 villages in China using indicators to assess coverage, equality, and effectiveness of rural public health services noting the most difficulties in noncommunicable disease management, especially in those with the lowest incomes. Implementation of health care reform to rectify access to public health services, which increased from 2008 to 2009, has still not corrected significant interregional and intraregional inequalities in health care access.

Yip and coworkers[31] noted difficulties in transforming money and insurance coverage into cost-effective services when the delivery of health care was hindered by waste, inefficiencies, poor quality of services, scarcity, and maldistribution of qualified providers. There seemed to be the need for reforming incentive structures for providers, improved governance of public hospitals, and institution of stronger regulatory systems efforts of which have been slowed by opposition from stakeholders and lack of implementation capacity.

Yip and Hsiao[12] studied China's 2009 health care reform proposal noting that, although expansion of insurance coverage was accomplished, the goal of affordable and equitable access to quality health care for all of its citizens might not be obtained because of wasteful and inefficient health care service provision. The privatization of profit-driven public hospital sectors combined with a fragmented for-profit system would result in an escalation of health care expenditures with patients bearing increasing costs and poor population outcome due to an eventual 2-tier care system. Reformed for the public's interest, public and private collaboration might be further expanded after an objective assessment of its effect on China's health policy goals. This reform would include the following factors: recreation of exemplary models of public hospitals to provide equal, accessible, and quality universal health care; creation of a board to which public hospitals would be accountable; and reasonable salaries to physicians.

In spite of leading the way for world progress in alleviating extreme poverty over the last 2 decades, the Chinese have been charged with active suppression of health information at home, contributing to initial failures during the severe acute respiratory syndrome (SARS) epidemic; however, Hesketh and Xing[32] argue that inadequacy of data collection systems and a target-driven culture were partly to blame. Health care reform for elderly Chinese citizens has included recommendations to accelerate development of community-based primary health care, educational programs to increase basic knowledge about health among the elderly and the promotion of healthy behaviors, as well as increasing the Social Security Fund of pension reserves, which is presently 2% of the GDP.[33]

The reemergence of selected infectious diseases, such as gonorrhea and syphilis, has been associated with a large increase in migrant populations and in commercial sex, whereas others, such as AIDS, SARS, highly pathogenic avian influenza, *Streptococcus suis*, and the zoonoses, present new microbial threats notably because of the increasing size and density of populations that present opportunities for large epidemics and the need for swift national responses to prevent international spread.[34] To address these and other future microbial threats, the Chinese government has promised to commit substantial resources to the implementation of new strategies, including the development of real-time monitoring systems as part of its infectious disease surveillance.

With increasing worldwide needs on the biomedicine center stage, the development of biomedical research in China has become a massive and unique challenge.[35] While encouraging researcher-initiated projects by increasing the budget of the National Natural Science Foundation nearly 5-fold over the past decade, China has been able to launch key programs and establish major scientific facilities in genomics, proteomics, gene therapy, and stem-cell research. With the move toward scientific development, China has placed public health at the top of its agenda, with the aim of Health for All by 2020. China is poised to boost accessibility and equal provision of health services with cutting-edge technology in a serve-all approach combined with drug innovation and prevention and control of major emerging infectious diseases.

GLOBAL BURDEN OF DISEASE 2013: IMPLICATIONS FOR NEUROLOGY

Following the methods of the Global Burden of Disease Study 2013,[36] investigators systematically analyzed all available demographic and epidemiologic data sources for China at the provincial level and developed methods to aggregate county-level surveillance data to inform provincial-level analysis; the investigators used local data to develop specific garbage code redistribution procedures for China. They assessed levels of and trends in all-cause mortality, causes of death, and YLL in all 33 province-level administrative units in Mainland China, all of which were referred to as provinces, for the years between 1990 and 2013.

All provinces in Mainland China have made substantial strides to improve life expectancy at birth between 1990 and 2013. Increases ranged from 4.0 years in Hebei province to 14.2 years in Tibet. Improvements in female life expectancy exceeded those in male life expectancy in all provinces except Shanghai, Macao, and Hong Kong. There was a significant heterogeneity among provinces in life expectancy at birth and probability of death at 0 to 14, 15 to 49, and 50 to 74 years of age. Such heterogeneity was also present in cause of death structures between sexes and provinces. From 1990 to 2013, leading causes of YLLs changed substantially. In 1990, 16 of 33 provinces had lower respiratory infections or preterm birth complications as the leading causes of YLLs. Fifteen provinces had cerebrovascular disease and 2 (Hong Kong and Macao) had ischemic heart disease. By 2013, 27 provinces had cerebrovascular disease as the leading cause, 5 had ischemic heart disease, and one had lung cancer (Hong Kong). Road injuries became a top 10 cause of death in all provinces in Mainland China. The most common noncommunicable diseases, including ischemic heart disease, stroke, chronic obstructive pulmonary disease, and cancers (liver, stomach, and lung), contributed much more to YLLs in 2013 compared with 1990.

REFERENCES

1. Wang H, Dwyer-Lindgren L, Lofgren KT, et al. Age-specific and sex-specific mortality in 187 countries, 1970-2010: a systematic analysis for the Global Burden of Disease Study 2010. Lancet 2012;380:2071–94.
2. Yang G, Wang Y, Zeng Y, et al. Rapid health transition in China, 1990-2010: findings from the Global Burden of Diseases Study 2010. Lancet 2013;381(9882):1987–2015.
3. Countdown Coverage Writing Group, Countdown to 2015 Core Group, Bryce J, Daelmans B, Dwivedi A, et al. Countdown to 2015 for maternal, newborn, and child survival: the 2008 report on tracking coverage of interventions. Lancet 2008;371:1247–58.
4. Han Q, Chen L, Evans T, et al. China and global health. Lancet 2008;372:1439–41.
5. Dong Z, Phillips MR. Evolution of China's health-care system. Lancet 2008;372:1715–6.
6. Blumenthal D, Hsiao W. Privatization and its discontents-the evolving Chinese health care system. N Engl J Med 2005;353:1165–70.
7. Hesketh T, Wei XZ. Health in China: from Mao to market reform. BMJ 1997;314:1543–5.
8. Yarkley J. Xinmin village journal: a deadly fever, once defeated, lurks in a Chinese lake. New York Times 2005;A4.
9. Liu Y, Rao K, Fei J. Economic transition and health transition: comparing China and Russia. Health Policy 1998;44:103–22.
10. Liu Y. China's public health-care system: facing the challenges. Bull World Health Organ 2004;82:532–8.
11. Hesketh T, Zhu W. Health in China: the healthcare market. BMJ 2004;314:1616–8.
12. Yip W, Hsiao W. Harnessing the privatization of China's fragmented health-care delivery. Lancet 2014;384:805–18.
13. Bhattacharyya O, Delu Y, Wong S, et al. Evolution of primary care in China 1997-2009. Health Policy 2011;100:174–80.
14. Pan X, Dib H, Wang X, et al. Service utilization in community health centers in China: a comparison analysis with local hospitals. BMJ 2006;6:93.
15. Yip WC, Hsiao W, Meng Q, et al. Realignment of incentives for health-care providers in China. Lancet 2010;375:1120–30.
16. Wang R, Henderson G. Medical research ethics in China. Lancet 2008;372:1867–8.
17. Yao L. Pilot study on separating revenues and expenditures accounting system. Beijing (China): Ministry of Health Project; 2007.
18. General Office of MoH. To carry out experiments in use of case-based payment systems. Beijing (China): Ministry of Health General Office; 2004.
19. Liu Y, Rao K, Hsiao WC. Medical spending and rural impoverishment in China. J Health Popul Nutr 2003;21:216–22.

20. Anand S, Fan V, Zhang J, et al. China's human resources for health: quality, quality and distribution. Lancet 2008;372:1774–81.
21. Liu Y, Rao K, Gakidou E. China's health system performance. Lancet 2008;372: 1914–23.
22. Yang G, Kong L, Zhao W, et al. Emergence of chronic non-communicable diseases in China. Lancet 2008;372:1697–705.
23. Xiao S, Kohrman M. Anthropology in China's health promotion and tobacco. Lancet 2008;372:1617–8.
24. Frieden TR, Bloomberg MR. How to prevent 100 million deaths from tobacco. Lancet 2007;369:1758–81.
25. Kohrman M. Depoliticizing tobacco's exceptionality: male sociality, death, and memory-making among Chinese cigarette smokers. China J 2007;58:85–109.
26. Liu Y. Reforming China's health care: for the people, by the people? Lancet 2009; 373:281–3.
27. Chen Z. Launch of the health-care reform plan in China. Lancet 2009;373:1322–4.
28. Eggleston K, Ling L, Qingyue M, et al. Health service delivery in China: a literature review. Health Econ 2008;17:149–65.
29. Wang H. China's new health department: progress and priorities. Lancet 2014; 384:733–4.
30. Tian M, Feng D, Chen X, et al. China's rural public health system performance: a cross-sectional study. PLoS One 2013;8:e83822.
31. Yip W, Hsiao W, Chen W, et al. Early appraisal of China's huge and complex health-care reforms. Lancet 2012;379:833–42.
32. Hesketh T, Xing Z. Human rights in China. Lancet 2006;368:27.
33. Wang X, Chen P. Population ageing challenges health care in China. Lancet 2014;383:870.
34. Wang L, Wang Y, Jin S, et al. Emergence and control of infectious diseases in China. Lancet 2008;372:1598–605.
35. Chen Z, Wang HG, Wen ZJ, et al. Life sciences and biotechnology in China. Philos Trans R Soc Lond B Biol Sci 2007;362:947–57.
36. Zhou M, Wang H, Zhu J, et al. Cause-specific mortality for 240 causes in China during 1990-2013: a systematic subnational analysis for the Global Burden of Disease Study 2013. Lancet 2016;387(10015):251–72.

Health Care in South Africa

David S. Younger, MD, MPH, MS[a,b,]*

KEYWORDS

• South Africa • Health care • Public health • Global health • Epidemiology

KEY POINTS

- The South African health care system is embedded in a background of racial subordination and sexual violence against girls and women, fostering vulnerability to HIV/AIDS and epidemic sexually transmitted disease.
- Hierarchical male authority from youth to adulthood has accentuated epidemic communicable disease through multiple sexual partners, polygamous marriage, and secret concurrent relationships.
- Low wages, unemployment, urban overcrowding, inadequate sanitation, malnutrition, crime, and violence all contribute to economic and health inequality.
- Unacceptable rates of infant mortality and mortality rates for children less than 5 years and increased age-standardized death rates from communicable diseases and noncommunicable diseases (NCDs) are highly prevalent.
- There is inequity between men and women in provinces, between urban and rural communities, and between the white and black races in South Africa.
- African countries are undergoing an epidemiologic transition driven by sociodemographic and lifestyle changes. The burden of NCDs, including cardiovascular risk factors, is increasing.
- The incidence of stroke, a cardinal complication of cardiovascular risk factors, seems to be rising in Africa and other low-income and middle-income country settings.

BACKGROUND

Brazil, Russia, India, China, and South Africa are members of the BRICS nations. Collectively, the BRICS are useful comparisons because of their size; racial, ethnic, and geographic diversity; and inherent problems of social inequality, making them more similar to the United States than their European counterparts. South Africa has experienced a remarkable epidemiologic and demographic transition during the past several decades. This article examines the health care system and the global burden of diseases of South Africa.

The author has nothing to disclose.
[a] Division of Neuroepidemiology, Department of Neurology, New York University School of Medicine, New York, NY, USA; [b] College of Global Public Health, New York University, New York, NY, USA
* Corresponding author. 333 East 34th Street, 1J, New York, NY 10016.
E-mail address: david.younger@nyumc.org

Neurol Clin 34 (2016) 1127–1136
http://dx.doi.org/10.1016/j.ncl.2016.06.004
0733-8619/16/$ – see front matter © 2016 Elsevier Inc. All rights reserved.

neurologic.theclinics.com

Coovadia and colleagues[1] described the social, political, and economic contexts of health in South Africa. The first European settlement brought permanent European settlers to the Cape of Good Hope in 1652. The indigenous Africans, whose ancestry dated back tens of millennia, were disposed of their land and later exported as slaves and became some of the ancestors of the people later designated as colored under apartheid. The country was transformed from an agricultural to an industrial and mining economy after discovery of diamonds and gold in the 1800s, leading to an indentured male black labor force that subsequently became the mainstay of social, economic, and political developments and a determinant of health and disease patterns. With the growth of the black population in the early 1900s and racial segregation of urban areas, communicable diseases, such as tuberculosis (TB), were present in more than 90% of black adults. Despite formation of the African National Congress in 1912 that opposed formation of the Union of South Africa, advocating for participation of the country's black majority for decades to come, the National Party of right-wing politicians consolidated the state policy of apartheid that excluded blacks from the political system, marginalized them economically, and separated blacks socially, reinforcing 3 decades of racial injustice. Pressure from resistance, reformists, and an easing of the white ruling class helped dismantle apartheid, allowing the country to hold to its first democratic election in 1994. Yet embedded in the background of racial discrimination were key contributors to the country's health problems, such as subordination and sexual violence against girls and women, which fostered vulnerability to HIV/AIDS and epidemic sexually transmitted disease, and culturally embedded hierarchical male authority, from youth to adulthood, that accentuated epidemic communicable disease through multiple sexual partners, polygamous marriage, and secret concurrent relationships.

Low wages, unemployment, urban overcrowding, inadequate sanitation, malnutrition, crime, and violence have all contributed to economic and health inequality, with sustained unacceptable rates of infant mortality, mortality rates for children under 5 years, age-standardized death rates from communicable and NCDs, and inequity between men and women in provinces, between urban and rural communities and between the white and black races in South Africa. To illustrate, the infant mortality of the black population was 67 per 1000 compared with 7 per 1000 in whites in 2002,[2] with an almost 3-fold difference between middle-class areas and squatter settlements within the Cape Town metropolitan area,[3] and the under 5-year mortality rate for children was 46 per 1000 live births in the Western Cape province compared with 116 in the KwaZulu-Natal province. Age-standardized death rates from asthma and TB in men in the Eastern Cape province were 4 times greater than in the Western Cape province or Gauteng province,[4] and despite the higher rate of HIV infection in women, mortality was 1.38-fold higher in men, with alcohol accounting for 7% of all deaths in South Africa in 2000 and 4 times as many alcohol-related deaths in men than women.

GEOGRAPHY

The map of South Africa is shown in **Fig. 1**. It occupies the southern tip of Africa with a coastline that stretches more than 2500 km from its desert border with Namibia on the Atlantic coast, southward around the tip of Africa, and north to the border, with subtropical Mozambique on the Indian Ocean. South Africa borders Namibia, Botswana, and Zimbabwe to the north and Mozambique to the east and curves around Swaziland before rejoining Mozambique's southern border. The coast lies low for most of its distance but gives way to mountainous regions. With a total land area of more than 1.2 million km², it is one-eighth the size of the United States, twice that of France, and

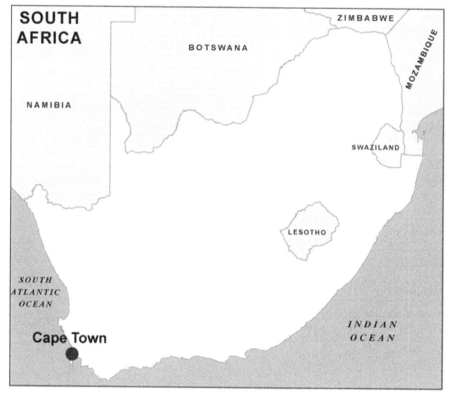

Fig. 1. Geography of South Africa. (*From* MapOpenSource. Available at: http://www.maps opensource.com/south-africa-capital-map-black-and-white.html.)

more than 3 times the size of Germany; South Africa has 9 provinces that vary in size from smaller Gauteng, Eastern Cape, North West, Free State, KwaZulu-Natal, Limpopo, Mpumalanga, and Western Cape to larger arid Northern Cape. In the interior is the small mountainous country of Lesotho surrounded by South African territory. The 3 capital cities are the legislative capital of Cape Town in the Western Cape, the judicial capital of Bloemfontein in the Free State; and the administrative capital city of Pretoria in Gauteng, home to the Union Buildings and a large proportion of the public service. The largest and most important city, however, is Johannesburg, the economic heartland of the country. Other important centers include Durban and Pietermaritzburg in KwaZulu-Natal and Port Elizabeth in the Eastern Cape.

SOCIAL DEMOGRAPHY AND VITAL STATISTICS

The vital statistics of South Africa area shown in **Table 1**. With a population of approximately 49,668, 000 in South Africa of 804,865,000 of the entire African region in 2008, according to the African Health Observatory (www.afro.who.int), a substantial portion of the population resides in the 20 to 30 years of age category, divided equally between men and women (**Fig. 2**); 61% of the population reside in urban communities, increased from 52% in 1990. In 2012, according to Motsoaledi,[5] 4 key health indicators, including life expectancy, maternal and child mortality, the burden of disease related to HIV and TB, and strengthening of the effectiveness of the health system,

Table 1 Vital statistics: South Africa	
Population	1.36 Billion (July 2014 estimated)
Life expectancy at birth	Total population: 75.2 y Male: 73.1 y Female: 77.4 y
Maternal mortality ratio	37 Deaths/100,000 live births (2010)
Infant mortality ratio	14.8 Deaths/1000 live births
Literacy rate	Total population: 95.1% Male: 97.5% Female: 92.7%
GDP	$13.39 Trillion (2013 estimated)
GDP per capita	$9800 (2013 estimated)
Population below poverty line	6.1%
Health expenditures	5.2% of GDP (2011)
Physician density	1.46 Physicians/1000 population (2010)
Hospital bed density	3.8 Beds/1000 population (2009)
HDI	0.629
Gini coefficient	65

Abbreviations: GDP, gross domestic product; HDI, Human Development Index.
From The world factbook 2016–17. Washington, DC: Central Intelligence Agency; 2016. Available at: https://www.cia.gov/library/publications/the-world-factbook/index.html.

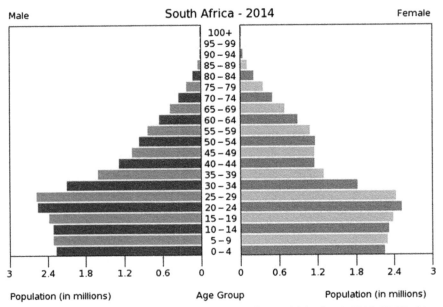

Fig. 2. Population pyramid of South Africa. (*From* The world factbook 2016–17. Washington, DC: Central Intelligence Agency; 2016. Available at: https://www.cia.gov/library/publications/the-world-factbook/index.html.)

have improved since the preceding 3 years. Life expectancy at birth increased from 56.5 to 60 years, child mortality decreased from 40 to 30 per 1000 children, and infant mortality fell from 40 to 30 per 1000 infants,[6] due largely to improved performance in the public health sector, with successes in mother-to-child transmission of HIV, provision of antiretroviral therapy, more HIV and TB tests, and medical male circumcisions than ever before. Child and infant mortality has been impacted by application of the rotavirus and pneumococcal vaccines introduced in 2009, and broad improvements were made in social determinants of health with the 2011 census, evidenced by more than three-quarters of South Africans having formal housing, access to running water, and electricity in their dwelling and more than one-half with flushing toilets.

Despite social grants, 45% of the population of South Africa lives in absolute poverty, surviving on $2 per day, and more than 10 million people on less than $1 per day, below which they are unable to purchase enough food for an adequate diet.[7] With a Gini coefficient increasing from 0.6 in 1995 to 0.7 in 2009, the top 10% of South Africans earn approximately 58% of the total annual national income whereas the bottom 70% combined earn only 17%. The annual per capita expenditure on health ranges from $140 in the public sector to $1400 in the private sector, with disparities in the provision of health care services. The national public health sector, staffed by approximately 30% of the country's physicians, provides care to approximately 40 million people, or 84% of the national population, who are uninsured. Approximately 16%, or 8 million Africans, who are privately insured, receive health care from the 70% of remaining physicians, as do 25% of uninsured people who pay out of pocket for private care.

INFRASTRUCTURE

Rapid economic growth of South Africa between 1960 and 1970, which gave rise to a strong private health sector supportive of academic medicine, consumed a third of the 5% of gross national product (GNP) devoted to health care; however, they were mainly hospital based, providing a mixture of community and tertiary health care.[8] With 60% of the country's physicians caring for 80% of the population and accounting for 70% of the national health expenditure in the late 1970s, one-half went to academic institutions, where the bulk of public medicine was practiced, and the ratio of private to public earnings was 2 to 3:1. Over the next 2 decades, private tertiary medical facilities expanded that were unsupportive of academic medicine. With 80% of whites insured compared with only 15% of blacks, the proportion of GNP spend on health care increased to 8%, two-thirds of which was consumed by the private sector. The cost of health insurance continued to rise to more than 3 times the rate of the consumer price index and academic medicine. The academic and public sectors suffered under the wave of privatization, with a further widening of the private to public physician salary ratio to 5:1 and emigration of medical, nursing, and technological staff to private institutions. Acknowledging the importance of the social basis of health, the new government has opted for a district-based primary care system; however, the process of reform was complicated by a nationalization process of redistribution that was unsuccessful and economic growth that fell short of expectations. With a government income 35% of GNP and 40% of expenditures, redistribution policies were coupled instead with fiscal discipline. Four major principles of reform to reach equity included reallocation of budgets in line with the populations in each of the 9 provinces, reshaping of the racial and gender compositions of the public health sector, change in ideology toward primary care, and a shift in the investigative thrust toward essential national health research. Hampered by stasis of the health management bureaucracy of the past decade, leadership by the Ministry of Health (MoH) and current managers have implemented policy and health system–level changes into the public service sector at a time when mortality has worsened because of HIV/AIDS, TB, and malaria[9-11]; NCDs[7,12]; childhood illness and malnutrition[13,14]; and interpersonal violence and accidents.[15]

REFORM

After approximately 7 previous attempts to introduce universal health coverage since 1928, National Health Service reform arrived to South Africa in 2009 with a phase-in period of approximately 14 years. It calls for tax funding of health services, merging of the well-resourced private and poorly resourced public sectors, and improvement in the balance between community-based and hospital-centered medical care. The experience of National Health Insurance piloted in 10 selected health districts[16] was harshly criticized for lack of compliance with quality standards, long wait times, and interruption of care due to unavailable resources.[17]

With use of both allopathic and traditional African healers for their ailments, the South African Traditional Health Practitioners Act[18] defined traditional health practice for South Africans using indigenous techniques and principles of traditional medicine, including physical and mental preparation for puberty, childbirth, and death. The number of new medical students enrolling annually increased by 34% between 2000 and 2012 during a period characterized by a demographic shift of greater black African and female enrollees.[7] Although the number of graduates increased by 18% between 2000 and 2012, the ratio of physicians per 1000 population was unchanged between 2004 (0.77) and 2011 (0.76), failing to keep up with population growth, at a rate less than Brazil's in 2008 (1.76), Russia's in 2006 (4.31), and China's in 2010 (1.46), although better than India's in 2009 (0.65). The emigration of health professionals to the United Kingdom, the United States (US), and Canada has resulted in loss of more than $2 billion in US dollars. The effort to strengthen existing public facilities and strive for high-quality teaching has coincided with the launch of a 10-year science and technology plan by the government.[19]

AFRICAN EBOLA OUTBREAK

The deadly virus, Ebola, is now the most feared because of the severe disease it causes and the high case-fatality rate of 90%.[20] It is caused by an enveloped, non-segmental RNA virus with characteristic filamentous particles that gives the virus family its name. First reported in the 2 African locations of southern Sudan and northern Zaire, now the Democratic Republic of the Congo,[21,22] by distinct species of the Ebola virus, namely Sudan ebolavirus and Zaire ebolavirus. A third African Ebola species was isolated from an infected ethnologist who worked in the Taï Forest reserve in the Ivory Coast after conducting a necropsy on an infected chimpanzee that had derived from a troop that lost several members to Ebola hemorrhagic fever.[23] The latest African Ebola species of human pathogenic Ebola virus was found in equatorial Africa.[24,25] Ebola virus disease (EVD) remains a plague for the population of equatorial Africa, with an increase in numbers and outbreaks since 2000 and almost all cases due to the emergence or re-emergence of known viral species. Contained in arboreal bat species with bat-to-bat and incidental human transmission through close contact with animals, human, outbreaks occur through close contact with infected tissues and body fluids, such as during preparation of bodies for burial, while spread is also amplified in hospitals with poor infection control practices. To date, there have been 2 cases of EVD in South Africa, 1 of which was a source patient, a physician, and the other a nurse who cared for him.[26] The latter died of thrombocytopenia and cerebral hemorrhage, and the diagnosis was confirmed retrospectively by the physician who survived. None of the other 300 contacts contracted the illness and the investigators concluded that identification of high-risk patients and use of universal blood and body fluid precautions decrease the risk of nosocomial spread. According to Polonsky and colleagues,[27] the increasing frequency of epidemics resulted from the combination of improvements in monitoring and diagnostic capabilities, increase among humans and natural reservoirs of the virus, and growth of the viral load and prevalence of the virus in reservoirs. Destruction of forests and human impact on broader areas also contribute to the increase in frequency and severity of outbreaks. Ebola virus infection can occur in the human population at a significant rate that does not always entail the emergence of epidemics. Ebola virus is detected in most patient secretions, including blood, saliva, feces, breast mild, tears, and genital secretion, but not from vomit, sputum, sweat, or urine.[28] The largest Ebola virus outbreak in West Africa, in particular New Guinea, Sierra Leone, and Liberia, resulted in 3, 338 deaths as of October 1, 2014.[29] With recognition that the index case patient had contracted Ebola virus in Liberia and had flown to Lagos, Nigeria, with a stopover in Lomé, Togo, where he became symptomatic and sought medical attention, it is not inconceivable that other cases could occur in South Africa similar to the occurrence of localized transmission in both Spain and the United States by infected travelers and health care workers.[30] The success of Nigeria and Senegal in halting the transmission of EVD highlights the critical importance of preparedness, including strong political leadership, early detection by a variety of rapid serologic tests, and the possession of a United Nations Mission for Ebola Emergency Response protocol for suspected cases. The treatment of Ebola virus commences with exclusion of other mimickers, such as malaria and typhoid fever, with prompt institution of supportive and symptomatic measures, such as isolation, malaria treatment, broad-spectrum antibiotics, antipyretics, and intravenous fluids, toward maintenance of blood volume and prevention of systemic shock, cerebral edema, and disseminated anticoagulation, all of which can be offered in field hospitals, as can treatment with human convalescent blood or serum for passive immunization. Prevention is forthcoming using one of several approaches, the likeliest of which is a live attenuated recombinant Ebola viral vaccine.

GLOBAL BURDEN OF DISEASE 2013: IMPLICATIONS FOR NEUROLOGY

African countries are undergoing an epidemiologic transition driven by sociodemographic and lifestyle changes. The burden of NCDs, including cardiovascular risk factors, is increasing. Consequently, the incidence of stroke, a cardinal complication of cardiovascular risk factors, seems to be rising in Africa and other low and middle-income country (LMIC) settings. Therefore, 86% of all stroke deaths around the world are contributed by LMICs in Africa and other continents. By contrast, the incidence of stroke seems to be declining in high-income countries. Ironically, there is insufficient information on the current epidemiology of stroke in African countries and other LMICs, where this knowledge is needed most. This is due to and contributes to deficient manpower and other resources to combat the epidemic. Accurate, up-to-date information on stroke burden is necessary for the development and evaluation of effective and efficient preventative acute care and rehabilitation programs for stroke patients.

In an attempt to fill this gap, the Global Burden of Diseases collaborators published data on the burden of stroke and stroke subtype, and 1 meta-analysis[31] focused solely on the prevalence and incidence of stroke in Africa, albeit with pooled data of uneven quality. From reported overall crude incidence and prevalence of stroke in a given cohort, a random effect of this meta-analysis was conducted with pooled effect of stroke expressed per 100,000 person years or population. The overall data estimates of age-specific and gender-specific prevalence and incidence from all studies were used and adjusted for mean ages and the crude prevalence and incidence rates of stroke from all studies and modeled corresponding to the given sample size. A fitted curve explained the largest proportion of variance (best fit). It estimated new cases of stroke and number of stroke survivors in populations across 5-year age groups.

There were more than 483,000 new cases of stroke in Africa in 2009 among people aged 15 years or more, equivalent to 81.2 (13.2–94.9)/100,000 per year, with approximately 305,000 and more than 178,000 new cases of stroke, equivalent to 103.3 (20.7–109.2)/100,000 per year and 59.5 (6.9–84.3)/100,000 per year among men and women, respectively. Comparable figures for the years 2010 and 2013 based on the same incidence rates were 496,000 (80.6–579.7 thousand) and 535,000 (87.0–625.3 thousand) new stroke cases, respectively, suggesting an increase of 10.8% between 2009 and 2013 that is attributable to growth and ageing of the African population alone.

The estimated number of stroke survivors in Africa in 2009 was 1.89 million among people aged 15 years or more, with a prevalence of 317.3 (314.0–748.2)/100,000 population. There were approximately 990,000 and 898,000 stroke survivors equivalent to 335.5 (302.3–702.7)/100,000 and 299.3 (268.4–579.0)/100,000 among men and women, respectively. Based on the same prevalence rates, comparable figures for the year 2010 and 2013 amount to 1.94 million (1.90–4.57 million) and 2.09 million (2.06–4.93 million) stroke survivors, respectively, suggesting an increase of 9.6% between 2009 and 2013 that is attributable to growth and ageing of the African population.

The prevention of stroke and many NCDs in Africa has been affected mainly by weak health systems and poor government response. To date, the priorities of many African countries remain infectious diseases, mainly HIV/AIDS, malaria, and TB. Despite the availability of affordable and cost-effective stroke prevention initiatives. African countries do not have national strategies to address smoking, alcohol, physical inactivity, and unhealthy diets, including reducing salt and fat contents of processed foods, and stroke units, where the awareness on these risk factors could have been raised, are rarely available. Hypertension is the main risk factor of all stroke subtypes, with odds of approximately 2.64, and this is more prominent among young Africans who present with stroke unaware of their high blood pressure status. There is an urgent need for more research on stroke and related vascular disease risk factors to appropriately quantify this burden. An investment in research capacity, basically to conduct and fund higher-quality research, may help raise awareness on stroke burden in Africa. An awareness and fair understanding of stroke burden and disease pattern in Africa may further prompt appropriate policy response and scale up current intervention programs.

REFERENCES

1. Coovadia H, Jewkes R, Barron P, et al. The health and health system of South Africa: historical roots and current public health challenges. Lancet 2009;374: 817–34.

2. Bradshaw D, Nannan N. Health status. In: Ijumba P, Day C, Ntuli A, editors. The South African health review 2003/2004. Durban (South Africa): Health Systems Trust; 2004.

3. Groenewald P, Bradshaw D, Daniels J, et al. Cause of death and premature mortality in Cape Town, 201–2006. Cape Town (South Africa): Medical Research Council; 2008.

4. Bradshaw D, Nannan N, Naubscher R, et al. South African national burden of disease study 2000. Estimates of provincial mortality. Cape Town (South Africa): Medical Research Council; 2007.

5. Motsoaledi A. Progress and changes in the South African health sector. Lancet 2012;380:1969–70.

6. Bradshaw D, Dorrington RE, Laubscher R. Rapid mortality surveillance report 2011. Cape Town (South Africa): South African Medical Research Council; 2012.

7. Mayosi BM, Benatar SR. Health and health care in South Africa-20 years after Mandela. N Engl J Med 2014;371:1344–53.

8. Kirsch R. Country profile. South Africa. Lancet 1997;349:1537–45.

9. Abdool SS, Churchyard GJ, Abdool Karim Q, et al. HIV infection and tuberculosis in South Africa: an urgent need to escalate the public response. Lancet 2009; 374:921–33.

10. Wagner B, Blower S. Costs of eliminating HIV in South Africa have been underestimated. Lancet 2010;376:953–4.

11. Tollman SM, Kahn K, Sartorius B, et al. Implications of mortality transition for primary health care in rural South Africa: a population-based surveillance study. Lancet 2008;372:893–901.

12. Baleta A, Mitchell F. Country in focus: diabetes and obesity in South Africa. Lancet Diabetes Endocrinol 2014;2:687–8.

13. Chopra M, Lawn JE, Sanders D, et al. Achieving the health Millennium Developmental Goals for South Africa: challenges and priorities. Lancet 2009;374: 1023–31.

14. Chopra M, Daviaud E, Pattinson R, et al. Saving the lives of South Africa's mothers, babies, and children: can the health system deliver? Lancet 2009; 374:835–46.

15. Seedat M, Van Niekerk A, Jewkes R, et al. Violence and injuries in South Africa: prioritizing an agenda for prevention. Lancet 2009;374:1011–22.

16. Baleta A. South Africa rolls out pilot health insurance scheme. Lancet 2012;379: 1185.

17. Harris B, Goudge J, Ataguba JE, et al. Inequities in access to health care in South Africa. J Public Health Policy 2011;32(Suppl 1):S102–23.

18. Peltzer K. Traditional health practitioners in South Africa. Lancet 2009;374:956–7.

19. Gevers W. Clinical research in South Africa: a core asset under pressure. Lancet 2009;374:760–1.

20. Weyer J, Blumberg LH, Paweska JT. Ebola virus disease in West Africa-an unprecedented outbreak. S Afr Med J 2014;104:555–6.

21. WHO. Ebola haemorrhagic fever in Sudan, 1976. Bull World Health Organ 1978; 56:247–70.

22. WHO. Ebola haemorrhagic fever in Zaire, 1976. Bull World Health Organ 1978;56: 271–93.

23. Le Gueeno B, Formenty P, Wyers M, et al. Isolation and partial characterization of a new strain of Ebola virus. Lancet 1995;345:1271–4.

24. Towner JS, Sealy TK, Khristova ML, et al. Newly discovered Ebola virus associated with hemorrhagic fever outbreak in Uganda. PLoS Pathog 2008;4:e1000212.

25. Jahrling PB, Geisbert TW, Johnson ED, et al. Preliminary report: isolation of Ebola virus from monkeys imported to USA. Lancet 1990;335:502–5.
26. Richards GA, Murphy S, Jobson R, et al. Unexpected Ebola virus in a tertiary setting: Clinical and epidemiological aspects. Crit Care Med 2000;28:240–4.
27. Polonsky JA, Warmala JF, de Clerk H, et al. Emerging filoviral disease in Uganda: proposed explanations and research directions. Am J Trop Med Hyg 2014;90: 790–3.
28. Chippaux J-P. Outbreaks of Ebola virus disease in Africa: the beginnings of a tragic saga. J Venom Anim Toxins Incl Trop Dis 2014;20:44.
29. Fasina FO, Shittu A, Lazarus D, et al. Transmission dynamics and control of Ebola virus disease outbreak in Nigeria, July to September 2014. Euro Surveill 2014; 19(40):20920.
30. WHO. Ebola response roadmap situation report. Global Alert and Response Bulletins. World Health Organization; 2014.
31. Adeloye D. An estimate of the incidence and prevalence of stroke in Africa: a systematic review and meta-analysis. PLoS One 2014;9(6):e100724.

Special Article

Quick Evidence Synopsis
Nonsteroidal Anti-Inflammatory Drugs for Alzheimer Disease

Authors: David R. Goldmann, MD, Tatyana A. Shamliyan, MD, MS

Clinical question this synopsis is addressing: What are the benefits and harms of nonsteroidal anti-inflammatory drugs (NSAIDs) for Alzheimer disease?

Intervention	Quality of Evidence	Balance Between Benefits and Harms
NSAIDs vs placebo	Low	Likely harmful Evidence suggests that traditional nonselective NSAIDs or selective cyclooxygenase-2 (COX-2) inhibitors do not improve patient or caregiver outcomes but can cause adverse effects in adults with mild to moderate Alzheimer disease

Quality of evidence: Quality of evidence scale (GRADE): high, moderate, low, and very low. For more information on the GRADE rating system, see http://www.gradeworkinggroup.org/.

Balance between benefits and harms: The Guideline Elements Model: beneficial, likely to be beneficial, unknown effectiveness, tradeoff between benefits and harms, likely harmful, and harmful. For more information, see http://gem.med.yale.edu/default.htm.

What are the parameters of our evidence search?

PICO	
Population	Adults with Alzheimer disease, diagnosed according to the Diagnostic and Statistical Manual of Mental Disorders or the World Health Organization classification of mental and behavioral disorders (*International Statistical Classification of Diseases, 10th Revision*) Patient demographics, disease severity
Intervention	NSAIDs, including selective COX-2 inhibitors (eg, nimesulide, rofecoxib, celecoxib) and traditional NSAIDs (eg, aspirin, naproxen, indomethacin, ibuprofen, piroxicam, diclofenac)
Comparator	Placebo
Primary Outcome(s)	Mortality, cognition, disability, quality of life All harms

What is the basis for the conclusion(s)?

Population: Adults with mild to moderate Alzheimer disease (Mini-Mental State Examination score of 13–26)
Settings: Any
Intervention: NSAIDs (any drug and dose)
Comparator: Placebo

Neurol Clin 34 (2016) 1137–1141
http://dx.doi.org/10.1016/j.ncl.2016.08.002
0733-8619/16

neurologic.theclinics.com

Table 1
Nonsteroidal anti-inflammatory drugs versus placebo for adults with Alzheimer disease

Outcome	Risk with Intervention per 1000	Risk with Comparator per 1000	Relative Measure of Association (95% CI)	Number of Participants (Studies)	Quality of the Evidence (GRADE)	Comments
All-cause mortality, 3 y	25	12	RR 1.6 (0.8; 3.3)	1930 (6 RCTs)[1,2]	Low	No difference
Cognitive performance as measured with ADAS-cog+ score,[a] 3 y	NR	NR	MD −1.1 (−2.6; 0.4) SMD −0.1 (−0.3; 0.1)	1964 (11 RCTs)[1,2]	Very low	No difference
Cognition as measured with MMSE score,[a] 3 y	NR	NR	**MD −1.08 (−2.21; 0.04) SMD −0.55 (−1.08; −0.03)**	**1268 (6 RCTs)[1]**	**Very low**	**Favors placebo**
Global clinical dementia rating as measured with CDR sum score,[a] 3 y	NR	NR	MD 0.03 (−0.25; 0.30) SMD 0.00 (−0.12; 0.12)	1124 (6 RCTs)[1]	Low	No difference
Behavioral disturbance measured with BEHAVE-AD score,[a] 3 y	NR	NR	MD 0.30 (−1.58; 2.19) SMD 0.08 (−0.30; 0.47)	479 (6 RCTs)[1]	Very low	No difference
Activities of daily living as measured with ADL score,[a] 3 y	NR	NR	MD −0.26 (−0.82; 0.30) SMD −0.22 (−0.48; 0.03)	1737 (6 RCTs)[1]	Very low	No difference
Quality of life as measured with PSMS score,[a] 3 y	NR	NR	MD 0.33 (−0.43; 1.09) SMD 0.08 (−0.14; 0.29)	382 (6 RCTs)[1]	Low	No difference
Caregiver burden as measured with GHQ score,[a] 3 y	NR	NR	MD −0.35 (−0.88; 0.18) SMD −0.36 (−0.64; −0.08)	201 (6 RCTs)[1]	Low	No difference
Bleeding (any), 3 y	10	0	RR 3.2 (0.4; 27.9)	644 (6 RCTs)[1,2]	Low	No difference
Gastrointestinal adverse effects (other than bleeding, eg, nausea and vomiting), 3 y	**81**	**44**	**RR 1.7 (1.1; 2.8)**	**1894 (10 RCTs)[1,2]**	**Low**	**Favors placebo**
Psychiatric side effects (eg, neuropsychiatric inventory measures, delusions), 3 y	64	57	RR 1.2 (0.5; 2.7)	805 (5 RCTs)[1,2]	Low	No difference
Cerebrovascular adverse effects (eg, cerebral ischemia or other events reported by investigators), 3 y	26	22	RR 1.2 (0.5; 3.3)	1774 (5 RCTs)[1,2]	Low	No difference

Between studies differences in continuous outcomes: MD, mean difference in absolute values of continuous outcomes between intervention and comparator; SMD, standardized mean difference between intervention and comparator where the magnitude of the effect is defined as small (SMD, 0–0.5 standard deviations), moderate (SMD, 0.5–0.8 standard deviations), and large (SMD >0.8 standard deviations).

Note: Boldface type denotes statistical significance.

[a] See Appendix 1 for more information about scales for measuring Alzheimer patient and caregiver outcomes.

WHAT DO THE CLINICAL GUIDELINES SAY?

American College of Physicians/American Academy of Family Physicians. Current Pharmacologic Treatment of Dementia, 2008.[3] (AGREE II Score: 66%)

- This guideline does not mention NSAIDs.

Alzheimer Association. Guideline for Alzheimer Disease Management, 2008.[4] (AGREE II Score: 55%)

- This guideline does not mention NSAIDs.

American Psychiatric Association. Practice Guideline for the Treatment of Patients with Alzheimer Disease and Other Dementias, 2007.[5] (AGREE II Score: 78%)

- This guideline recommends against using NSAIDs, because of a lack of efficacy and safety in placebo-controlled trials in patients with Alzheimer disease.

European Federation of Neurological Societies. Recommendations for the Diagnosis and Management of Alzheimer Disease and Other Disorders Associated With Dementia, 2010.[6] (AGREE II Score: 64%)

- This guideline states that aspirin should not be used as a treatment for Alzheimer disease (Level A), although it can be used in those with Alzheimer disease who also have other indications for its use (eg, to prevent cardiovascular events).
- This guideline does not mention other NSAIDs.

Scottish Intercollegiate Guidelines Network. Management of Patients with Dementia, 2006.[7] (AGREE II Score: 89%)

- This guideline states that aspirin is only recommended in people with vascular dementia who have a history of vascular disease.
- This guideline does not mention other NSAIDs.

AUTHOR COMMENTARY

This synopsis focuses on a clinical question about benefits and harms of NSAIDs for treatment of Alzheimer disease. Our comprehensive search in PubMed, Embase, the Cochrane Library, and clinicaltrials.gov in April 2015 and March 2016 identified a high-quality Cochrane review of 13 randomized controlled trials (RCTs) of aspirin and other NSAIDs and an additional unpublished double-blind RCT.[1,2] Primary studies enrolled adults with mild to moderate Alzheimer disease and examined the effects of aspirin, traditional NSAIDs, and selective COX-2 inhibitors.

Low-quality evidence suggests that traditional nonselective NSAIDs or selective COX-2 inhibitors do not improve patient or caregiver outcomes but cause adverse effects (**Table 1**). Treatment benefits are similar to placebo for individual drugs and for pharmacologic classes of traditional NSAIDs or selective COX-2 inhibitors.[1,2]

The quality of evidence was lowered due to risk of bias in the body of evidence, inconsistency, and imprecision of treatment estimates.

Current clinical practice guidelines either do not mention using NSAIDs for the treatment of Alzheimer disease or recommend against using these drugs because of a lack of efficacy.[3–7] Cost-effectiveness analysis has concluded that use of NSAIDs in adults with Alzheimer disease is not justified.[8]

The balance between the benefits and harms of aspirin for preventing cerebrovascular events contributing to cognitive decline in adults with mixed dementia (vascular dementia and Alzheimer disease) is unknown.

GLOSSARY

ADAS-cog, Alzheimer Disease Assessment Scale Cognitive Subscale; ADL, activities of daily living; AGREE II, Appraisal of Guidelines for Research and Evaluation; BEHAVE-AD, Behavioral Pathology in Alzheimer Disease; CDR, Clinical Dementia Rating; CI, confidence interval; COX-2, cyclooxygenase-2; DAD, Disability Assessment for Dementia; GHQ, General Health Questionnaire; GRADE, Grading of Recommendations Assessment, Development, and Evaluation; MD, mean difference; MMSE, Mini-Mental State Examination; NR, not reported; PSMS, Physical Self-Maintenance Scale; RCT, randomized controlled trial; RR, relative risk; SMD, standardized mean difference.

REFERENCES

1. Jaturapatporn D, Isaac MG, McCleery J, et al. Aspirin, steroidal and non-steroidal anti-inflammatory drugs for the treatment of Alzheimer's disease. Cochrane Database Syst Rev 2012;(2):CD006378.
2. Lifesciences JSW. Efficacy and safety of lornoxicam in patients with mild to moderate probable Alzheimer's disease. In: ClinicalTrials.gov [Internet]. Bethesda (MD): National Library of Medicine (US); 2011. Available at: http://clinicaltrials.gov/show/NCT01117948. NLM Identifier: NCT01117948.
3. Qaseem A, Snow V, Cross JT Jr, et al. Current pharmacologic treatment of dementia: a clinical practice guideline from the American College of Physicians and the American Academy of Family Physicians. Ann Intern Med 2008;148(5):370–8.
4. California Workgroup on Guidelines for Alzheimer's Disease Management; Alzheimer's Association. Guideline for Alzheimer's disease management. 2008. Available at: https://www.cdph.ca.gov/programs/alzheimers/Documents/professional_GuidelineFullReport.pdf. Accessed September 9, 2016.
5. APA Work Group on Alzheimer's Disease and other Dementias, Rabins PV, Blacker D, et al. American Psychiatric Association practice guideline for the treatment of patients with Alzheimer's disease and other dementias. 2nd edition. Am J Psychiatry 2007;164(Suppl 12):5–56.
6. Hort J, O'Brien JT, Gainotti G, et al. EFNS guidelines for the diagnosis and management of Alzheimer's disease. Eur J Neurol 2010;17(10):1236–48.
7. Scottish Intercollegiate Guidelines Network. Management of patients with dementia. 2006. Available at: http://www.sign.ac.uk/guidelines/fulltext/86/index.html. Withdrawn in June 2016.
8. Topinkova E, Baeyens JP, Michel JP, et al. Evidence-based strategies for the optimization of pharmacotherapy in older people. Drugs Aging 2012;29(6):477–94.
9. Raina P, Santaguida P, Ismaila A, et al. Effectiveness of cholinesterase inhibitors and memantine for treating dementia: Evidence review for a clinical practice guideline. Ann Intern Med 2008;148(5):379–97.

APPENDIX 1: SCALES FOR MEASURING ALZHEIMER PATIENT AND CAREGIVER OUTCOMES

	Direction of Improvement
Disability	
ADL score, higher score = improvement	Positive
DAD instrumental activities of daily living—any (eg, 1 score improvement) positive changes indicate improvement	Positive
Cognition	
MMSE—any positive changes indicate improvement. Minimal clinically important improvement in MMSE was defined as an increase by 3 or more score[9]	Positive
ADAS-cog—any negative changes indicate improvement. Minimal clinically important changes in ADAS-cog scale were defined as a reduction by 4 or more scores[9]	Negative
BEHAVE-AD score—any increase in score indicates worsening (0–75); lower score = improvement	Negative
CDR-SB—any negative changes indicate improvement	Negative
Quality of life	
PSMS—lower score = improvement	Negative
Caregiver burden	
Caregiver burden (GHQ for caregiver 0–30)—lower score = improvement	Negative

Index

Note: Page numbers of article titles are in **boldface** type.

Moving?

Make sure your subscription moves with you!

To notify us of your new address, find your **Clinics Account Number** (located on your mailing label above your name), and contact customer service at:

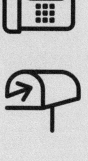

Email: **journalscustomerservice-usa@elsevier.com**

800-654-2452 (subscribers in the U.S. & Canada)
314-447-8871 (subscribers outside of the U.S. & Canada)

Fax number: 314-447-8029

Elsevier Health Sciences Division
Subscription Customer Service
3251 Riverport Lane
Maryland Heights, MO 63043

*To ensure uninterrupted delivery of your subscription, please notify us at least 4 weeks in advance of move.

Printed and bound by CPI Group (UK) Ltd, Croydon, CR0 4YY

07/10/2024

01040505-0008